theclinics.com

# MAGNETIC RESONANCE IMAGING CLINICS of North America

## MR Imaging of the Hip

Zehava Sadka Rosenberg, MD
Guest Editor

November 2005 • Volume 13 • Number 4

SAUNDERS

An Imprint of Elsevier, Inc.
PHILADELPHIA LONDON TORONTO MONTREAL SYDNEY TOKYO

**W.B. SAUNDERS COMPANY**
*A Divison of Elsevier Inc.*

Elsevier, Inc. • 1600 John F. Kennedy Boulevard • Suite 1800 • Philadelphia, Pennsylvania 19103-2899

http://www.mri.theclinics.com

**MRI CLINICS OF NORTH AMERICA**
**November 2005**
Editor: Barton Dudlick

**Volume 13, Number 4**
**ISSN 1064-9689**
**ISBN 1-4160-2730-0**



*Magnetic Resonance Imaging Clinics of North America* (ISSN 1064-9689) is published quarterly by the W.B. Saunders Company. Corporate and editorial offices: Elsevier, Inc., 1600 John F. Kennedy Boulevard, Suite 1800, Philadelphia, PA 19103-2899. Accounting and circulation offices: 6277 Sea Harbor Drive, Orlando, FL 32887-4800. Periodicals postage paid at Orlando, FL 32862, and additional mailing offices. Subscription prices are $205.00 per year (US individuals), $305.00 per year (US institutions), $100.00 (US students and residents), $230.00 per year (Canadian individuals), $375.00 per year (Canadian institutions), $280.00 per year (foreign individuals), and $375.00 per year (foreign institutions). To receive student and resident rate, orders must be accompanied by name of affiliated institution, date of term, and the *signature* of program/residency coordinator on institution letter-head. Orders will be billed at individual rate until proof of status is received. Foreign air speed delivery is included in all *Clinics* subscription prices. All prices are subject to change without notice. POSTMASTER: Send address changes to *Magnetic Resonance Imaging Clinics of North America*, W.B. Saunders Company, Periodicals Fulfillment, Orlando, FL 32887-4800. **Customer Service: 1-800-654-2452 (US). From outside of the US, call 1-407-345-4000. E-mail: hhspcs@harcourt.com.**

*Magnetic Resonance Imaging Clinics of North America* is covered in the *RSNA Index of Imaging Literature, Index Medicus, MEDLINE*, and *EMBASE/Excerpta Medica*.

Printed in the United States of America.

# GUEST EDITOR

**ZEHAVA SADKA ROSENBERG, MD,** Professor of Radiology, New York University School of Medicine; and Department of Radiology, New York University—Hospital for Joint Diseases, New York, New York

# CONTRIBUTORS

**ANDREW ABELES, BS,** University of Missouri—Columbia School of Medicine, Columbia, Missouri

**RITIKA ARORA, MD,** Assistant Professor of Radiology, Department of Radiology, New York University, Hospital for Joint Diseases Orthopaedic Institute, New York, New York

**LAURA W. BANCROFT, MD,** Assistant Professor, Department of Radiology, Mayo Clinic College of Medicine, Jacksonville, Florida

**JAVIER BELTRAN, MD,** Director of Medical Education, Franklin & Seidelmann, Inc.; Clinical Professor of Radiology, Mount Sinai School of Medicine, New York; and Chairman, Department of Radiology, Maimonides Medical Center, Brooklyn, New York

**JENNY T. BENCARDINO, MD,** Head—Musculoskeletal Radiology, Medical Arts Radiology Group, PC; and Department of Radiology, Huntington Hospital, North Shore Long Island Jewish Health System, Huntington, New York

**MARCELO BORDALO-RODRIGUES, MD,** Director, Department of Radiology, Instituto de Ortopedia e Traumatologia, Hospital das Clinicas, University of Sao Paulo Medical School, Sao Paulo, Brazil

**MIRIAM A. BREDELLA, MD,** Instructor in Radiology, Harvard Medical School; and Division of Musculoskeletal Radiology, Department of Radiology, Massachusetts General Hospital, Boston, Massachusetts

**CONRADO F.A. CAVALCANTI, MD,** Research Fellow, Department of Radiology, Hospital for Joint Diseases, New York, New York

**DEEP S. CHATHA, MD,** Department of Radiology, New York University, Hospital for Joint Diseases Orthopaedic Institute, New York, New York

**CHRISTINE B. CHUNG, MD,** Department of Radiology, University of California—San Diego and Veterans Affairs Health Care System, La Jolla, California

**LEONARD P. CONNOLLY, MD,** Staff Radiologist, Division of Nuclear Medicine, Children's Hospital Boston, Boston, Massachusetts

**SUSAN A. CONNOLLY, MD,** Staff Radiologist, Department of Radiology, Children's Hospital Boston, Boston, Massachusetts

**JOHANNE E. DILLON, MD,** Assistant Radiologist, Department of Radiology, Massachusetts General Hospital, Boston, Massachusetts

**JERRY DWEK, MD,** Department of Radiology, Children's Hospital, San Diego; and Department of Radiology, University of California—San Diego and Veterans Affairs Health Care System, La Jolla, California

**DIEGO JARAMILLO, MD,** Radiologist-in-Chief and Chairman of Radiology, Children's Hospital of Philadelphia, Philadelphia, Pennsylvania

**ARA KASSARJIAN, MD, FRCPC,** Assistant Professor of Radiology, Division of Musculoskeletal Radiology, Massachusetts General Hospital, Boston, Massachusetts

**YOUNG-JO KIM, MD, PhD,** Orthopedic Surgeon, Department of Orthopaedic Surgery, Children's Hospital Boston, Boston, Massachusetts

**GEORGE KOULOURIS, MD,** Musculoskeletal Imaging Fellow, Division of Musculoskeletal and General Diagnostic Imaging, Thomas Jefferson University Hospital, Philadelphia, Pennsylvania

**MARK J. KRANSDORF, MD,** Professor, Department of Radiology, Mayo Clinic College of Medicine, Jacksonville, Florida; and Professor, Department of Radiologic Pathology, Armed Forces Institute of Pathology, Walter Reed Army Medical Center, Washington, District of Columbia

**ROBERT MEISLIN, MD,** Assistant Professor of Orthopedic Surgery, New York University—Hospital for Joint Diseases, New York, New York

**JOSÉ M. MELLADO, MD,** Institut de Diagnostic per la Imatge, Hospital Universitari de Tarragona Joan XXIII, Tarragona, Spain

**THEODORE T. MILLER, MD,** Chief, Division of Musculoskeletal Imaging, Department of Radiology, North Shore University Hospital and LIJ Medical Center, Great Neck; and Associate Professor of Radiology, New York University School of Medicine, New York, New York

**WILLIAM B. MORRISON, MD,** Director and Associate Professor, Division of Musculoskeletal and General Diagnostic Imaging, Thomas Jefferson University Hospital, Philadelphia, Pennsylvania

**ERIK N. NELSON, MD,** Instructor, Harvard Medical School; and Assistant Radiologist, Division of Musculoskeletal Radiology, Massachusetts General Hospital, Boston, Massachusetts

**OLEG OPSHA, MD,** Resident, Department of Radiology, Maimonides Medical Center, Brooklyn, New York

**WILLIAM E. PALMER, MD,** Chief of Musculoskeletal Imaging, Division of Musculoskeletal Radiology, Massachusetts General Hospital, Boston, Massachusetts

**MINI PATHRIA, MD,** Department of Radiology, University of California—San Diego and Veterans Affairs Health Care System, La Jolla, California

**CHERYL PETERSILGE, MD,** Assistant Clinical Professor of Radiology and Orthopedic Surgery, Case Western Reserve University, Cleveland, Ohio

**JEFFREY J. PETERSON, MD,** Assistant Professor, Department of Radiology, Mayo Clinic College of Medicine, Jacksonville, Florida

**CHRISTIAN PFIRRMANN, MD,** Department of Radiology, University Hospital Balgrist, Zurich, Switzerland

**ZEHAVA SADKA ROSENBERG, MD,** Professor of Radiology, New York University School of Medicine; and Department of Radiology, New York University—Hospital for Joint Diseases, New York, New York

**NOGAH SHABSHIN, MD,** Chief of Musculoskeletal Radiology, Department of Diagnostic Imaging, Chaim Sheba Medical Center, Tel-Hashomer, Israel

**ANTHONY STANLEY, MD,** Department of Diagnostic Imaging, National University Hospital, Singapore

**DAVID W. STOLLER, MD, FACR,** Director of Magnetic Resonance Imaging, California Pacific Medical Center, San Francisco, California

**ADAM C. ZOGA, MD,** Assistant Professor of Radiology; and Director of Musculoskeletal MRI, Department of Radiology, Thomas Jefferson University Hospital, Philadelphia, Pennsylvania

# CONTENTS

## FORTHCOMING ISSUES

February 2006

**3T MR Imaging**
Mark C. DeLano, MD, *Guest Editor*

May 2006

**Breast MR Imaging**
Christiane Kuhl, MD, *Guest Editor*

## RECENT ISSUES

August 2005

**MR-Guided Interventions**
Jonathan S. Lewin, MD, *Guest Editor*

May 2005

**Abdominal MR Imaging**
Diego R. Martin, MD, PhD, *Guest Editor*

## GOAL STATEMENT

The goal of *Magnetic Resonance Imaging Clinics of North America* is to keep practicing radiologists and radiology residents up to date with current clinical practice in radiology by providing timely articles reviewing the state of the art in patient care.

## ACCREDITATION

The *Magnetic Resonance Imaging Clinics of North America* is planned and implemented in accordance with the Essential Areas and Policies of the Accreditation Council for Continuing Medical Education (ACCME) through the joint sponsorship of the University of Virginia School of Medicine and Elsevier. The University of Virginia School of Medicine is accredited by the ACCME to provide continuing medical education for physicians.

The University of Virginia School of Medicine designates this educational activity for a maximum of 60 category 1 credits per year, 15 category 1 credits per issue, toward the AMA Physician's Recognition Award. Each physician should claim only those credits that he/she actually spent in the activity.

The American Medical Association has determined that physicians not licensed in the US who participate in this CME activity are eligible for AMA PRA category 1 credit.

Category 1 credit can be earned by reading the text material, taking the CME examination online at http://www.theclinics.com/home/cme, and completing the evaluation. After taking the test, you will be required to review any and all incorrect answers. Following completion of the test and evaluation, your credit will be awarded and you may print your certificate.

## FACULTY DISCLOSURE/CONFLICT OF INTEREST

The University of Virginia School of Medicine, as an ACCME accredited provider, endorses and strives to comply with the Accreditation Council for Continuing Medical Education (ACCME) Standards of Commercial Support, Commonwealth of Virginia statutes, University of Virginia policies and procedures, and associated federal and private regulations and guidelines on the need for disclosure and monitoring of proprietary and financial interests that may affect the scientific integrity and balance of content delivered in continuing medical education activities under our auspices.

The University of Virginia School of Medicine requires that all CME activities accredited through this institution be developed independently and be scientifically rigorous, balanced and objective in the presentation/discussion of its content, theories, and practices.

All authors/editors participating in an accredited CME activity are expected to disclose to the readers relevant financial relationships with commercial entities occurring within the past 12 months (such as grants or research support, employee, consultant, stock holder, member of speakers bureau, etc). The University of Virginia School of Medicine will employ appropriate mechanisms to resolve potential conflicts of interest to maintain the standards of fair and balanced education to the reader. Questions about specific strategies can be directed to the Office of Continuing Medical Education, University of Virginia School of Medicine, Charlottesville, Virginia.

***The authors/editors listed below have identified no financial or professional relationships for themselves or their spouses/partners:***
Andrew Abeles, BS; Ritika Arora, MD; Laura W. Bancroft, MD; Javier Beltran, MD; Jenny T. Bencardino, MD; Marcelo Bordalo-Rodriques, MD; Miriam A. Bredella, MD; Conrado F.A. Cavalcanti, MD; Deep S. Chatha, MD; Leonard P. Connolly, MD; Susan A. Connolly, MD; Johanne E. Dillon, MD; Barton Dudlick, Acquisitions Editor; Diego Jaramillo, MD, MPH; Ara Kassarjian, MD, FRCPC; Young-Jo Kim, MD, PhD; George Koulouris, MD, MBBS, FRANZCR, MMed (Radiology); Mark J. Kransdorf, MD; Robert Meislin, MD; José M. Mellado, MD; Theodore T. Miller, MD; William B. Morrison, MD; Erik N. Nelson, MD; Oleg Opsha, MD; William E. Palmer, MD; Cheryl Petersilge, MD; Jeffrey J. Peterson, MD; Zehava Sadka Rosenberg, MD; Nogah Shabshin, MD; David W. Stoller, MD, FACR; and Adam C. Zoga, MD.

***The authors listed below have not provided disclosures for themselves or their spouses/partners:***
Christine B. Chung, MD; Jerry Dwek, MD; Mini Pathria, MD; Christian Pfirrmann, MD; and Anthony Stanley, MD.

*Disclosure of discussion of non-FDA approved uses for pharmaceutical and/or medical devices:*
**The University of Virginia School of Medicine, as an ACCME provider, requires that all authors identify and disclose any "off label" uses for pharmaceutical and medical device products. The University of Virginia School of Medicine recommends that each physician fully review all the available data on new products or procedures prior to clinical use.**

## TO ENROLL

To enroll in the *Magnetic Resonance Imaging Clinics of North America* Continuing Medical Education program, call customer service at 1-800-654-2452 or visit us online at http://www.theclinics.com/home/cme. The CME program is available to subscribers for an additional fee of $175.00.

ELSEVIER
SAUNDERS

Magn Reson Imaging Clin N Am
13 (2005) xiii

MAGNETIC
RESONANCE
IMAGING CLINICS
of North America

# Dedication

To my mother, Tova Murad Sadka, with love.

1064-9689/05/$ - see front matter 
doi:10.1016/j.mric.2005.10.002

ELSEVIER
SAUNDERS

Magn Reson Imaging Clin N Am
13 (2005) xv–xvi

MAGNETIC
RESONANCE
IMAGING CLINICS
of North America

# Preface

# MR Imaging of the Hip

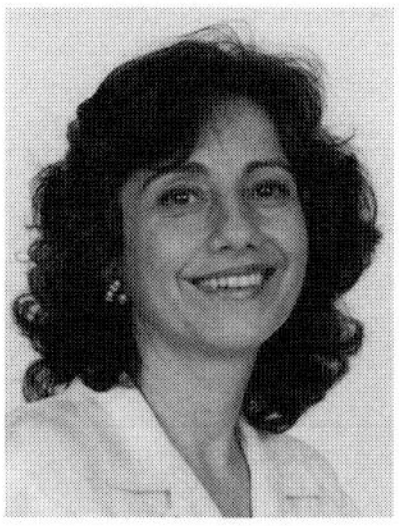

Zehava Sadka Rosenberg, MD
*Guest Editor*

It is surprising that, to date, there has not been an issue of the *Magnetic Resonance Imaging Clinics of North America* or a textbook on MR imaging of the hip, considering that one of the earliest musculoskeletal MR applications was assessment of marrow hip disorders. The early detection of avascular necrosis of the femoral head, transient osteoporosis of the hip, and occult hip fracture engaged much of the early MR literature. Subsequently, though, hip MR imaging has significantly lagged behind that of other joints. Recently there has been a heightened awareness of the diverse disorders affecting the hip, partly because of the increasing athletic demands placed on the hip as well as the advent of hip arthroscopy. This has led to a more intense appraisal of MR imaging's role in evaluating this joint.

The hip is a challenging joint to image. The neighboring three-dimensional bony anatomy is complex; a myriad of tendons, ligaments, and an intricate intra-articular anatomy must be considered; and a full MR assessment mandates inclusion of the pelvis, sacrum, and contralateral hip. This necessitates careful attention to MR protocols, an in-depth familiarity with the normal anatomy, and an understanding of the many disease processes affecting the hip joint. The excellent article on technical considerations in this issue reviews many of the above difficulties. In addition to a dedicated article on the normal MR anatomy of the hip, most of the articles in this issue begin with a detailed discussion of the pertinent normal MR anatomy and potential pitfalls. The subjects covered range from well-established topics such as marrow disorders and tumors to newer concepts such as deep musculotendinous injuries, the interplay between bony anatomy and labral and cartilaginous disease, femoro-acetabular impingement, and the complementary roles of ultrasound and MR imaging.

I am indebted to the distinguished group of authors who so graciously contributed their time and expertise into the making of this issue. I would also like to thank the innumerable residents, fellows, and musculoskeletal colleagues, who, in their unrelenting, sometimes exasperating quest for knowledge, have kept me humble, on my toes, and always striving.

Our knowledge of MR imaging of the hip is still in its infancy; it is precisely for that reason that

1064-9689/05/$ - see front matter 
doi:10.1016/j.mric.2005.10.001

editing this issue was such an exciting endeavor. There remain numerous topics whose MR characteristics are still relatively unfamiliar to us, such as MR imaging of disorders of the capsular and intra-articular ligaments and MR imaging of entrapment neuropathies. It is my hope that this issue will serve both as a comprehensive and instructive summary of our present knowledge of MR imaging of hip disorders and as a springboard for further work on this challenging topic.

Zehava Sadka Rosenberg, MD
*Department of Radiology*
*New York University—Hospital for Joint Diseases*
*Bernard Aronson Plaza*
*301 East 17th Street*
*6th Floor*
*New York, NY 10003, USA*

*E-mail address:* Zehava@RAMtoGO.com

ELSEVIER
SAUNDERS

Magn Reson Imaging Clin N Am
13 (2005) 605–615

MAGNETIC RESONANCE IMAGING CLINICS of North America

# MR Imaging of the Normal Hip

Deep S. Chatha, MD, Ritika Arora, MD*

*Department of Radiology, New York University, Hospital for Joint Diseases Orthopaedic Institute, 301 East 17th Street, Room 600, New York, NY 10003, USA*

The construct of the hip joint is unique in that it is designed to support the entire body weight and shifting mechanical loads during ambulation and activity. When considering normal ambulation, this translates to four to seven times the body weight being transmitted through each hip joint. The hip joint accomplishes this via its unique structure as a ball and socket, or enarthrodial, joint, where the sphere of the femoral head moves freely within the rounded cavity of the acetabulum [1].

In contradistinction to the shoulder joint, the hip joint is designed for stability. The femoral head is tightly apposed to the acetabulum, and the shapes of the acetabulum and femoral head are designed to complement one another. The apposition is further accentuated by the addition of a surrounding fibrocartilaginous ring, the glenoidal labrum, which lends even further stability. Surrounding capsular and ligamentous structures provide additional support. The proximal femur and adjacent pelvis and acetabulum allow tendinous attachments for all the muscles involved in ambulation. These surrounding structures are divided into static and dynamic stabilizers of the hip. The hip capsule and ligaments, primarily the iliofemoral ligament, act as static stabilizers. The dynamic stabilizers are composed of the surrounding muscles and their tendinous attachments, with the most significant group being the abductors [2].

## Hip imaging protocols

The pelvis should be imaged using a pelvic or torso phased-array coil. At our institution, dedicated pelvic imaging includes a T1-weighted sequence and a short tau inversion recovery (STIR) sequence in the coronal plane, an axial T1-weighted sequence, and an axial T2-weighted sequence with fat saturation. For any suspected marrow process or patients older than 40 years of age, coronal opposed phase imaging can be added. The field of view is large enough to cover the skin surfaces overlying both hips, and the axial images are obtained from the top of the iliac crest to below the lesser trochanters.

If there is a specific complaint regarding one hip, a local surface coil should be used over the symptomatic side, usually a shoulder coil. A side-to-side comparison may be performed with a coronal or axial sequence of the entire pelvis. Again, at our institution, dedicated hip imaging includes a T1-weighted sequence and a STIR sequence in the coronal plane, an oblique axial proton density–weighted sequence, and a sagittal T2-weighted sequence with fat saturation (Table 1).

If there is suspicion of labral pathologic findings, an MR arthrogram is useful in evaluating the detailed articular structures. Initially, a fluoroscopically guided arthrogram is performed just before MR imaging. Again, a surface coil is used, because only one hip is of interest. Our MR hip arthrogram protocol includes a coronal T1-weighted sequence, an axial T2-weighted sequence with fat saturation, and triplane (axial, sagittal, and coronal) T1-weighted sequences with fat saturation (Table 2). A T2-weighted sequence is useful for identifying extra-articular fluid collections, such as paralabral cysts, as well as subtle bone marrow edema [3]. The axial plane is an oblique axial sequence that is oriented along the axis of the femoral neck.

* Corresponding author.
*E-mail address:* ritika.arora@nyumc.org (R. Arora).

1064-9689/05/$ - see front matter 
doi:10.1016/j.mric.2005.08.012

Table 1
Routine hip protocol

| Sequence | FOV | Matrix | TR | TE | TI | Bandwidth | Echo train length |
|---|---|---|---|---|---|---|---|
| Coronal T1-weighted SE | 18 | 256×192 | 400–800 | Minimum | — | 16 | — |
| Coronal STIR | 18 | 256×192 | >2000 | 20–40 | 150 | 16 | 16 |
| Oblique axial PD-weighted TSE | 14–16 | 256×256 | >2000 | 30–40 | — | 32/64 | 8 |
| Sagittal T2-weighted fat-sat TSE | 18 | 256×256 | 2000–6000 | 45 | — | 32 | 16 |

Routine hip MR imaging should be performed with a phased array coil.

*Abbreviations:* fat-sat, fat-saturated; FOV, field of view; PD, proton density; SE, spin echo; TE, echo time; TI, inversion time; TR, repetition time; TSE, turbo spin echo.

## Marrow

The appearance of marrow signal on MR imaging is dependent on the age of the patient, specifically the relation of yellow or fatty marrow to that of red or hematopoietic marrow. On T1-weighted images, predominantly fatty or yellow marrow appears hyperintense, whereas on T2-weighted images, it demonstrates intermediate signal intensity. Hematopoietic marrow demonstrates intermediate signal on both T1- and T2-weighted images because of its higher water content [4,5]. Conversely, cortical and trabecular bone has significantly lower water content and thus is markedly hypointense on T1- and T2-weighted images [6,7].

The signal changes related to the conversion of marrow in the proximal femur are quite organized and well recognized. In a fetus and at the time of birth, all bone marrow is hematopoietic; thus, uniform intermediate signal is present in the femur and pelvis. Subsequently, there is organized conversion to yellow marrow, beginning in apophyses and epiphyses of the femur, which generally occurs by 1 year of age. The femoral diaphysis is the next region to undergo conversion, and there is progression of conversion toward the metaphyseal regions. In the adult, most of the marrow within the femur is fatty; however, if hematopoietic marrow is present, it is generally restricted to the proximal femoral metaphysis (Fig. 1).

In the pelvis, there is usually widely distributed hematopoietic marrow throughout childhood. The conversion pattern here is much less predictable than in the femur, and although there may be fatty marrow replacement as the patient ages, there is often patchy red marrow distribution throughout adulthood as well.

## Osseous and articular anatomy

The femoral head forms two thirds of a sphere, and its articular surface is thicker along the mediocentral aspect and thinnest along the periphery. The femoral head is directed upward, slightly anteriorly and medially. Conversely, the acetabular cavity faces obliquely forward, lateral, and downward to create close apposition of the two articular surfaces. The acetabulum itself is

Table 2
Routine direct hip arthrogram

| Sequence | FOV | Matrix | TR | TE | TI | Bandwidth | Echo train length |
|---|---|---|---|---|---|---|---|
| Coronal T1-weighted fat-sat | 18 | 256×256 | 400–800 | Minimum | — | 16 | — |
| Sagittal T1-weighted fat-sat | 20 | 256×192 | 400–800 | Minimum | — | 16 | — |
| Oblique axial T1-weighted fat-sat | 18 | 256×256 | 400–800 | Minimum | — | 16 | — |
| Coronal T1-weighted | 18 | 256×256 | 400–800 | Minimum | — | 16 | — |
| Axial T2-weighted fat-sat TSE | 18 | 256×256 | >2000 | 20–40 | — | 16 | 16 |

*Abbreviations:* fat-sat, fat-saturated; FOV, field of view; TE, echo time; TI, inversion time; TR, repetition time; TSE, turbo spin echo.

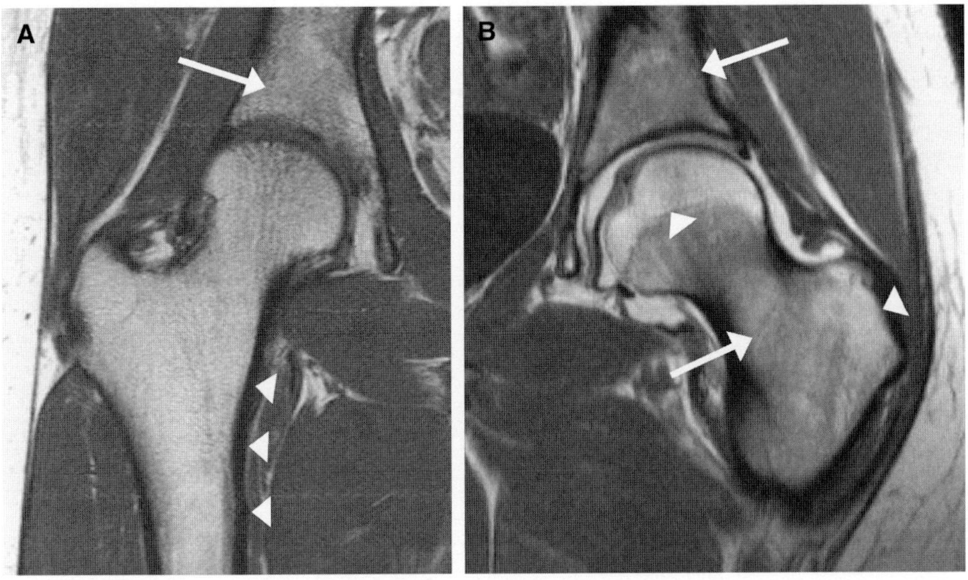


Fig. 1. (*A*) Coronal T1-weighted image of the hip in an adult demonstrates normal marrow distribution in a skeletally mature individual. The medullary cavity is predominantly hyperintense, corresponding to fatty marrow replacement. The cortical bone demonstrates hypointense signal on all pulse sequences (*arrowheads*). Note the intermediate signal in the supra-acetabular region, indicating patchy red marrow (*arrow*). The marrow conversion pattern within the pelvis is less predictable than that of the femur. (*B*) Coronal T1-weighted image from an MR arthrogram in a young adult with preservation of red marrow throughout much of the proximal femur and pelvis (*arrows*). There is fatty marrow replacement within the femoral head and greater trochanter, an apophysis (*arrowheads*). This is also a normal marrow pattern in adults.

composed of all three bones of the pelvis and is hemispheric in shape. Medially, the acetabulum is formed by the pubis; laterally and inferiorly, it is formed by the ischium; and superiorly, it is formed by the ilium [1]. There is a normal cortical articular ridge along the superior acetabulum that is often seen on coronal images, which should not be mistaken for osseous pathologic change (Fig. 2).

There is also a surrounding fibrocartilaginous rim, termed the *acetabular labrum* or *cotyloid ligament*, that acts to deepen the hip joint and provide further stability. At the anteroinferior aspect of the acetabulum, there is a focal deficiency of the bony acetabulum, termed the *acetabular notch*. This notch is bridged by the transverse ligament. The remaining opening deep to the ligament is referred to as the acetabular foramen, which is filled with fat. It is through this structure that nutrient vessels and nerves perforate to enter the joint (Fig. 3). The periphery of the notch subsequently acts as an attachment site for the ligamentum teres.

The construct of the hip is further strengthened by attachments to surrounding osseous structures,

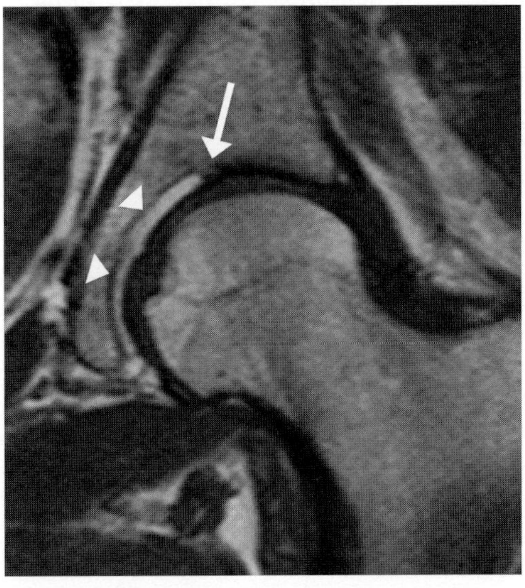

Fig. 2. Coronal T1-weighted image of the hip demonstrating the normal cortical articular ridge (*arrow*) along the superior acetabulum. This is a normal finding and should not be mistaken for osseous pathologic change. Normal fat signal (*arrowheads*) is seen within the acetabular fossa.

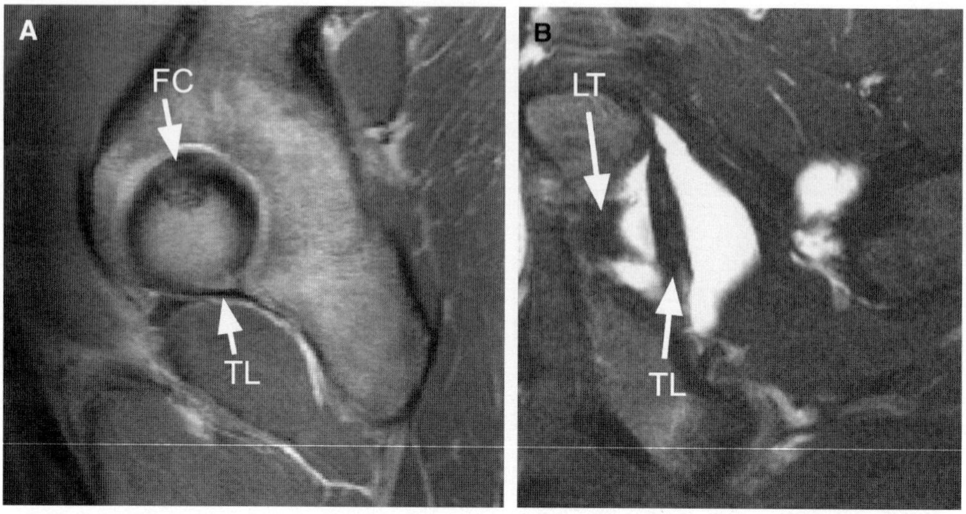


Fig. 3. (*A*) Sagittal proton density–weighted image at the medial aspect of the hip joint demonstrates the roughened depression of the femoral head, the fovea capitis (FC), as a rounded low-signal irregularity devoid of articular cartilage. Along the inferior aspect of the joint, the linear low-signal transverse ligament (TL) is seen spanning the acetabular notch and serves as the attachment site for the ligamentum teres. (*B*) Axial T2-weighted fat-saturated image after intra-articular administration of gadolinium at the level of the inferior acetabulum clearly shows the transverse ligament (TL) spanning the acetabular notch. The two bands of the ligamentum teres (LT) are seen as they extend inferiorly to attach to the transverse ligament.

namely, the greater and lesser trochanters. The greater trochanter is a quadrilateral bony eminence at the superior aspect of the junction of the femoral neck and proximal shaft. The surface of the greater trochanter has four distinct facets for tendinous attachments and sites for bursae [2,8]. The lesser trochanter is more of a triangular or conical eminence that arises at the inferior aspect of the junction of the femoral neck and the proximal femur and projects posteriorly. Again, there are three distinct facets along its bony margins that allow for tendinous insertions.

It is important to examine the surrounding osseous structures of the hip carefully, because they are often the cause of cryptic hip pain. The field of view for an examination of the pelvis should include the anterior superior iliac spine, an anterior protrusion at the junction of the iliac crest and the anterior border of the pelvis, whereas a dedicated hip examination is not likely to include this area. Along the superior margin of the acetabulum is the second anterior protrusion, the anterior inferior iliac spine. The anterior superior iliac spine and anterior inferior iliac spine serve as important attachment sites for muscles of the anterior quadrant of the hip, and avulsion injuries from these sites are not uncommon. The superior and inferior pubic rami should also be included in all examinations of the hip, as should the symphysis pubis, to exclude an insufficiency fracture or arthritic process of the symphysis. The most posterior and inferior extent of the ischium is a roughened prominence, the ischial tuberosity, that allows for the attachment of the hamstring tendons. Avulsive injuries from this location are also a common cause of occult hip pain and should be included in the field of view for dedicated hip MR imaging.

## Cartilage

The acetabulum is lined by a nearly circumferential region of articular cartilage known as the lunate cartilage because of its moon-shaped appearance en face. The cartilage does not extend over the acetabular fossa. The fovea capitis is the only aspect of the femoral head that is not covered with articular cartilage. The thickest cartilage is located along the superior margin of the femoral head, corresponding to the greatest region of weight bearing. The posterior margin of the femoral head contains the thinnest region of articular cartilage [9,10]. On routine MR imaging of the hip, the articular cartilage of the femoral head and acetabulum is identified as a thin zone

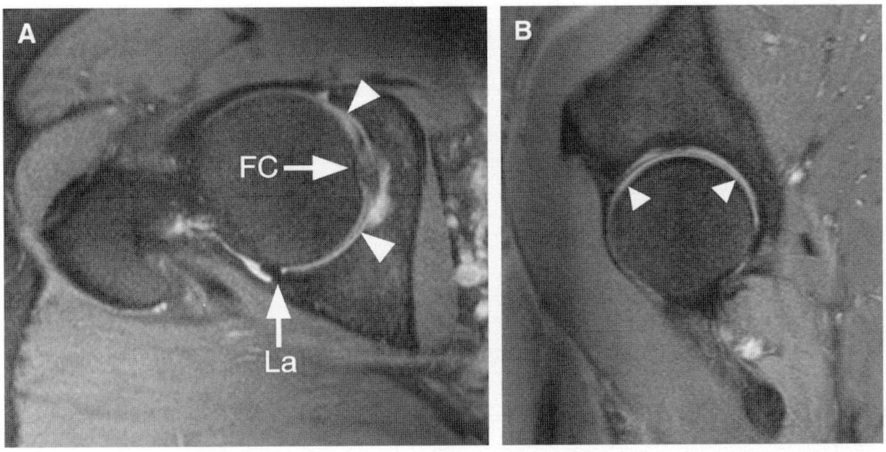


Fig. 4. Axial (*A*) and sagittal (*B*) proton density–weighted fat-saturated images with articular cartilage appearing as a thin zone of intermediate signal (*arrowheads*) between the femoral head and acetabulum. Note the absence of articular cartilage at the fovea capitis (FC) of the femoral head, allowing for the insertion of the ligamentum teres. The low-signal triangular labrum (La) is well delineated posteriorly.

of intermediate signal on spin echo and gradient echo images (Fig. 4) [11–13].

With the subsequent evolution of high resolution MR imaging techniques, bilaminar and trilaminar appearances of the articular cartilage have been described [14–16]. On routine imaging, these are not often discernible, however.

## Capsular and ligamentous anatomy

An inelastic fibrous capsule envelops the hip joint and attaches proximally to the acetabulum, labrum, and transverse ligament and extends distally to surround most of the femoral neck with attachment at the base of the trochanters. Anteriorly, the capsule extends further laterally over the femoral neck compared with the posterior aspect (Fig. 5). Most of the fibers of the capsule are oriented longitudinally from the pelvis to the femur. There is a deep layer of circularly oriented fibers termed the *zona orbicularis* that encircles the capsule at the base of the femoral neck, however (Fig. 6A, B). These fibers do not directly attach to bone and may be mistaken for the acetabular labrum at arthroscopy [17].

The fibrous capsule is reinforced by several ligaments, namely, the ischiofemoral, iliofemoral, and pubofemoral ligaments, which are discernible thickenings of the capsule. The iliofemoral ligament is the thickest and strongest ligament and extends from the anterior inferior iliac spine to the intertrochanteric line of the femur with an inverted Y shape anteriorly, thus lending to its lesser used name, the Y ligament of Bigelow (see Fig. 6C, D). The pubofemoral ligament extends horizontally from the superior pubic ramus and obturator crest to the undersurface of the femoral neck and blends in with the fibers of the capsule and deep surface of the iliofemoral ligament. There is an inherent weakening or hole between the vertical band of the iliofemoral ligament and

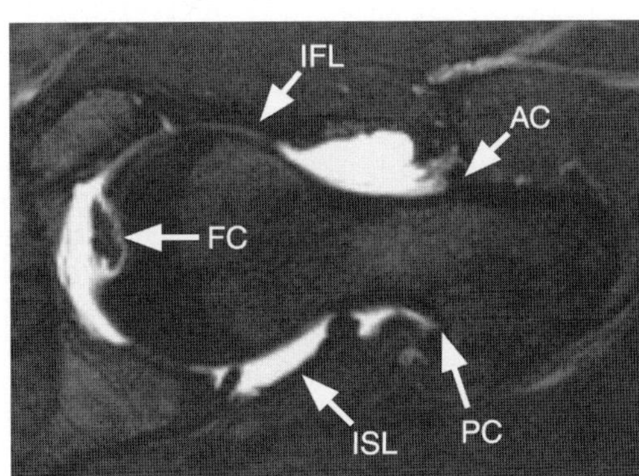


Fig. 5. Axial T2-weighted fat-saturated image after intra-articular gadolinium administration demonstrates the anterior (AC) and posterior (PC) capsular insertions on the femoral neck. The fovea capitis (FC) and insertion of the ligamentum teres are well outlined by the intra-articular contrast. Anteriorly and posteriorly are thickenings of the capsule and the iliofemoral (IFL) and ischiofemoral (ISL) ligaments, demonstrated as low signal intensity bands.

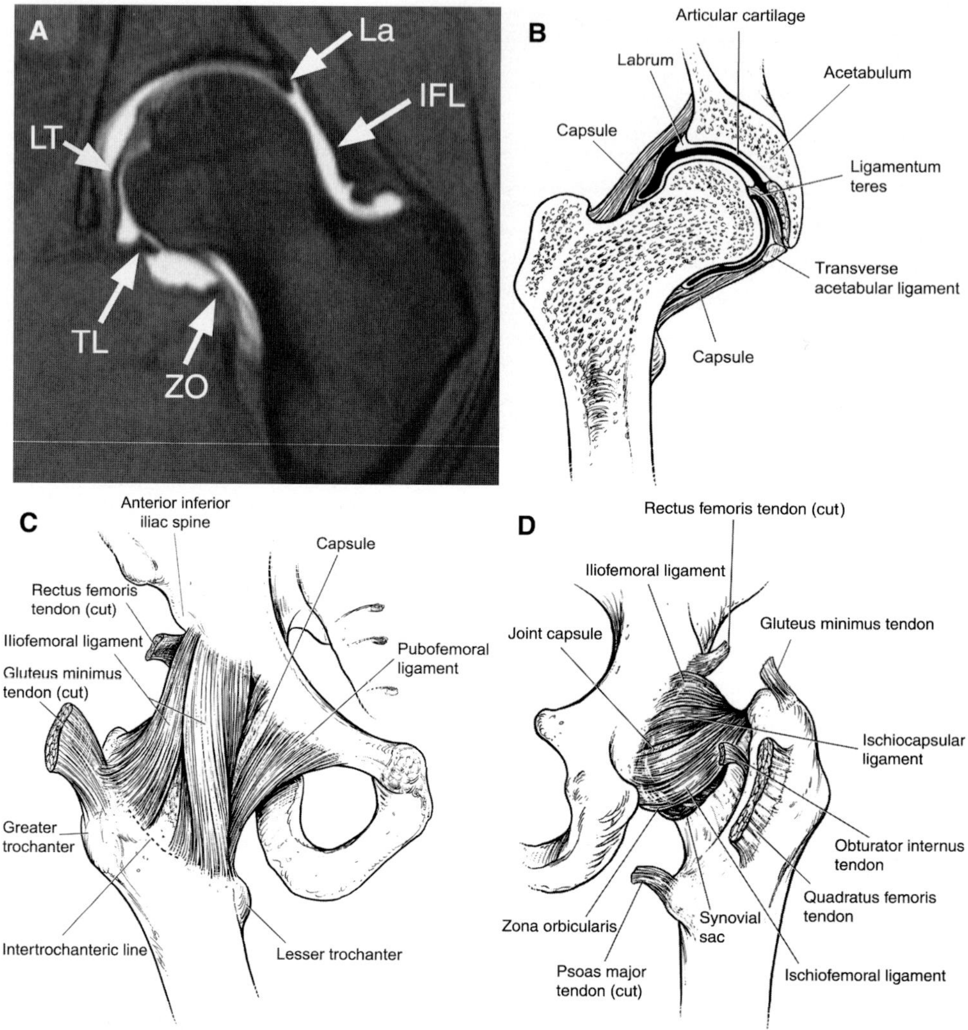


Fig. 6. (*A*) Coronal T1-weighted fat-saturated image from an MR arthrogram delineates the ligamentum teres (LT) and its attachment to the femoral head at the fovea capitis. The ligamentum teres extends inferiorly to attach along the transverse ligament (TL). At the base of the femoral neck, the zona orbicularis (ZO) is identified as a region of circumferential fibers surrounding the capsule. The superior margin of the iliofemoral ligament (IFL) is well demonstrated as a low-signal region of capsular thickening. The triangular low-signal acetabular labrum (La) is visualized superolaterally. (*B*) Line drawing of coronal section of the hip demonstrates the capsule along with the ligamentum teres and transverse ligament. (*C*) Line drawing of anterior view of the hip demonstrates the iliofemoral and pubofemoral ligaments as thickenings of the capsule anteriorly. (*D*) Line drawing of posterior view of the hip demonstrates the ischiofemoral ligament and zona orbicularis fibers of the posterior joint capsule.

the pubofemoral ligament anteriorly that can allow communication of the joint with the iliopsoas tendon bursa, which is present in 10% to 15% of individuals [2]. On MR arthrograms in these patients, the iliopsoas bursa distends with contrast and is readily visualized on axial images (Fig. 7) [18,19]. There are several other smaller bursae surrounding the hip joint; however, these are not routinely visualized in the normal hip. The ischiofemoral ligament extends superolaterally from the ischium along the posterior aspect of the femoral neck to combine with the fibers of the zona orbicularis and insert on the greater trochanter [19,20].

The ligamentum teres is a weak intra-articular ligament with a pyramidal morphology. It is

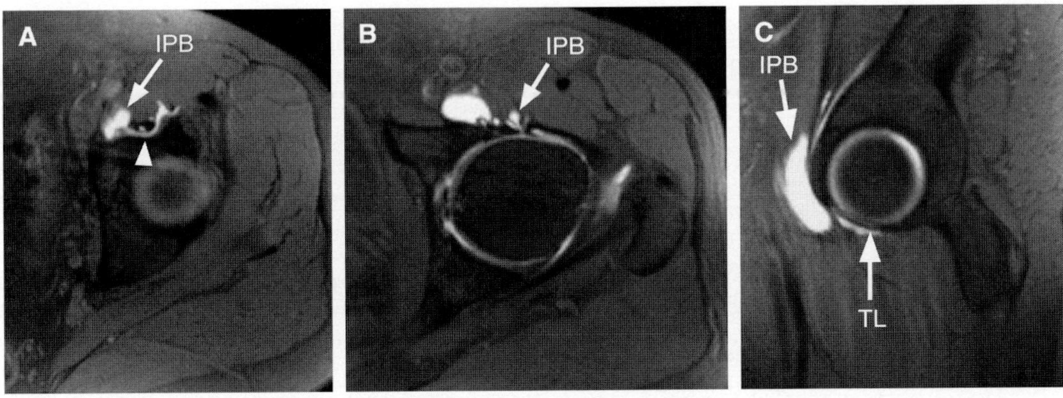


Fig. 7. (*A*) Axial T1-weighted fat-saturated image after intra-articular administration of gadolinium demonstrates a normal iliopsoas bursa (IPB) filling with contrast, which is present in 10% to 15% of individuals. The bursa can be seen to extend around the adjacent iliopsoas tendons (*arrowhead*). (*B*) Axial T1-weighted fat-saturated image of the same patient at a slightly more inferior level delineates a communication (*arrow*) with the joint space via an inherent weakening or hole between the vertical band of the iliofemoral ligament and the pubofemoral ligament anteriorly. (*C*) Sagittal T1-weighted fat-saturated image of the same patient shows the anterior relation of the IPB with the hip joint. The transverse ligament (TL) is well appreciated.

covered by a synovial membrane and extends from its basal attachment as two bands on the acetabular notch and transverse ligament to its apex at the fovea capitis, a centrally located roughened depression on the femoral head, which, incidentally, is the only region of the femoral head that is not covered by articular cartilage [21]. In some individuals, only the synovial sheath is present without a discernible ligament, and in a small percentage of the population, neither can be identified [17]. The ligamentum teres transmits the foveal artery, which provides a minimal contribution of the blood supply to the femoral head [22]. The ligamentum teres does not provide significant structural integrity to the hip joint, and other than surrounding this small nutrient artery to the femoral head, its function is not known.

The acetabular labrum is a fibrocartilaginous rim that serves to deepen the acetabular cavity. The transverse ligament is a part of the acetabular labrum, which bridges over the acetabular notch at the inferolateral acetabulum to form a complete circle and blends in with the labrum [17,23]. It consists of strong flattened fibers that differ from the labrum because they do not contain cartilage and transform the acetabular notch into a foramen through which nutrient vessels enter the joint. The fibrocartilaginous labrum is most often triangular in cross-section and is thicker posterosuperiorly [18,19]. The normal labrum is most often seen as a well-defined triangular structure of homogeneous low signal intensity [24–26]. The superior aspect of the joint capsule inserts several millimeters above the labrum, which creates a normal perilabral recess (Fig. 8) [23,24]. In addition, the joint capsule inserts directly at the base of the labrum along the anterior and posterior margins of the joint, thus creating smaller perilabral recesses.

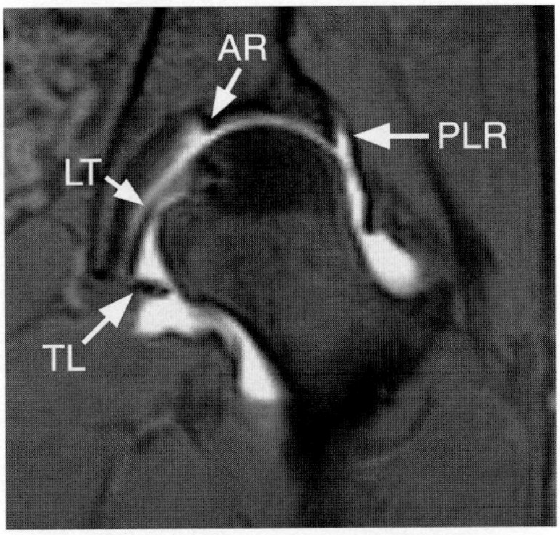


Fig. 8. Coronal T1-weighted fat-saturated image from an MR arthrogram demonstrates gadolinium invaginating into a focal cleft, the perilabral recess (PLR) between the labrum, seen as a triangular hypointense structure arising from the acetabulum, and the low-signal linear capsule superiorly. Again noted is the ligamentum teres (LT) extending from the fovea capitis to attach to the transverse ligament (TL). A normal cortical articular ridge (AR) is identified.

## Muscle and tendon anatomy

The hip musculature is well identified on T1- or proton density–weighted images, where the muscles demonstrate intermediate signal and are separated by high signal intensity fat along the fascial divisions. In addition to the muscles surrounding the hip and their tendinous attachments, the sciatic nerve is a structure that should be routinely identified on all imaging of the pelvis or hip. The sciatic nerve is the largest nerve in the body and measures approximately 2 cm in width. It begins as a continuation of the sacral plexus and travels laterally through the pelvis and out the greater sciatic foramen just anterior and inferior to the piriformis muscle, where it is generally seen as an isointense rounded structure or grouping of neural fascicles surrounded by fat (Fig. 9B).

The muscles in the anterior quadrant of the hip, including the iliopsoas, sartorius, rectus femoris, and pectineus, act as the primary flexors of the hip. The iliopsoas muscle is seen anterior to the femoral head at the 12 o'clock position on axial images and traverses the pelvis and exits anteriorly over the superior pubic ramus to insert on the lesser trochanter (see Fig. 9A, B). The pectineus arises from the iliopubic ramus and inserts just distal to the lesser trochanter. The sartorius muscle arises from the anterior superior iliac spine and runs inferiorly and medially along the thigh to insert on the proximal tibia as part of the pes anserinus tendon group. The rectus femoris muscle arises as two tendons: the anterior, or straight, tendon arises from the anterior inferior iliac spine, and the posterior, or reflected, tendon is anterolateral to the iliofemoral ligament and follows the lateral brim of the acetabulum (Fig. 10C) [1,2]. The adductor muscles of the hip lay anteromedially and include the adductor longus, brevis, and magnus as well as the gracilis and pectineus and arise from the pubic bone (see Fig. 10D). The obturator externus arises from the ramus of the pubis and ischium as well as from the external surface of the obturator membrane. Its tendon extends posterolaterally and inserts into the trochanteric fossa on the medial aspect of the greater trochanter (Fig. 11A, B).

The lateral quadrant contains the abductor muscles, including the gluteus medius and minimus and the tensor fascia latae more superficially (see Fig. 10A). The gluteus medius muscle arises laterally from the ilium and inserts onto the lateral and superoposterior facet of the greater

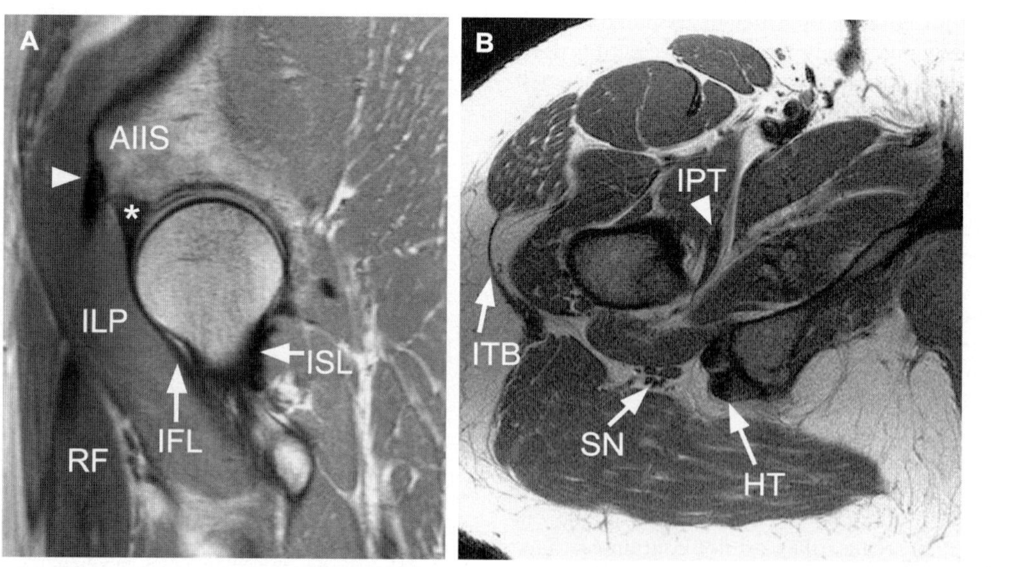


Fig. 9. (*A*) Sagittal proton density–weighted image demonstrates the origin of the straight tendon of the rectus femoris (RF) muscle (*arrowhead*) from the anterior inferior iliac spine (AIIS). The iliopsoas muscle (ILP) runs anterior to the hip joint as it descends to insert on the lesser trochanter. The iliofemoral ligament (IFL) is clearly seen anteriorly from its insertion on the anterior labrum (*) as well as a portion of the ischiofemoral ligament (ISL) posteriorly. (*B*) Axial T1-weighted image at the level of the inferior pubic ramus demonstrates the iliopsoas tendon (IPT) inserting onto the lesser trochanter. The origin of the hamstring muscles from the ischial tuberosity is appreciated as well as the iliotibial band (ITB) laterally. The sciatic nerve (SN) is clearly seen and surrounded by fat. HT, hamstring tendons.

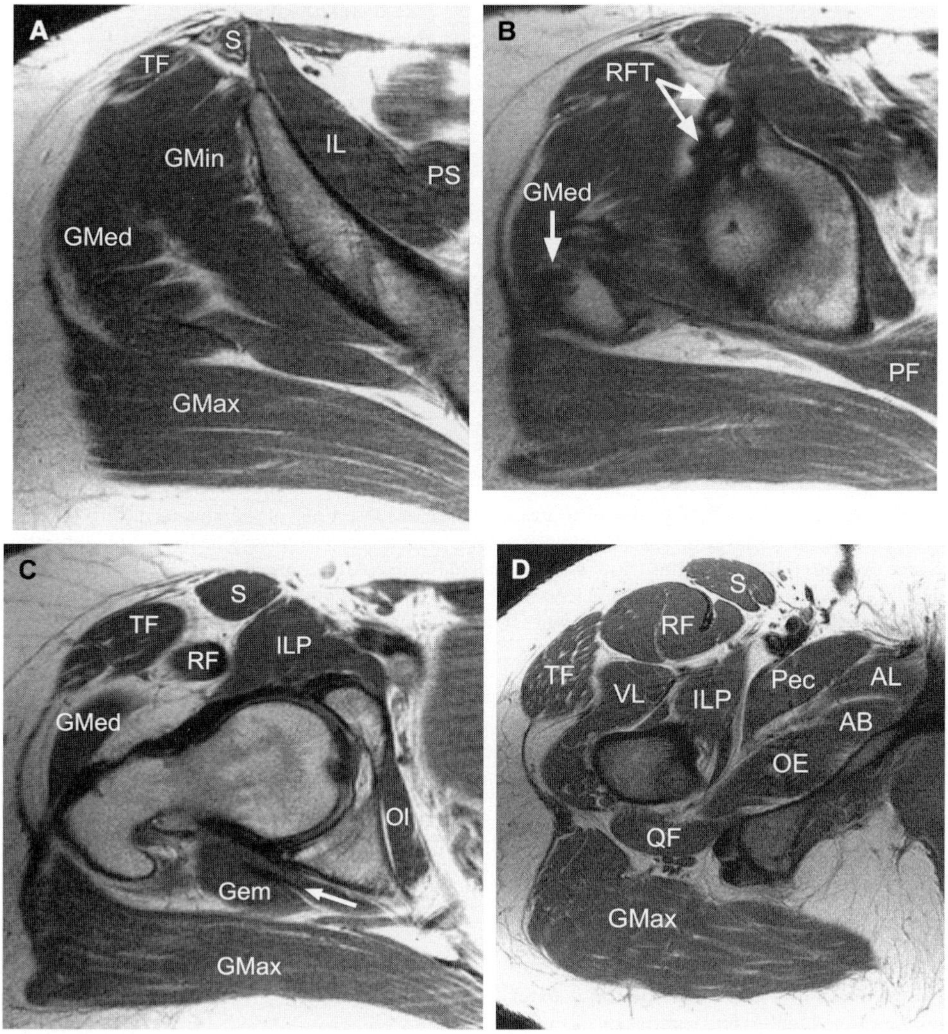


Fig. 10. Axial oblique T1-weighted images at various levels through the hip joint. (*A*) Level immediately inferior to the anterior superior iliac spine. The iliacus (IL) and psoas (PS) muscles are now identified as separate entities. GMax, gluteus maximus; GMed, gluteus medius; GMin, gluteus minimus; S, sartorius; TF, tensor fascia latae. (*B*) Level of the superior acetabulum. The two tendons of the rectus femoris (RFT) are identified. The straight head, which arises from the anterior inferior iliac spine, is seen more anterior to the reflected head, which follows the lateral brim of the acetabulum. The GMed tendon is seen inserting on the lateral and superoposterior facets of the greater trochanter. The piriformis muscle (PF) courses out of the pelvis through the greater sciatic notch, and its tendon is visualized inserting on the upper border of the greater trochanter. (*C*) Level of the femoral head. The tendon of the obturator internus (*arrow*) is seen as it courses through the lesser sciatic notch and joins the superior and inferior gemelli muscles to insert onto the greater trochanter. Gem, gemelli; ILP, iliopsoas; OI, obturator internus muscle; RF, rectus femoris. (*D*) Level of the lesser trochanter. The muscles surrounding the hip are clearly demarcated by high signal intensity fat. AB, adductor brevis; AL, adductor longus; OE, obturator externus; Pec, pectineus; QF, quadratus femoris; VL, vastus lateralis.

trochanter, which can be well visualized on sagittal images. The gluteus minimus muscle lies deep to the gluteus medius and inserts onto the anterior facet of the greater trochanter (see Fig. 10C, D) [8].

The muscles in the posterior quadrant include the extensors and external rotators, consisting of the gluteus maximus, piriformis, obturator internus, superior gemellus, inferior gemellus, and quadratus femoris. The gluteus maximus is a large superficial muscle that inserts into the iliotibial band. The piriformis muscle originates from the anterior sacrum and passes out of the pelvis

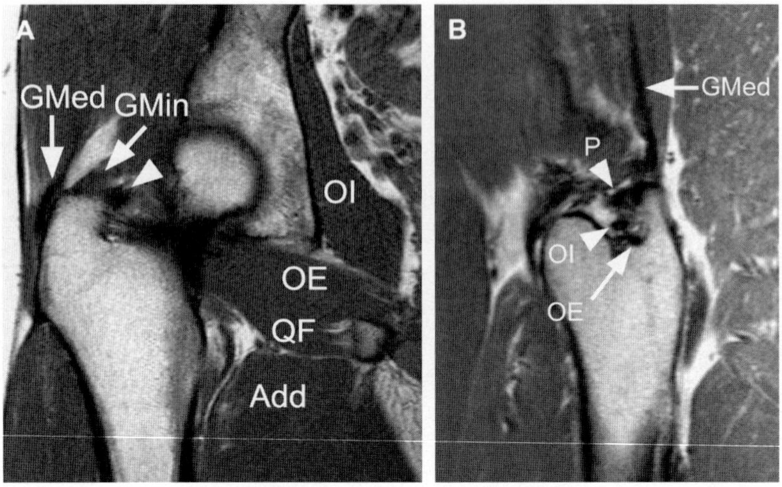


Fig. 11. (*A*) Coronal T1-weighted image demonstrates the tendinous insertions of the gluteus medius (GMed), gluteus minimus (GMin), and piriformis (*arrowhead*) onto the greater trochanter. The muscle bellies of the obturator internus (OI), obturator externus (OE), quadratus femoris (QF), and adductors (Add) are well seen. (*B*) Sagittal T1-weighted image through the greater trochanters. The GMed tendon inserts onto the lateral and superoposterior facets of the greater trochanter. The tendons of the piriformis (P), OI, and OE are seen proximal to their insertions on the greater trochanter and intertrochanteric fossa.

through the greater sciatic notch to insert on the upper border of the greater trochanter between the iliofemoral ligament anteriorly and the gluteus medius tendon posteriorly (see Fig. 10B). Lying inferior to the piriformis, the obturator internus muscle also arises from the medial surface of the pubis, passes by the lesser sciatic notch, and joins the superior and inferior gemelli muscles to insert onto the greater trochanter laterally. The tendinous insertions of these muscles can be well seen on sagittal images along the facets of the greater trochanter (see Fig. 11) [8]. The quadratus femoris lies inferior to the gemelli muscles and inserts onto the posterior aspect of the greater trochanter.

The hamstring tendons originate at the ischial tuberosity and can be evaluated using all three imaging planes. The semimembranosus tendon arises from the superolateral aspect of the ischial tuberosity, whereas the conjoined tendon of the semitendinosus and long head of the biceps femoris arise from a medial impression on the superior aspect of the ischial tuberosity [27]. It should also be noted that the adductor magnus has a curvilinear attachment to the lateral surface of the ischiopubic ramus and the inferolateral aspect of the ischial tuberosity.

## Summary

This article reviews the complex normal anatomy of the hip joint and its surrounding structures on MR imaging, including MR arthrography. Thorough knowledge of the normal appearance of the marrow and osseous and articular anatomy as well as the ligaments, tendons, and surrounding muscles of the hip is essential for imaging diagnosis.

## Acknowledgments

The authors thank Hugh Nachamie for his illustrations.

## References

[1] Williams PL, Warwick R, editors. Arthrology: the joints of the lower limb—the hip (coxal) joint. In: Gray's anatomy. 36th edition. Philadelphia: WB Saunders; 1980. p. 477–82.
[2] Resnick D. Diagnosis of bone and joint disorders. Philadelphia: WB Saunders; 2002.
[3] Steinbach LS, Palmer WE, Schweitzer ME. MR arthrography. Radiographics 2002;22:1223–46.
[4] Moore SG, Dawson KL. Red and yellow marrow in the femur: age-related changes in appearance at MR imaging. Radiology 1990;175:219–23.
[5] Andrews C. Evaluation of the marrow space in the adult hip. Radiographics 2000;20(Suppl):S27–42.
[6] Vogler JB III, Murphy WA. Bone marrow imaging. Radiology 1988;168:679–93.
[7] Vande Berg BC, Malghem J, Lecouvert FE, et al. Magnetic resonance imaging of the normal bone marrow. Skeletal Radiol 1998;27:471–83.

[8] Pfirrmann CWA, Chung CB, Theumann NH, et al. Greater trochanter of the hip: attachment of the abductor mechanism and a complex of three bursa—MR imaging and MR bursography in cadavers and MR imaging in asymptomatic volunteers. Radiology 2001;221:469–77.
[9] Maroudas A, Venn M. Chemical composition and swelling of normal and osteoarthritic femoral head cartilage. II. Swelling. Ann Rheum Dis 1977;36:399–406.
[10] Cova M, Toffanin R, Frezza F, et al. Magnetic resonance imaging of articular cartilage: ex vivo study on normal cartilage correlated with magnetic resonance microscopy. Eur Radiol 1998;8:1130–6.
[11] Konig H, Sauter R, Deinling M, et al. Cartilage disorders: comparison of spin echo, CHESS and FLASH sequence MR images. Radiology 1987;164(3):753–8.
[12] Gylys-Morin VM, Hajek PC, Sartoris DJ, et al. Articular cartilage defects: detectability in cadaver knees with MR. AJR Am J Roentgenol 1987;148(6):1153–7.
[13] Reicher MA, Basset LW, Gold RH. High resolution MR imaging of the knee joint: pathologic correlations. AJR Am J Roentgenol 1985;145(5):903–9.
[14] Modl JM, Sether LA, Haughton VM, et al. Articular cartilage: correlation of histologic zones with signal intensity at MR imaging. Radiology 1991;181(3):853–5.
[15] Recht MP, Kramer J, Marcelis S, et al. Abnormalities of articular cartilage in the knee: analysis of available MR techniques. Radiology 1993;187(2):473–8.
[16] Rubenstein JD, Kim JK, Morava-Protzner I, et al. Effects of collagen orientation on MR imaging characteristics of bovine articular cartilage. Radiology 1993;188(1):219–26.
[17] Stoller DW. Magnetic resonance imaging in orthopaedics and sports medicine. Philadelphia: Lippincott-Raven; 1997.
[18] Petersilge CA, et al. Acetabular labral tears: evaluation with MR arthrography. Radiology 1996;200:231–5.
[19] Ghebontni L, Roger B, Brasseur JL, et al. Intraarticular pathology of the hip: MR arthrographic findings [abstract]. Radiology 1996;201:532.
[20] Petersilge CA. From the RSNA Refresher Courses. Radiological Society of North America. Chronic adult hip pain: MR arthrography of the hip. Radiographics 2000;20(Spec No):S43–52.
[21] Keene GS, Villa RN. Arthroscopic anatomy of the hip: an in vivo study. Arthroscopy 1994;10:392–9.
[22] Fang C, Teh J. Imaging of the hip. Imaging 2003;15:205–16.
[23] Petersilge CA. MR arthrography for evaluation of the acetabular labrum. Skelet Radiol 2001;30:423–30.
[24] Ghebontni L, Roger B, El-Khoury J, et al. MR arthrography of the hip: normal intra-articular structures and common disorders. Eur Radiol 2000;10:83–8.
[25] Czerny C, Hofmann S, Neuhold A, et al. Lesions of the acetabular labrum: accuracy of MR imaging and arthrography in detection and staging. Radiology 1996;200:225–30.
[26] Hodler J, Yu JS, Goodwin D, et al. MR arthrography of the hip: improved imaging of acetabular labrum with histologic correlation. AJR Am J Roentgenol 1995;165:887–91.
[27] Kouloris G, Connell D. Hamstring muscle complex: an imaging review. Radiographics 2005;25:571–86.

ELSEVIER
SAUNDERS

Magn Reson Imaging Clin N Am
13 (2005) 617–634

MAGNETIC
RESONANCE
IMAGING CLINICS
of North America

# Technical Considerations in MR Imaging of the Hip

Adam C. Zoga, MD*, William B. Morrison, MD

*Department of Radiology, Thomas Jefferson University Hospital, 111 South 11th Street, Suite 3390 Gibbon, Philadelphia, PA 19107, USA*

Without question, MR imaging of joints has become an integral and even indispensable tool in the diagnosis and treatment of musculoskeletal disease. Through the 1980s and 1990s, hip MR imaging did not begin to approach the level of knee, shoulder, or even ankle MR imaging in popularity for clinician referral. In 2000, our musculoskeletal section generated 3107 reports for MR imaging of the knee, and only 433 reports were dedicated to the hip for an identical segment of imaging centers. Over the past 2 years, however, this trend has shown strong indications of long-term change. For a slightly different segment of centers in 2004 we generated 490 hip MR imaging reports compared with 2845 knee reports. Knees, along with 1869 shoulders and 1145 ankles, were the most frequently referred and imaged joints at these centers. This change in referral patterns is reflected strongly in the radiology literature and scientific meeting programs. A simple Pubmed search of "hip MRI" at the time of this writing generated 1137 citations (a similar search for "knee MRI" yielded 2772 citations), but nearly half of them are from 2000 through early 2004. This clear evidence that MR imaging of the hip is a thriving and advancing science serves as our foundation for this discussion on technical considerations in MR imaging of the hip. It stands to reason that an increase in referrals has generated new interest in improving study quality. In the case of the hip, however, it may be the evolution of orthopedic treatment algorithms and surgical interventions that has provided us with the knowledge base and incentive to improve our imaging techniques. Whatever combination of these two factors truly exists, we are in a sort of Renaissance regarding MR imaging of the hip, and the technical considerations and the opportunities for improvement remain abundant.

* Corresponding author.
*E-mail address:* adam.zoga@jefferson.edu (A.C. Zoga).

## General, noncontrast protocol issues

Creating functional protocols for MR imaging of the hip is a challenging endeavor, with inherent difficulties rarely encountered in joint imaging. In general, protocols for hip imaging should allow for adequate evaluation not only of the hip itself but also of surrounding regional muscle insertions and other structures that may cause symptoms artifactually attributed to the hip itself. These structures include but are not limited to the lower lumbar disc levels, the sacroiliac joints, the lumbar plexus nerve roots, and even the entirety of the bony pelvis. At the same time, hip MR imaging protocols must allow for high resolution of small cartilaginous structures, including the acetabular labrum and articular cartilage on the acetabulum and the femoral head. Consider the challenge of creating a shoulder protocol adequate to evaluate rotator cuff impingement, instability related to labral pathology, the pectoralis musculature, cervical radiculopathy, and even arthropathies that involve bilateral glenohumeral joints. These are, in essence, analogous expectations to those we need to have for each MR imaging examination of the hip (Table 1).

As a weight-bearing articulation of the lower extremity, osteoarthritis should be a primary consideration in nearly every hip examination in skeletally mature patients. When considering osteoarthritis and other hip arthropathies, symmetry should serve as a discriminating characteristic. It is one of the motivating factors behind inclusion of

1064-9689/05/$ - see front matter 
doi:10.1016/j.mric.2005.08.008

Table 1
MR imaging protocol: hip general noncontrast

| Primary sequences | Plane | Sequence | Coil | FOV | Slice | Matrix NEX | TR | TE | TI | Flip angle | Band | ETL | Fat suppression? | Other | Estimated time (min) |
|---|---|---|---|---|---|---|---|---|---|---|---|---|---|---|---|
| Localizer | 3 plane | FSPGR | Torso | 36–48 | — | — | — | — | — | — | — | — | — | Parameters set by system | 2 |
| 1 | Coronal | T1 SE | Torso | 36–48 | 4/1 | 256×256 2 | 400–800 | 10–20 | — | — | 16 | — | No | — | 3–4 |
| 2 | Coronal | STIR | Torso | 36–48 | 4/1 | 256×192 2 | 2000–6000 | 25–40 | 150 | — | 16 | 8 | — | — | 5–6 |
| 3 | Sagittal | T2 FSE | Torso | 16 | 3/1 | 256×256 2 | 2000–6000 | 70–80 | — | — | 16 | 8 | Yes | Consider obliquity with acetabular rim off coronal localizer | 3–4 |
| 4 | Axial | T2 FSE | Torso | 36–48 | 4/1 | 256×256 2 | 2000–6000 | 70–80 | — | — | 16 | 8 | Yes | Image entire pelvis | 3–4 |
| 5 | Axial | PD FSE | Torso or local surface | 16 | 3/1 | 256×256 2 | 2000–6000 | 30–40 | — | — | 16 | 8 | No | Optimize for labrum signal | 4 |
| Optional for labrum, cartilage | Coronal | T2 FSE | Torso or local surface | 16 | 3/1 | 256×256 2 | 2000–6000 | 70–80 | — | — | 16 | 8 | Yes | Signal may be best in setting of effusion | 3–4 |

Special instructions: If patient is too big for the torso coil on series 1 and 2, use body coil.

*Abbreviations:* ETL, echo train length; FOV, field of view; FSPGR, fast spoiled gradient echo; NEX, number of excitations; PD, proton density; TE, echo time; TI, time to inversion; TR, repetition time.

coronal or axial sequences of the entire pelvis in hip MR imaging protocols. A second consideration that supports the acquisition of lower resolution, large field-of-view sequences of the entire pelvis is the high incidence of pelvic metastases and infiltrating bone marrow processes, in which asymmetry of bone marrow signal or diffuse abnormal bone marrow signal in a large imaging field of view may lead to the ultimate diagnosis. If more support is needed for the inclusion of these large field-of-view sequences acquired with a phased array body or torso coil, musculotendinous injuries about the pelvis can be difficult to diagnose without the contralateral structure for comparison.

With this reasoning as motivation, we include at least two coronal sequences of the entire pelvis in most of our hip MR imaging protocols. One sequence should be fluid sensitive, and the nicely homogeneous fat suppression achieved with inversion recovery and the inherent signal richness that accompanies such a large field of view (36–48 cm) generally makes short tau inversion recovery (STIR) a preferred choice on most of our high field strength and low field strength systems. For the second, we most often chose a spin echo (SE) T1-weighted sequence, which allows for optimal sensitivity to abnormal bone marrow patterns. Aberrant bone marrow signal on this sequence without a clearly delineated lesion can be a difficult issue. When possible, the addition of a sequence acquired at an echo time when fat and water are out of phase but with otherwise identical parameters may help discriminate between atypical but benign variant bone marrow patterns and infiltrative bone marrow processes or foci of metastasis (Figs. 1 and 2). Another benefit of these large field-of-view coronal sequences is quick identification of other clinical confounders for hip pain, including sacral insufficiency fractures, muscle injuries, and lumbar plexus lesions (Fig. 3) [1–3].

In the interest of imaging center efficiency, we try to restrict noncontrast joint protocols to five sequences after a three plane localizer. Staying within these confines, we can select one sagittal and two axial series to accompany our two large field-of-view coronal sequences. The sagittal sequence should be dedicated to the hip in question with a field of view in the range of 16 cm, which allows for high resolution for labral tears and articular cartilage defects and should be fluid sensitive for optimal identification of cystic lesions, bone marrow edema, and muscle injuries. We find that a fast spin echo (FSE) T2-weighted sequence with fat suppression serves these purposes well, because it provides optimal fluid sensitivity and better signal at a smaller field of view than would inversion recovery. If there is clinical concern for a sacroiliac pathologic condition, the sagittal sequence should be extended through the sacrum and contralateral hip.

The axial sequences allow for more patient-specific leeway. For the purposes of detecting labral tears and early osteoarthritis, we generally choose an intermediate weighted (proton density) FSE with a 15- or 16-cm field of view. Non–fat-suppressed images allow for optimal assessment of the cortex and subchondral bone. The second axial sequence can be omitted for a shorter protocol or can be used as an adjunct to our imaging of the entire pelvis. An FSE T2-weighted sequence

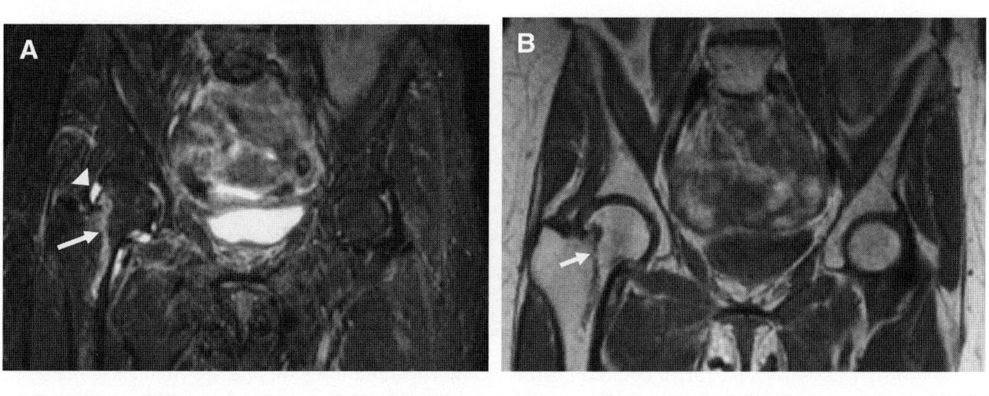


Fig. 1. (*A*) STIR and T1-weighted large field-of-view coronal images from a limited hip fracture protocol MR image acquired at 1.5 T demonstrate an acute intertrochanteric fracture. (*B*) The nondisplaced fracture (*arrow*) was occult on hip radiographs. Note the asymmetric right hip effusion (*A*, *arrowhead*).

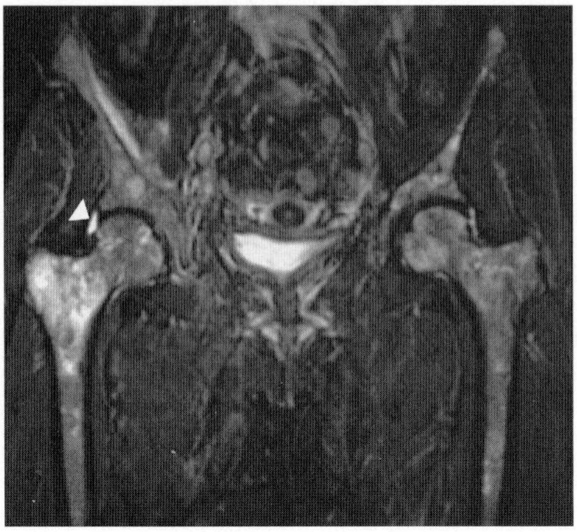

Fig. 2. STIR image from a limited hip fracture protocol without fracture demonstrates extensive metastatic bone marrow infiltration. Although bone pain related to the metastases may have been the cause of pain, note the asymmetric right hip effusion (*arrowhead*), which suggests a potential mechanical cause for the pain.

of the entire pelvis (field of view, 26–38 cm) can prove valuable in its fluid sensitivity (bursitis, paralabral cysts, geodes) and in its symmetry (muscle injury or atrophy, joint effisions). Aquiring all five sequences should allow for diagnosis of most lesions that cause outpatient hip pain and dysfunction and should occupy the scanner for 22 to 25 minutes per patient, which is optimal for 30-minute scheduling blocks. Using smaller surface coils for these small field-of-view sequences has received consideration, but the abundance of soft tissue surrounding the hip joint and the inherent size of the pelvic girdle create difficulties in acquiring homogeneous signal with small surface coils. This reasoning and acknowledgment of logistical difficulties in changing coils during a single examination have led us to use the built-in torso coil for the entirety of our noncontrast hip protocol and for almost all hip imaging in general.

## Direct and indirect arthrography: to inject or not to inject

In musculoskeletal imaging, general indications for MR arthrography include suspicion of injury involving signal poor structures, small cartilaginous structures, and structures that compartmentalize (eg, intra-articular bodies). MR imaging examinations of hip and pelvis structures are inherently signal rich. That is, an imager generally need not go to extreme lengths to acquire acceptable signal to noise when compared with other musculoskeletal examinations, such as wrist, ankle, and even shoulder. The hip joint itself pales in capacity when compared with the knee or shoulder, and labral-capsular structures may appear redundant and contiguous on noncontrast sequences. Small cartilaginous defects in the setting of hyaline cartilage on the articular surface or fibrocartilage in the labrum also may be occult on routine images without joint distension. Keeping these strengths and shortcomings of the noncontrast hip protocol in mind, we recommend MR arthrography of the hip in select clinical scenarios.

In the setting of a suspected acetabular labrum injury, we strongly recommend direct MR arthrography (Table 2). A fluoroscopy-guided hip joint injection of dilute gadopentate dimeglumine contrast medium is a quick and reliable mechanism

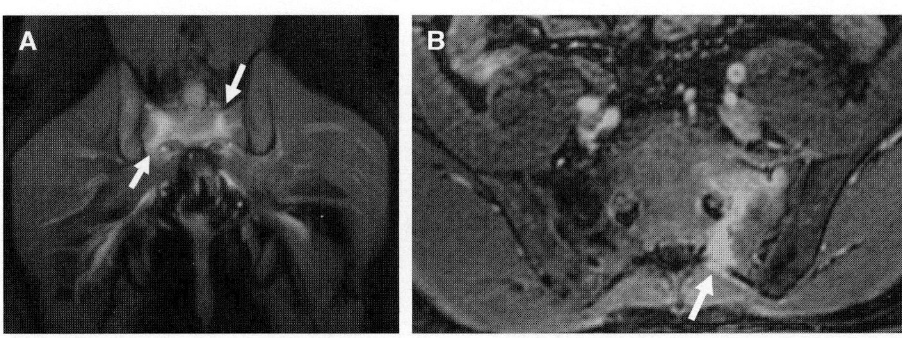


Fig. 3. Sacral insufficiency fractures are a common cause of low back and hip pain and are frequently bilateral. (*A*) A coronal large field-of-view STIR image shows bilateral insufficiency fractures with the classic "Honda sign" configuration (*arrows*). (*B*) An axial T2 FSE image with fat suppression demonstrates a unilateral fracture of the left sacral ala (*arrow*).

Table 2
MR imaging protocol: hip (Gad arthrogram)

| Primary sequences | Plane | Sequence | Coil | FOV | Slice | Matrix NEX | TR | TE | TI | Flip angle | Band | ETL | Fat suppression? | Other | Estimated time (min) |
|---|---|---|---|---|---|---|---|---|---|---|---|---|---|---|---|
| Localizer | 3 plane | FSPGR | Torso | 36–48 | — | — | — | — | — | — | — | — | — | Parameters set by system | 2 |
| 1 | Axial | T2 FSE | Torso | 14–16 | 4/1 | 256×256 2 | 2000–4000 | 50–60 | — | — | 16 | 8 | Yes | Consider enlarging FOV if symptoms nonspecific | 3–4 |
| 2 | Coronal | T1 SE | Torso | 14–16 | 3/1 | 256×256 3 | 400–600 | 10–20 | — | — | 16 | — | Yes | — | 5 |
| 3 | Coronal | T2 FSE | Torso | 36–48 | 4/1 | 256×192 2 | 2000–4000 | 70–80 | — | — | 16 | 8 | No | Bone marrow sequence | 3–4 |
| 4 | Axial | T1 SE | Torso | 14–16 | 3/1 | 256×256 3 | 400–600 | 10–20 | — | — | 16 | — | Yes | Increase slice thickness if too much time | 5 |
| 5 | Sagittal | T1 SE | Torso | 14–16 | 3/1 | 256×256 3 | 400–600 | 10–20 | — | — | 16 | — | Yes | Specific for anterior labrum | 5 |
| Optional sequences | | | | | | | | | | | | | | | |
| 1 | Radial Sagittal Oblique | T1 SE | Torso | 14–16 | 12 equal segments like "clock face" | 256×256 3 | 400–600 | 10–20 | — | — | 16 | — | Yes | Tech can likely take slice selection from MRCP protocol | 4 |
| 2 | Axial | 3D FSPGR | Torso | 14–16 | 1.2/0 | 256×128 2 | 30–40 | min | — | 15 | 16 | 8 | 3D FSPGR | Consider for bodies, ossicles, capsular injury | 5–6 |

Special instructions: Use respiratory compensation if breathing artifact is present.

*Abbreviations:* ETL, echo train length; FOV, field of view; FSPGR, fast spoiled gradient echo; MRCP, magnetic resonance cholangiopancreatography; NEX, number of excitations; TE, echo time; TI, time to inversion; TR, repetition time.

to distend the hip joint and provide for optimal MR contrast [4]. With the patient supine and the leg in a neutral position, the hip joint can be accessed easily, even without the presence of a joint effusion, by passing a spinal needle to the periosteum at the superolateral cortical border of the femoral head-neck junction. Pitfalls to this approach include needle tip locations in the iliopsoas tendon, iliopsoas bursa, or femoral periosteum. Infusion of a small quantity of iodinated contrast (1–2 mL) confirms either an intra-articular position or one of three misplaced positions. I have found that a periosteal needle tip position can be adjusted to an intra-articular position easily in most cases simply by twisting the needle hub a half turn and rotating the bevel 180°. Iliopsoas tendon and bursa locations generate a characteristic elongated pattern of contrast after the long axis of the tendon and can be adjusted easily with direct needle advancement to the periosteum (Fig. 4).

We recommend a solution of 0.1 mL of a 0.5 mM gadolinium contrast diluted in 20 mL of

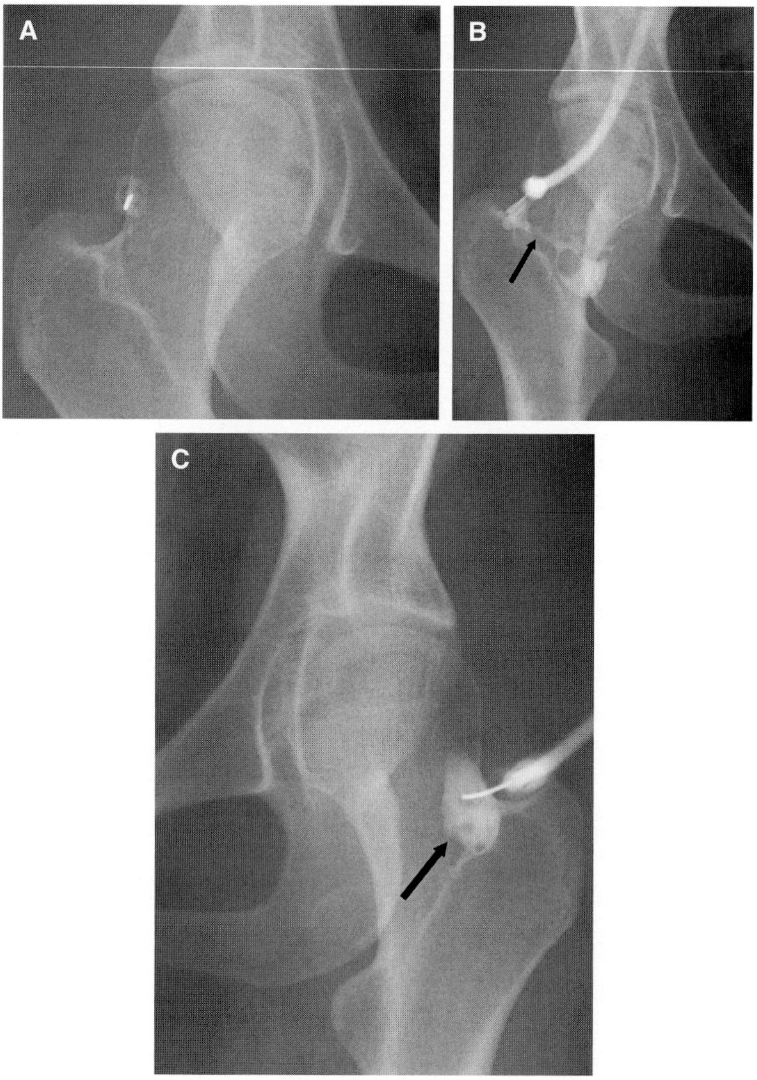


Fig. 4. Fluoroscopic spot images from a hip arthrogram. (*A*) Optimal needle position at the superolateral cortex at the head-neck junction. (*B*) At the right hip, iodinated contrast immediately encircles the femoral neck (*arrow*) and confirms an intra-articular position. (*C*) At the left hip, contrast remains focal with a globular configuration that suggests a suboptimal, extra-articular position, likely within the iliopsoas tendon (*arrow*).

normal saline, ultimately generating a 2.5 mOsm solution for injection [5]. In general, a nonarthritic hip is distended nicely with 7 to 10 mL of the dilute gadolinium solution, which allows for optimal visualization of labrocapsular structures. Postsurgical and arthritic hip joints can be decidedly more capacious, however. In these cases, experience of the arthrographer in sensing a distended, tense joint without overdistending and extravasating contrast can be valuable. MR imaging should be undertaken within 1 hour of contrast injection.

Direct MR arthrogram hip protocols should take advantage of inherent signal strength and maximize resolution of labral and articular structures by using a small field of view (14–16 cm) and a large matrix (at least 256×256). Adding chemically selective fat suppression to SE T1-weighted sequences provides for optimal demonstration of small cartilage defects and labral tears. Our protocol includes small field-of-view T1 SE sequences in sagittal, axial, and coronal planes. Gradient echo sequences with fat suppression offer superior contrast and allow for thin slices, as small as 1 mm on many high field strength systems. One should consider adding an axial thin slice spoiled gradient echo sequence if there is suspicion of intra-articular bodies or if labral structures are equivocal for tear on the other sequences (Fig. 5). Some musculoskeletal specialists advocate an axial oblique fat-suppressed sequence perpendicular to the transverse ligament to optimize labral resolution. Recently, we have been adding a series of 12 radial slices with T1 weighting and fat suppression acquired tangential to the acetabular rim for a circumferential view of the labrum. It is important to remember, however, that these high-resolution sequences are relatively insensitive to bone marrow abnormalities. We include at least one non–fat-suppressed sequence of the entire pelvis, generally a T2 FSE axial or a T1 SE coronal sequence, and a fat-suppressed T2 FSE sequence (coronal or axial) dedicated to the affected hip. This sequence allows for some leeway should technical problems related to the arthrogram (eg, extravasation or poor contrast signal) occur (Fig. 6).

In our experience, indirect arthrography of the hip falls short of direct MR arthrography in the setting of labral tears. Although an intravenous contrast injection readily finds its way to the hip joint with only a short delay, we have had little success in achieving adequate distention by indirect arthrography without a pre-existing joint effusion. We reserve indirect arthrography of the hip for postoperative patients and for patients who have suspected labral tears when a direct arthrogram is logistically impractical. If performing an indirect arthrogram for a suspected acetabular labral tear, we recommend a delay of approximately 20 minutes between intravenous contrast injection and imaging, with at least 5 minutes of passive motion involving the affected joint before imaging. Our hip indirect arthrogram

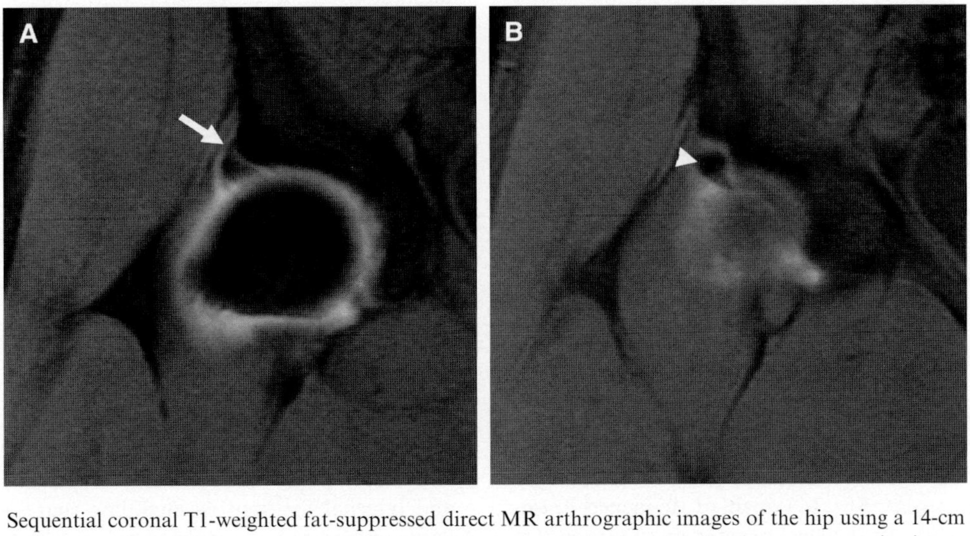


Fig. 5. Sequential coronal T1-weighted fat-suppressed direct MR arthrographic images of the hip using a 14-cm field of view in a hockey player with a recurrent, painful hip click during abduction. (*A*) On the more posterior image, a full-thickness defect allows passage of contrast (*arrow*) through the anterior, superior labrum. (*B*) On the most anterior image, a large ossicle is evident at the anterior labrum and capsule (*arrowhead*).

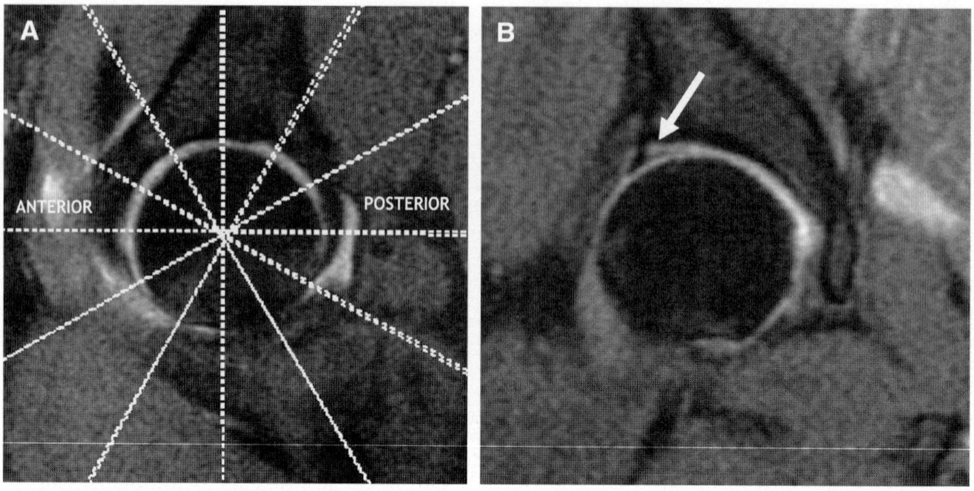


Fig. 6. Radial imaging of the acetabular labrum during direct MR arthrography. (*A*) Localizer grid for the 12 radial images prescribed at equal intervals from a sagittal oblique image (angled with the acetabulum). (*B*) T1-weighted fat-suppressed direct MR arthrographic image from the radial sequence demonstrates a tear of the anterior labrum (*arrow*).

protocol combines some of the positive attributes of the direct MR arthrogram protocol and the noncontrast protocol. That is, we include a coronal T2-weighted FSE fat-suppressed small field-of-view sequence early in the protocol and coronal and axial T1-weighted SE sequences dedicated to the hip at the end of the protocol, which allows maximum time for accumulation of contrast in the joint. We acquire an SE non–fat-suppressed T1-weighted sequence of the entire pelvis and an axial T2 FSE with fat suppression, also with a large field of view. As always, it is important to acquire a small field-of-view sagittal sequence (T1 or T2 with fat suppression) to evaluate anterior labral structures.

Pre- and postcontrast imaging of the hip can be valuable in a select set of patients, and indications for enhancement are similar to those used when imaging other joints. Bony and soft tissue tumors do occur about the hip, and we recommend pre- and postcontrast images in all such cases, even if the tumor appears simple on noncontrast images. To measure enhancement of tissues accurately, it is important to acquire sequences with identical parameters before and after intravenous contrast injection. A fat-suppressed gradient echo sequence can provide for an excellent measure of enhancement with a rapid acquisition time. Alternatively, fat-suppressed SE T1-weighted sequences also provide for excellent assessment of enhancement but allow for better resolution with a cost of increased imaging time. We routinely acquire postcontrast images in at least two planes based on lesion morphology. Other indications for which pre- and postcontrast imaging should be considered include infection, inflammatory arthropathies, vascular lesions, periarticular processes, and certain postsurgical patients [6–9].

## Injury-specific imaging

Using this general protocol for patients who undergo routine outpatient hip MR imaging should serve the interpreting radiologist well for most hip maladies, but certain differential diagnoses either require more specific protocols or can be resolved with a shorter, limited MR imaging examination. As in all imaging, pretest suspicion guides protocol. The following conditions are considerations specific to some of the most common indications for hip MR imaging.

### *Occult hip fracture*

In the setting of a radiographic examination equivocal for hip fracture or negative radiographs with a persistent high clinical suspicion for occult hip fracture, we use a semi-emergent limited hip fracture protocol (Table 3). Because the results of such a study may lead to emergent open reduction and internal fixation, we mandate that such hip fracture studies be completed and interpreted urgently, even after hours and on weekends. The protocol can be completed in approximately 12

Table 3
MR imaging protocol: hip fracture

| Primary sequences | Plane | Sequence | Coil | FOV | Slice | Matrix NEX | TR | TE | TI | Flip angle | Band | ETL | Fat suppression? | Other | Estimated time (min) |
|---|---|---|---|---|---|---|---|---|---|---|---|---|---|---|---|
| 1 | Coronal | STIR | Torso | 36–48 | 4/1 | 256×192 2 | 2000–6000 | 25–40 | 150 | — | 16 | 8 | — | Acquire as first sequence | 5–6 |
| 2 | Coronal | T1 SE | Torso | 36–48 | 4/1 | 256×192 2 | 400–800 | 10–20 | — | — | 16 | — | No | — | 3–4 |
| 3 | Axial | T2 FSE | Torso | 36–48 | 5/1 | 256×192 2 | 2000–4000 | 70–80 | — | — | 16 | 8 | Yes | Consider no fat saturation if pathologic fracture | 3–4 |
| Optional sequences | | | | | | | | | | | | | | | |
| 4 | Sagittal | T2 FSE | Torso | 30–40 | 4/1 | 256×192 2 | 2000–4000 | 70–80 | — | — | 16 | 8 | Yes | May help with subcapital fracture alignment | 3–4 |

Special instructions: Coverage: front of crest through sacrum for coronals; top of crest past ischium for axials.
*Abbreviations:* ETL, echo train length; FOV, field of view; NEX, number of excitations; TE, echo time; TI, time to inversion; TR, repetition time.

minutes and includes large field-of-view coronal STIR and T1-weighted SE sequences and a non–fat-suppressed T2 FSE axial sequence. A sagittal FSE sequence can be added in more difficult cases but is most often unnecessary. The STIR should be acquired first as a cautionary measure for cases in which a patient cannot tolerate the full study. This sequence alone is generally enough to make a diagnosis of fracture versus no fracture [10,11]. Acute and subacute fractures are readily apparent on the STIR sequence by virtue of its sensitivity to bone marrow edema, even if the T1 is necessary for description and classification [12–15].

*Arthropathies*

Although bilateral and symmetric osteoarthritis remains an important finding, it is rarely the primary diagnostic impetus behind obtaining an MR image of the hip. First, radiographs remain the workhorse imaging study to support physical examination findings and guide therapeutic algorithms for osteoarthritis of the hips. Second, if MR imaging is the chosen imaging modality for evaluation of an arthropathy involving the hips, protocols dedicated to the bony pelvis may provide more information per imaging dollar than would MR imaging of the hip or bilateral hip MR imaging examinations. With atypical arthropathies, MR imaging of the hip may be the most valuable single imaging modality. For the hip in question, a small field-of-view axial or coronal T2 FSE with fat suppression may be of value in discerning cortical erosion from subchondral geode. An asymmetric hip joint effusion may serve as an indicator for the presence of an atypical arthropathy. When a joint effusion is present, the T1-weighted and the fat-suppressed FSE sequences are valuable in identifying synovitis and pannus. If MR imaging is to be used as a discriminating tool between arthropathies, however, pre- and postcontrast sequences using the same slice selection and parameters are strongly suggested. On high field strength systems, fast spoiled gradient echo or T1-weighted SE fat-suppressed sequences are favorite choices for the pre- and postcontrast imaging. T1 SE may provide more homogeneous signal, but gradient echo generally costs less imaging time [16–18].

*Labral tears*

The preferred technique for imaging the acetabular labrum is detailed in the section on direct MR arthrography, but it seems awkward to discuss impingement syndromes without including the often associated labral tear. Isao and colleagues [19] nicely described variants in acetabular labrum morphology in asymptomatic patients in 2000. The sublabral sulcus at the posterior labrum has been described as analogous to the sublabral recess seen frequently at the anterior glenoid labrum [20]. It seems indisputable that any defect that extends from the labral undersurface to its superior surface would classify as a tear, however. This diagnosis is strengthened by imbibition of contrast into the defect on direct MR arthrography. Smaller undersurface tears also can be differentiated from normal recesses by configuration of imbibed contrast. Most variant labral morphologies seem to be present in older patients with at least early findings of osteoarthritis. In young patients with no hip arthropathy, the normal anterior and superior labrum should be sharply defined, triangular, and hypointense on all sequences. Defects in these locations, especially those that allow for contrast imbibition, should raise strong suspicion for tears. On noncontrast images, a paralabral cyst can be the imager's friend in establishing this diagnosis [21]. Even in the absence of a visible defect, a multilobulated paralabral cystic structure combined with any abnormal labral morphology should be regarded as indicative of a tear (Fig. 7) [22–24].

*Impingement syndromes*

Femoral acetabular impingement has evolved into a favorite group of biomechanical pathologies in orthopedic journals over the past 3 years. The two patterns of impingement have been termed cam type and pincer type, and a multitude of new therapeutic techniques have been described for each in recent years. Cam type is more frequently described and is believed to be a more common cause of the clinical impingement syndrome. The femoral head articulates asymmetrically in the acetabulum with a configuration likened to the cam on the camshaft of a combustion engine [25]. Several scientific papers presented at the major radiology meetings over the past 2 years have described imaging appearances of cam type femoral acetabular impingement, but the most accepted criteria to date are based on radiographic studies [26]. A pattern of MR imaging findings is emerging as a reliable indicator of impingement. Capsular hypertrophy, anterior labral injury, productive change at the anterosuperior acetabulum, and a characteristic hyperostotic bump at the anterolateral femoral head-neck junction have been described in multiple series investigating the MR imaging appearance of cam type femoral acetabular impingement [27,28]. Although this constellation of findings can be identified with the standard noncontrast hip protocol, we are currently using a direct arthrographic protocol in the clinical setting suspicious for impingement. In the setting of suspected impingement, the addition of a coronal sequence with the patient positioned for abduction and external rotation of the hip may be of additional value (Fig. 8) [29].

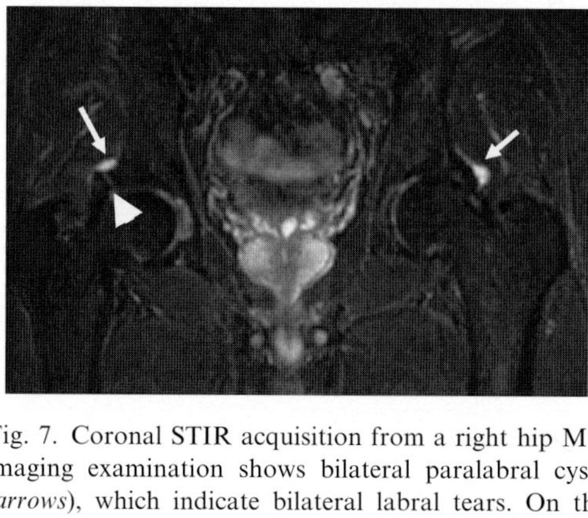

Fig. 7. Coronal STIR acquisition from a right hip MR imaging examination shows bilateral paralabral cysts (*arrows*), which indicate bilateral labral tears. On the right, a labral tear is apparent (*arrowhead*), even on this large field-of-view image.

*Osteonecrosis*

The standard noncontrast MR imaging protocol is highly sensitive and specific for femoral head osteonecrosis [30]. The high frequency of bilateral osteonecrosis supports our large field-of-view imaging sequences of the entire pelvis. When describing osteonecrosis, we believe it is important to acknowledge that the Ficat classification system for femoral head osteonecrosis is the one most frequently used by orthopedists in guiding treatment and is based on radiographic findings [31]. Even so, several of the stage-identifying traits in the Ficat classification can be identified on MR imaging and should be included in the report. We typically include T1 signal, T2 signal, any subchondral hypointense lines, and presence or absence of cortical collapse and fragmentation in the MR imaging report of osteonecrosis. As with all osteochondral defects, any evidence for an unstable fragment in the form of fluid signal partitioning the fragment from the remainder of the bone should be reported. Because of its propensity

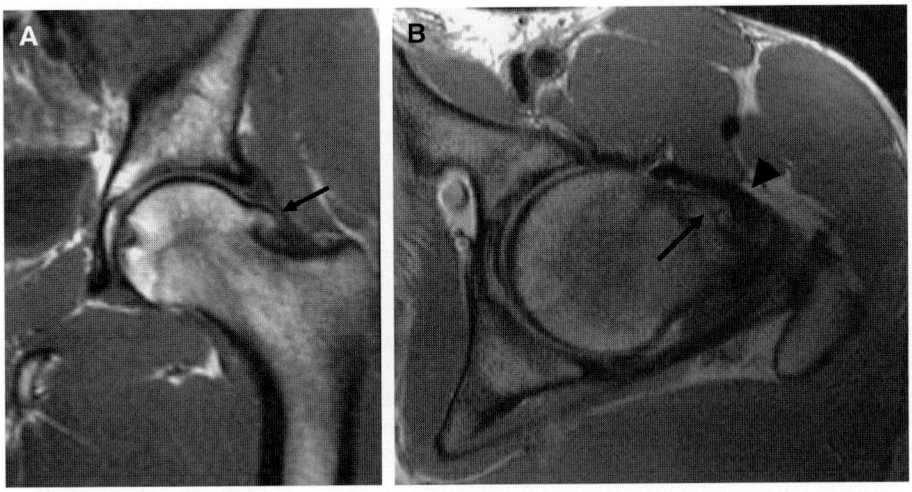


Fig. 8. Coronal T1-weighted (*A*) and axial proton density FSE (*B*) images of the left hip in a 26-year-old basketball player with chronic pain during abduction. These high-resolution sequences demonstrate a large, hyperostotic excrescence at the femoral head-neck junction typical of cam type impingement (*arrow*). Note the resultant anterior capsular hypertrophy (*arrowhead*).

for bilaterality, the importance of imaging the contralateral hip in patients with femoral head osteonecrosis cannot be overstated [32]. Although not included in our standard hip osteonecrosis protocol, additional information can be obtained with a dynamic postcontrast sequence. This sequence can be achieved on most 1.5 T systems using a fast, spoiled gradient echo sequence and acquiring signal before intravenous contrast injection and then at five sequential 20-second intervals after the injection (Fig. 9) [33,34].

A potential confounder for the diagnosis of acute femoral head osteonecrosis is the entity termed "transient osteoporosis of the hip." Because of the overlap in imaging findings with these two diagnoses, we suggest short interval follow-up MR imaging in cases with both entities remaining on the differential after one study. Striking and extensive subchondral bone marrow edema in the femoral head with recent onset of pain and no cortical collapse or findings of osteoarthritis are features typical for acute osteonecrosis and transient osteoporosis. A subchondral hypointense line can be seen in both conditions, so serial MR imaging may play an important role in discriminating between early-stage avascular necrosis and transient osteoporosis. A seemingly growing faction of orthopedists and radiologists consider transient osteoporosis, in the appropriate clinical setting, in the spectrum of disease that includes subchondral insufficiency fractures. Because these cases may resolve spontaneously, as in the setting of transient osteoporosis, or progress to cortical collapse and late-stage osteonecrosis, we believe that follow-up noncontrast MR imaging 3 to 6 weeks after the initial study can be an important tool in guiding therapy (Fig. 10) [35,36].

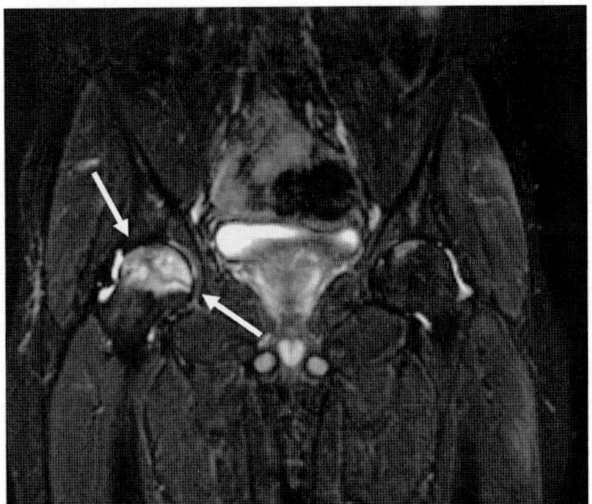

Fig. 9. Bilateral femoral head osteonecrosis in a patient on long-term steroid use for inflammatory bowel disease. The large region of involvement on the right is outlined by the linear hypointensity (*arrows*) and is supported by the striking bone marrow edema. A smaller region of subchondral involvement is visible on the left.

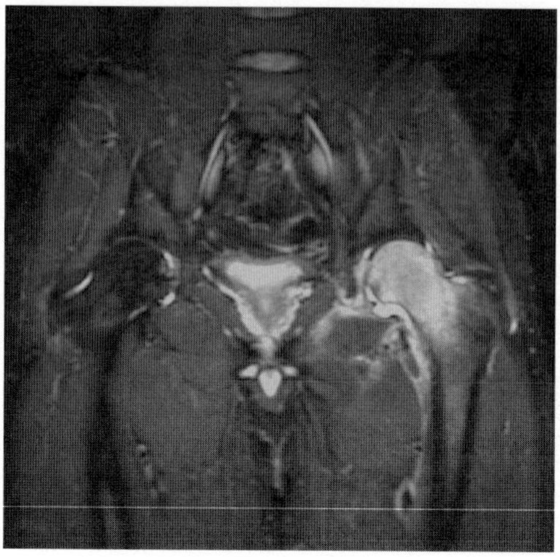

Fig. 10. The striking bone marrow edema involving the proximal femur on this STIR image was almost completely resolved on a follow-up study 8 weeks later. This 55-year-old man had a clinical and imaging scenario most consistent with transient osteoporosis of the hip.

### *Muscle injuries*

The numerous muscles that originate and insert about the hip and pelvis lend to an enormous number of myopathies that may be encountered on a routine hip MR imaging examination. In general, it is best to keep an atlas of pelvic musculature handy for proper identification of injured internal rotator, external rotator, abductor, adductor, and pelvic floor muscles. One muscle frequently identified as abnormal in the setting of hip pain is the gluteus medius. It originates from the middle iliac fossa, inserts on the greater trochanter of the femur, and has been called the rotator cuff of the hip because of tapered oblique configuration, analogous to the supraspinatous at the shoulder. The gluteus medius can be partially or completely torn or can be diffusely fatty atrophied, with patterns of injury similar to those seen in the rotator cuff musculature of the shoulder. Diffuse processes, such as a grade I gluteus medius strain or gluteus medius atrophy, may be seen best on the coronal sequences noting any asymmetry, but the sagittal FSE sequence may be the most specific for insertional strains and tears at its trochanteric insertion [37].

Pubalgia refers to groin pain without a clear cause on physical examination, and it is a common indication for MR imaging in athletic patients [38]. In these cases, careful evaluation of not only the hip joint is warranted but also the pubic symphysis, rectus abdominus insertions, internal and external oblique musculature, and inguinal rings [39].

Finally, one must remember the less common causalgias of muscle injuries about the pelvis. A multitude of snapping tendon or snapping hip syndromes have been described. Internal and external snapping hip syndromes and intra-articular and extra-articular snapping hip syndromes indicate a muscle or tendon snapping over an inciting structure, which can range from bursitis to normal bony protuberances. Whichever muscle or tendon is involved, the imager's responsibility is to identify the inflammation and consider potential biomechanical causes. Again, fat suppression is integral to identifying the muscle or tendon edema and any reactive bone marrow edema (Fig. 11) [40,41].

### *Bursitis*

A multitude of anatomic bursae exist about the hip, but the iliopsoas and several of the trochanteric bursae are most frequently identified as sources of pain and decreased range of motion. An abnormally enlarged, fluid distended bursa should be readily identifiable on fluid-sensitive sequences, especially those with fat suppression. Any organized collection of fluid that lifts the psoas tendon off the anterior hip capsule can be termed iliopsoas bursitis, but distension in the anteroposterior plane may be the best predictor of symptomatology [42,43]. The diagnosis of trochanteric bursitis is more complicated, because there are actually six anatomic bursae about the insertions of the gluteus maximus, medius, and minimus tendons about the greater trochanter. A sliver of fluid about the greater trochanter is present in most obese patients and may be normal. We reserve the term "trochanteric bursitis" for patients with fluid that measures more than 2 mm in a transverse plane adjacent to the greater trochanter or asymmetric fluid in this location with corresponding unilaterality of symptoms. Remember that distended bursae occasionally may become superinfected, and pre- and postcontrast sequences should be acquired if there is a suspicion for septic bursitis (Fig. 12) [44].

### *Sacroiliac pathology*

Although sacroiliac diseases should be imaged with a dedicated sacroiliac protocol, one can be prepared to adjust for incidental sacroiliac pathologies seen "on the fly" while imaging the hip. By tailoring the coronal sequences to the normal

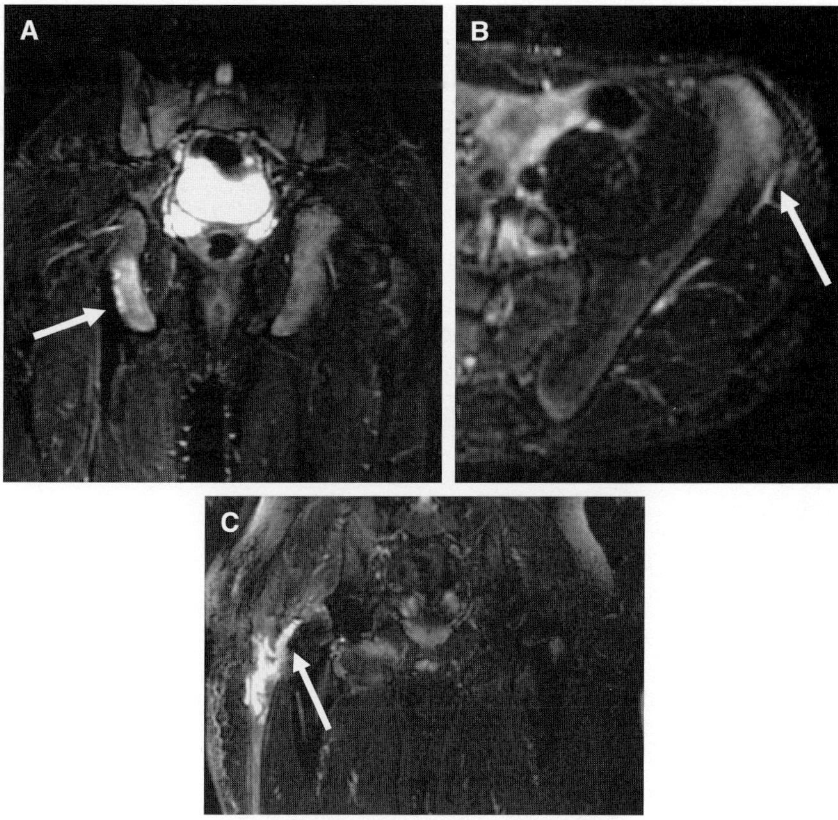


Fig. 11. Muscle avulsions about the pelvis mimicking hip pain. (*A*) Reactive bone marrow edema that involves the ischial tuberosity (*arrow*) from hamstring avulsive stress in a 14-year-old soccer player. (*B*) Avulsive injury at the anterior superior iliac spine that involves the tensor fascia lata (*arrow*) in a 29-year-old runner. (*C*) Complete or near complete gluteus medius avulsion (*arrow*) in a 62-year-old patient with loss of external rotator strength, imaged on a 0.3 T system.

sacroiliac configuration, angling with the sacrum based on a sagittal localizer, and decreasing the field of view to approximately 24 cm, a hip MR image can be optimized for sacroiliac arthropathies. A similar principle may be used to optimize protocols for lumbosacral plexopathies. A T2-weighted FSE fat-suppressed sequence angled with the sacrum may provide imagers with their best chance of finding lumbosacral plexus lesions, including cysts, neuromas, and nerve sheath tumors. If a mass is suspected, contrast-enhanced sequences are indicated. One important neural structure to identify in patients with hip pain and radiculopathic symptoms is the sciatic nerve. Occasionally, one division of the sciatic nerve can take an anomalous course and pass between bellies of the piriformis muscle. In these patients, contraction of the piriformis can cause impingement of the sciatic division involved, which is the clinical entity termed piriformis syndrome.

## Low field strength considerations

Open low field strength systems present a unique set of obstacles to the imager who is attempting to diagnose internal derangements of joints. The balance between signal to noise and resolution is becomes more delicate as field strength and gradient strength decrease, and typical applications common in 1.5 T protocols may not be available. Some patients imaged on open systems may not be candidates for imaging on high field strength systems with closed designs because of their body morphology, which makes acquisition of diagnostic images even more difficult. With attention to protocol and parameter detail and the ability to make patient-specific adjustments, most diagnoses

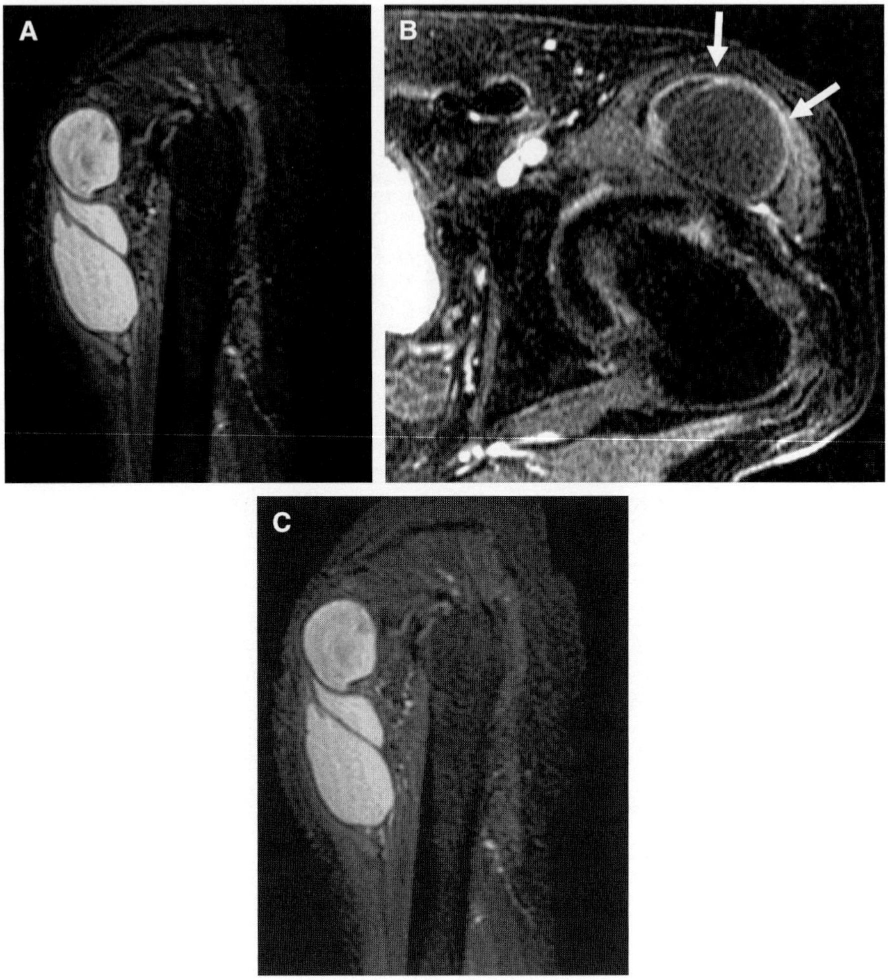


Fig. 12. Sagittal STIR (*A*) and postcontrast axial spoiled gradient echo (*B*) images of severe iliopsoas bursitis. Only a thin rind of peripheral enhancement of the fluid is evident (*arrows*), which is typical for an aseptic bursal collection.

we have reviewed should be made on open MR imaging systems (Table 4).

Inversion recovery becomes the workhorse mechanism for fat suppression on many low field strength systems. STIR sequences with parameters routinely used at 1.5 T may yield suboptimal fat suppression when field strength is lowered. We decrease the time to inversion for low field strength protocols, with optimal fat suppression and signal homogeneity achieved at a time to inversion of 80 to 90 msec on our 0.3 T systems. An echo time (TE) of 25 to 40 msec works well with this shorter time to inversion to provide homogeneous fat suppression, acceptable fluid sensitivity, and diagnostic resolution for these open, low field strength systems. We acquire a STIR sequence of the entire pelvis on all open hip MR imaging examinations and a T1-weighted SE using the same field of view. For the sequences dedicated to the affected hip, we enlarge the field of view compared with our high field strength protocols to maximize signal. Unless a patient's morphology dictates otherwise, we find a 22-cm field of view to provide a harmonious compromise of signal and contrast for the sagittal and coronal sequences. A sagittal T2 FSE with a matrix of 256×256 allows for diagnostic assessment of anterior labral structures and surrounding bursae and the gluteus medius insertion. An axial proton density FSE provides nice labral resolution but is inherently signal poor, which often necessitates a decrease in matrix to 192×256. In larger

Table 4
MR imaging protocol: 0.3 T open hip

| Primary sequences | Plane | Sequence | Coil | FOV | Slice | Matrix NEX | TR | TE | TI | Flip angle | Band | ETL | Fat suppression? | Other | Estimated time (min) |
|---|---|---|---|---|---|---|---|---|---|---|---|---|---|---|---|
| Localizer | 3 plane | FSPGR | Torso | 40–48 | — | — | — | — | — | — | — | — | — | Parameters set by system | 2 |
| 1 | Coronal | T1 SE | Torso | 40–48 | 5/1 | 256×192 2 | 400–800 | 10–20 | — | — | 16 | — | No | — | 3–4 |
| 2 | Coronal | STIR | Torso | 40–48 | 5/1 | 256×192 2 | 2000–6000 | 25–40 | 90 | — | 16 | 8 | — | — | 5–6 |
| 3 | Sagittal | T2 FSE | Torso | 24 | 4/1 | 256×192 3 | 2000–6000 | 60–80 | — | — | 16 | 8 | No | Consider obliquity with acetabular rim off coronal localizer | 3–4 |
| 4 | Axial | T2 FSE | Torso | 40–48 | 4/1 | 256×256 3 | 2000–6000 | 60–80 | — | — | 16 | 8 | No | Image entire pelvis | 3–4 |
| 5 | Axial | T1 SE | Torso | 40–48 | 4/1 | 256×192 2 | 400–800 | 10–20 | — | — | 16 | — | No | Image entire pelvis | 3–4 |

Special instructions: Maximize signal to noise as necessary with smaller matrix, larger FOV, thicker slices.

*Abbreviations:* ETL, echo train length; FOV, field of view; FSPGR, fast spoiled gradient echo; NEX, number of excitations; TE, echo time; TI, time to inversion; TR, repetition time.

patients, the paucity of signal may require that a T1 SE be substituted as the axial sequence.

An advantage of MR imaging at lower field strengths is decreased signal distortion and degradation associated with many of the described artifacts inherent to higher field strength systems. This is certainly the case with susceptibility artifact related to many orthopedic hardware devices. For this reason, we often find studies acquired on open, 0.3 T systems preferable in the setting of total joint and open reduction internal fixation devices about the hip. In addition to the significant drop in susceptibility artifact inherent to the lower field strength, our metal protocols are adjusted from the general protocols to minimize degradation of signal in bone and soft tissue by the adjacent hardware. Increasing the band width of most sequences should decrease susceptibility artifact with a linear relationship. Doubling the band width from 1.5 to 3 on a T2 FSE sequence should reduce metal-related artifact by approximately 50%. Any gradient echo sequences maximize susceptibility artifact related to orthopedic hardware and should be replaced when protocolling such studies. On fluid-sensitive long TE sequences, FSE acquisitions create less susceptibility artifact than SE sequences and are preferred with metal. Finally, decreasing the field of view and increasing the TE help decrease metal-associated artifact but also lower signal in general. These metal artifact–reducing techniques also can be applied to high field strength protocols, but an additional consideration at 1.5 T should be removal of chemically selective fat suppression from the FSE sequences. Using these general techniques, diagnostic images often can be acquired even in the setting of orthopedic hardware [45].

Arthrography on low field strength systems generally does not reach the resolution of similar studies acquired at 1.5 T, but diagnostic quality studies can be produced. Some vendors offer an alternative method of fat suppression in the form of either two-point or three-point Dixon fat/water separation. On our 0.3 T systems, we acquire a three-point Dixon sequence in the plane of most interest: axial if there is suspicion for anterior labral tear and coronal if there is suspicion for superior labral tear. The homogeneously fat suppressed out of phase to fat portion of the Dixon sequence frequently confirms or refutes findings suspicious for small labral tears on other sequences. One difficulty with MR arthrography at low field strengths has proved to be loss of intra-articular contrast signal on inversion recovery sequences. The Dixon and other opposed phase applications may be an imager's best bet for fat suppression in these cases.

High field strength imaging of joints on 3 T systems has generated interest in recent years. As coils and protocols improve, these systems may provide advantages over traditional 1.5 T systems, especially in imaging articular cartilage injury. To date, however, not enough studies have made it to

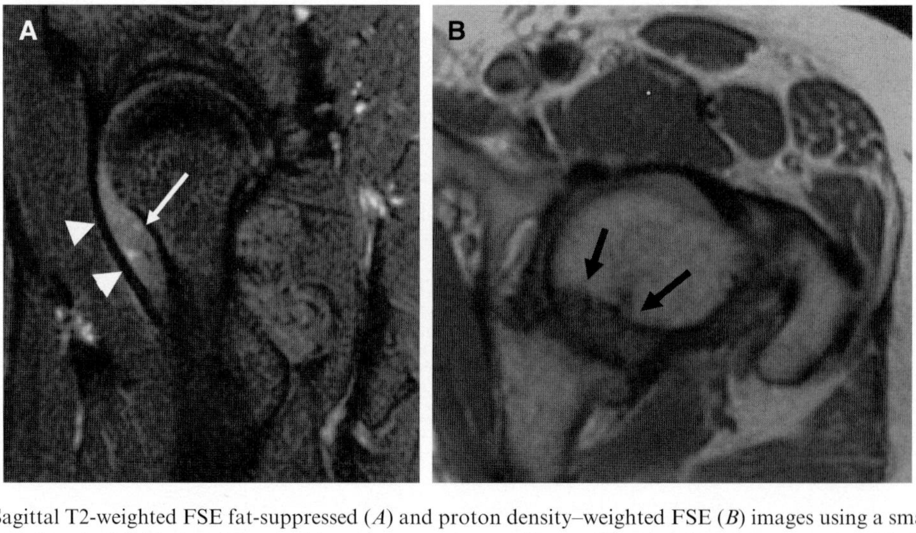


Fig. 13. Sagittal T2-weighted FSE fat-suppressed (*A*) and proton density–weighted FSE (*B*) images using a small field of view dedicated to the left hip in a 35-year-old postpartum woman. The proliferative, hypointense material (*white arrow*) suggests a synovitis. Note the anteriorly displaced iliopsoas tendon (*arrowheads*). A large pressure erosion (*black arrows*) on the posterior femoral head solidifies the diagnosis of pigmented villonodular synovitis.

the literature for 3 T imaging to be considered a standard of care. We look forward to embracing the imminent advances that will accompany further development of 3 T protocols for joint-specific pathology. Currently, the hip remains among the most challenging of joints to image effectively. With each examination, a balance must be struck between achieving the necessary resolution for diagnosing small lesions and evaluating distant structures that may cause pain or dysfunction attributed to the hip. With attention to detail directed to each individual examination, MR imaging of the hip can be a rewarding endeavor, frequently diagnosing previously unexpected sources of pathology (Fig. 13).

## References


[1] Lecouvet FE, Vande Berg BC, Malghem J, et al. Magnetic resonance and computed tomography imaging in multiple myeloma. Semin Musculoskelet Radiol 2001;5:43–55.

[2] May DA, Purins JL, Smith DK. MR imaging of occult traumatic fractures and muscular injuries of the hip and pelvis in elderly patients. AJR Am J Roentgenol 1996;166:1075–8.

[3] Zampa V, Cosottini M, Michelassi C, et al. Value of opposed-phase gradient-echo technique in distinguishing between benign and malignant vertebral lesions. Eur Radiol 2002;12:1811–8.

[4] Petersilge CA, Haque MA, Petersilge WJ, et al. Acetabular labral tears: evaluation with MR arthrography. Radiology 1996;200:231–5.

[5] Montgomery DD, Morrison WB, Schweitzer ME, et al. Effects of iodinated contrast and field strength on gadolinium enhancement: implications for direct MR arthrography. J Magn Reson Imaging 2002; 15(3):334–43.

[6] Nomikos GC, Murphey MD, Kransdorf MJ, et al. Primary bone tumors of the lower extremities. Radiol Clin North Am 2002;40:971–90.

[7] Lee SK, Suh KJ, Kim YW, et al. Septic arthritis versus transient synovitis at MR imaging: preliminary assessment with signal intensity alterations in bone marrow. Radiology 1999;211:459–65.

[8] Huang AB, Schweitzer ME, Hume E, et al. Osteomyelitis of the pelvis/hips in paralyzed patients: accuracy and clinical utility of MRI. J Comput Assist Tomogr 1998;22:437–43.

[9] Czerny C, Krestan C, Imhof H, et al. Magnetic resonance imaging of the postoperative hip. Top Magn Reson Imaging 1999;10:214–20.

[10] Meyers SP, Wiener SN. Magnetic resonance imaging features of fractures using the short tau inversion recovery (STIR) sequence: correlation with radiographic findings. Skeletal Radiol 1991;20:499–507.

[11] Lim KB, Eng AK, Chng SM, et al. Limited magnetic resonance imaging (MRI) and the occult hip fracture. Ann Acad Med Singapore 2002;31:607–10.

[12] Haramati N, Staron RB, Barax C, et al. Magnetic resonance imaging of occult fractures of the proximal femur. Skeletal Radiol 1994;23:19–22.

[13] Oka M, Monu JU. Prevalence and patterns of occult hip fractures and mimics revealed by MRI. AJR Am J Roentgenol 2004;182:283–8.

[14] Pandey R, McNally E, Ali A, et al. The role of MRI in the diagnosis of occult hip fractures. Injury 1998; 29:61–3.

[15] Bogost GA, Lizerbram EK, Crues JV III. MR imaging in evaluation of suspected hip fracture: frequency of unsuspected bone and soft-tissue injury. Radiology 1995;197:263–7.

[16] Tehranzadeh J, Ashikyan O, Dascalos J. Advanced imaging of early rheumatoid arthritis. Radiol Clin North Am 2004;42:89–107.

[17] Gupta KB, Duryea J, Weissman BN. Radiographic evaluation of osteoarthritis. Radiol Clin North Am 2004;42:11–41.

[18] Murray JG, Ridley NT, Mitchell N, et al. Juvenile chronic arthritis of the hip: value of contrast-enhanced MR imaging. Clin Radiol 1996;51:99–102.

[19] Isao A, Yoshitada H, Kazuhiro O, et al. Acetabular labrum: abnormal findings at MRI in asymptomatic hips. Radiology 2000;216:576–81.

[20] Dinauer PA, Murphy KP, Carroll JF. Sublabral sulcus at the posteroinferior acetabulum: a potential pitfall in MR arthrography diagnosis of acetabular labral tears. AJR Am J Roentgenol 2004;183(6): 1745–53.

[21] Schnarkowski P, Steinbach LS, Tirman PF, et al. Magnetic resonance imaging of labral cysts of the hip. Skeletal Radiol 1996;25:733–7.

[22] McCarthy JC, Noble PC, Schuck MR, et al. The Otto E. Aufranc award: the role of labral lesions to development of early degenerative hip disease. Clin Orthop 2001;393:25–37.

[23] Czerny C, Hofmann S, Urban M, et al. MR arthrography of the adult acetabular capsular-labral complex: correlation with surgery and anatomy. AJR Am J Roentgenol 1999;173:345–9.

[24] Leunig M, Werlen S, Ungersbock A, et al. Evaluation of the acetabular labrum by MR arthrography. J Bone Joint Surg Br 1997;79:230–4.

[25] Ito K, Minka MA II, Leunig M, et al. Femoroacetabular impingement and the cam-effect: an MRI-based quantitative anatomical study of the femoral head-neck offset. J Bone Joint Surg Br 2001;83:171–6.

[26] Leunig M, Podeszwa D, Beck M, et al. Magnetic resonance arthrography of labral disorders in hips with dysplasia and impingement. Clin Orthop 2004;418: 74–80.

[27] Jager M, Wild A, Westhoff B, et al. Femoroacetabular impingement caused by a femoral osseous head-neck bump deformity: clinical, radiological, and experimental results. J Orthop Sci 2004;9:256–63.

[28] Notzli HP, Wyss TF, Stoecklin CH, et al. The contour of the femoral head-neck junction as a predictor for the risk of anterior impingement. J Bone Joint Surg Br 2002;84:556–60.
[29] Ganz R, Parvizi J, Beck M, et al. Femoroacetabular impingement: a cause for osteoarthritis of the hip. Clin Orthop 2003;417:112–20.
[30] Glickstein MF, Burk DL Jr, Schiebler ML, et al. Avascular necrosis versus other diseases of the hip: sensitivity of MR imaging. Radiology 1988;169: 213–5.
[31] Ficat RP. Idiopathic bone necrosis of the femoral head—early diagnosis and treatment. J Bone Joint Surg (Br) 1985;67:3–9.
[32] Mitchell DG, Rao VM, Dalinka MK, et al. Femoral head avascular necrosis: correlation of MR imaging, radiographic staging, radionuclide imaging, and clinical findings. Radiology 1987;162:709–15.
[33] Lang P, Mauz M, Schorner W, et al. Acute fracture of the femoral neck: assessment of femoral head perfusion with gadopentetate dimeglumine-enhanced MR imaging. AJR Am J Roentgenol 1993;160: 335–41.
[34] Nadel SN, Debatin JF, Richardson WJ, et al. Detection of acute avascular necrosis of the femoral head in dogs: dynamic contrast-enhanced MR imaging vs spin-echo and STIR sequences. AJR Am J Roentgenol 1992;159:1255–61.
[35] Malizos KN, Zibis AH, Dailiana Z, et al. MR imaging findings in transient osteoporosis of the hip. Eur J Radiol 2004;50:238–44.
[36] Cheng EY, Thongtrangan I, Laorr A, et al. Spontaneous resolution of osteonecrosis of the femoral head. J Bone Joint Surg Am 2004;86-A(12): 2594–9.
[37] Robinson G, Hines AL, Richards PJ, et al. MRI abnormalities of the external rotators of the hip. Clin Radiol 2005;60(3):401–6.
[38] Albers SL, Spritzer CE, Garrett WE Jr, et al. MR findings in athletes with pubalgia. Skeletal Radiol 2001;30:270–7.
[39] Overdeck KH, Palmer WE. Imaging of hip and groin injuries in athletes. Semin Musculoskelet Radiol 2004;8(1):41–55.
[40] Vacarro JP, Sauser DD, Beals RK. Iliopsoas bursa imaging: efficacy in depicting abnormal iliopsoas tendon motion in patients with internal snapping hip syndrome. Radiology 1995;197:853–6.
[41] Pelsser V, Cardinal E, Hobden R, et al. Extraarticular snapping hip: sonographic findings. AJR Am J Roengenol 2001;176:67–73.
[42] Wunderbaldinger P, Bremer C, Schellenberger E, et al. Imaging features of iliopsoas bursitis. Eur Radiol 2002;12:409–15.
[43] Kozlov DB, Sonin AH. Iliopsoas bursitis: diagnosis by MRI. J Comput Assist Tomogr 1998;22: 625–8.
[44] Walsh G, Archibald CG. MRI in greater trochanter pain syndrome. Australas Radiol 2003;47:85–7.
[45] Olsen RV, Munk PL, Lee MJ, et al. Metal artifact reduction sequence: early clinical applications. Radiographics 2000;20(3):699–712.

ELSEVIER
SAUNDERS

Magn Reson Imaging Clin N Am
13 (2005) 635–640

MAGNETIC
RESONANCE
IMAGING CLINICS
of North America

# Role of Hip MR Imaging in the Management of Sports-Related Injuries

Robert Meislin, MD[a,*], Andrew Abeles, BS[b]

[a]*New York University—Hospital for Joint Diseases, 301 East 17th Street, 14th Floor, New York, NY 10003, USA*
[b]*University of Missouri-Columbia School of Medicine, One Hospital Drive, MA215, Columbia, MO 65212, USA*

MR imaging of the hip has provided the treating physician with an imaging modality that can better determine a more specific diagnosis for acute and chronic hip pain in the athlete. Intra- and extra-articular processes can be evaluated with MR imaging. Soft tissue and osseous injury around the hip can be assessed. In addition, the pelvis and contralateral hip are often included in the scanned images.

After a complete history and physical examination, plain radiographs of the hip and pelvis are taken. If direct or indirect trauma has occurred, radiographs must be carefully reviewed for an underlying fracture. Importantly, an acute stress fracture of the femoral neck may not be readily apparent on radiographs. Underlying hip dysplasia must be excluded by measuring the center edge (CE) angle of Wiberg. With the performance of saline or gadolinium MR imaging, intra-articular conditions, such as acetabular labral tears, osteochondral injury to the femoral head, a ruptured ligamentum teres (LT), or loose bodies, can be detected.

In this article, we discuss the various soft tissue and osseous conditions for which MR imaging can be helpful in the workup of the painful hip after and during athletic play.

* Corresponding author.
*E-mail address:* robert.meislin@med.nyu.edu (R. Meislin).

## Soft tissue conditions

### *Acetabular labral tears*

Clinically, labral tears of the acetabulum may present with nonspecific hip pain. Occasionally, the tear can be associated with painful snapping and clicking within the hip joint. Although labral tears can be associated with posterior hip dislocations and hip dysplasia ("the inverted labrum"), golfers and runners may present with an insidious onset of hip pain whose source is a torn labrum. MR arthrography has been shown to have improved sensitivity compared with plain MR imaging for labral tears [1–3]. With joint distention by the injected fluid, labral tears are delineated by displacing the capsule from the abutting labrum and underlying bone. This is similar to MR arthrography of the shoulder, which better outlines glenoid labral tears compared with conventional MR imaging.

Tears are often found at the anterior and anterosuperior aspects of the acetabular rim (Fig. 1). The introduction of saline or dilute gadolinium into the joint does not always allow for differentiation between a normal sublabral sulcus and a partially torn labrum. One group reported that a posteroinferior sublabral groove is a relatively normal anatomic hip variation [4]. No sublabral sulcuses were found anteriorly or anterosuperiorly on the acetabulum. Tears of the acetabular labrum can be similar to morphologic tears of the meniscus in the knee and have been characterized as radial flap, radial fibrillated, and longitudinal peripheral [5]. On occasion, a bucket-handle tear occurs. Tears may also be

1064-9689/05/$ - see front matter 
doi:10.1016/j.mric.2005.08.014

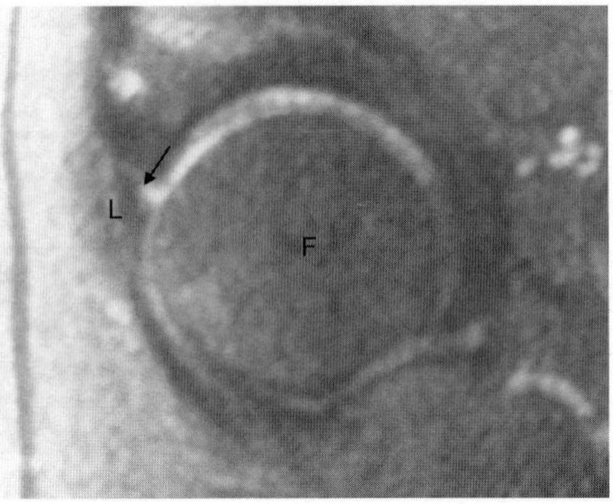


Fig. 1. MR coronal image of a tear (*arrow*) in the anterior labrum (L). F, femoral head.

classified based on cause: idiopathic, traumatic, or dysplastic [6].

In chronic situations, a paralabral cyst may develop (akin to a popliteal cyst in the knee secondary to a meniscal tear) with leakage of joint fluid through a rent in the capsule. A paralabral cyst on MR imaging should thus further one's suspicion for an underlying labral tear.

*Ruptured ligamentum teres*

The LT connects the fovea of the femoral head to the posteroinferior portion of the acetabular fossa, carries blood supply to the femoral head, and provides some stability to the hip. Similar to the torn labrum, mechanical symptoms can occur with a ruptured LT, including painful clicking and giving way. Tears of the LT may arise from major and minor trauma [7]. LT tears have been characterized as partial, complete, and degenerative [8]. Most apparent on axial and coronal MR images, abnormal enlargement, thickening, and deformity of the LT with intrasubstance cystic signal changes are seen.

*Osteochondral or chondral injuries, loose bodies, and synovial diseases*

Osteochondral and chondral injuries occur after hip dislocation and subluxation. In addition, fragmentation with ensuing loose body(ies) can occur. Use of MR arthrography greatly enhances staging of grade II through IV lesions [9]. Contrast material can track into osteochondral defects, indicating whether a lesion is stable or unstable. The articular cartilage surface can be best delineated, and articular cartilage deficiencies can be seen. Interestingly, there is a correlation between labral tears and chondral damage [6,10]. On fat-suppressed, T2-weighted, and short tau inversion recovery (STIR) sequences, bone marrow edema adjoining the cartilaginous surface can be best evaluated. Differentiation from osteonecrosis or avascular necrosis (AVN) can be accomplished by noting additional low signal intensity on all pulse sequences, which suggests nonviable bone and osteonecrosis. If increased intensity is seen on T2-weighted images, bone marrow should be considered alive. If subchondral cysts are viewed on MR imaging, there should be concern for underlying osteoarthritis.

Loose bodies may be cartilaginous, ossified, or a combination thereof. They may be solitary or multiple. MR imaging and MR arthrography are fine for detecting ossified loose bodies; however, cartilaginous loose bodies may be difficult to detect by MR imaging and MR arthrography. Multiple loose bodies secondary to synovial chondromatosis can often be adherent to the surrounding synovium. This condition represents metaplasia of the synovium and should be thought of when there are more than five or six loose bodies in the hip joint.

A second synovial condition is pigmented villonodular synovitis (PVNS), which is characterized by low signal intensity foci of T1- and T2-weighted MR imaging sequences relating to hemosiderin deposits associated with the disease. PVNS can present with a focal nodular or diffuse pattern involving proliferation of synovial fibroblasts and histiocytes. PVNS can be highly aggressive, with vascular erosion of the articular surfaces of the acetabulum and femoral head.

*Musculotendinous injuries about the hip*

The iliopsoas, hamstring, quadriceps, adductor, and gluteal muscle groups about the hip can be evaluated with MR imaging. Fat-suppressed T2-weighted images can demonstrate edematous changes within the muscle and/or tendon groups, whereas T1-weighted images can demonstrate hemorrhagic changes in acute injury and atrophy in more long-standing injuries. Chronic intramuscular hematoma is evident by hypointense signal on T1-weighted and T2-weighted and/or STIR images.

Acute tendinous avulsion injuries can be seen with the sartorius tendon at its origin at the anterior superior iliac spine, the rectus femoris at the anterior inferior iliac spine, the conjoined hamstring group at the ischial tuberosity, and the adductor group at the symphysis pubis. Avulsion injuries involving the sartorius and rectus femoris occur after forceful extension of the hip. This may be seen during a baseball swing or during a soccer kick. Avulsion injuries involving the hamstring occur during the forceful hip flexion that can occur during running and gymnastics. The degree of retraction and location of the tear allow the physician to determine if there is a need for surgery and time to recovery. Currently, orthopedists are taking a more aggressive approach in surgically repairing proximal hamstring avulsions. A nonoperative approach is still the mainstay for midsubstance hamstring tears. In general, hamstring injury tends to take longer to recover than sartorial and quadriceps injury. This is validated by the number of calendar days that a baseball or football player misses in his or her respective sport because of hamstring strains that seem innocuous at first. MR imaging also allows for viewing of associated bony avulsion fragments.

Injury surrounding the adductor muscle group can be seen well with MR imaging. Involvement may include stress reaction at the pubis (osteitis pubis) and is seen as subchondral bony marrow edema at the adductor origin. In osteitis pubis, pain can be seen radiating to the suprapubic and groin regions. This entity can be especially seen in runners, soccer, and ice or field hockey players who perform repetitive twisting and kicking motions. This may also be seen in the "sports hernia." Both are thought to be secondary to an imbalance of tension of the adductor musculature relative to the rectus abdominus, transversalis, and conjoined tendon musculature [11].

Actual muscle strain can be classified on MR imaging by determining the degree of muscle fiber injury. In first-degree muscle strain, a feathery MR imaging appearance is seen with interstitial edema at the musculotendinous junction. Second-degree muscle strain is more involved with a partial tear of the actual musculotendinous fibers. Increased fluid and hematoma are often seen. Third-degree muscle strain is characterized by complete tearing at the musculotendinous junction. Grading of musculotendinous tears is critical, because this determines the prognosis of the injury and dictates appropriate therapy and eventual return to sport.

MR imaging has been found to be effective in confirming abnormalities surrounding the iliopsoas tendon and/or muscle, bursa, and anterior capsule in three professional athletes with the internal snapping hip syndrome (coxa saltans) [12]. Snapping hip in the hip can be attributable to external, internal, or intra-articular causes. External sources include the iliotibial band, the greater trochanteric bursa, and the gluteus maximus. Internal causes include the iliopsoas tendon snapping over the iliopectineal eminence, iliopsoas capsule and/or bursal thickening, and the iliofemoral ligament. Intra-articular causes, some of which have been described previously, include acetabular labral and/or ligamentum tears, loose bodies, synovial chondromatosis, osteochondral lesions, and capsular instability.

Specific to internal snapping, physical examination of these athletes (two football players and one soccer player) found an anterior snap as the athlete's hip was brought from a position of flexion, abduction, and external rotation (FABER) to a position of extension, adduction, and internal rotation (EADIR). Axial and sagittal T1- and T2-weighted MR images consistently demonstrated hyperintensity of signal along the iliopsoas tendon. In addition, hypertrophic changes were noted in the iliopsoas tendon.

### *Piriformis syndrome*

The piriformis muscle is an external rotator of the hip and is clinically significant, because the sciatic nerve generally exits underneath its tendon insertion as it travels down the posterior thigh [13]. When the piriformis MT unit is irritated, compression of the sciatic nerve can occur, thus producing radicular type symptoms and making it difficult to differentiate the compression from sciatica of a lower lumbar or sacral disk injury. MR imaging of the lumbar or sacral spine may quickly rule out an underlying disk herniation. MR imaging of the piriformis region may demonstrate hyperintensity of the sciatic nerve on coronal T2-weighted images with edema.

## Osseous injury about the hip

### *Stress fractures*

A stress fracture in the femoral neck is a common cause of unexplained hip pain. A stress fracture generally occurs when normal bone is subjected to abnormal activity, which usually happens in a young patient. An example of this type of fracture is the result of a patient performing an activity that he or she is unaccustomed to. Another occurrence of a stress fracture may be when an abnormal bone is subjected to normal activity, which may occur in an elderly patient with osteoporosis. The femoral neck is one of the most common areas for this type of injury because of its weight-bearing function. This type of fracture may be asymptomatic until it eventually advances and leads to mechanical failure over time.

Diagnosis of stress injuries can be made with a clinical history and characteristic radiographic findings. At the initial clinical presentation during the early stages of femoral neck stress fractures, the plain radiographs may be normal. Because most stress fractures are not displaced, the fractures tend to be occult. The earliest changes seen may be a linear area of sclerosis or new bone formation, which is characteristic of increased bone turnover common to stress lesions.

MR imaging is more sensitive than radiographs in picking up early changes caused by stress fractures. This increased sensitivity is attributable to its ability to demonstrate bone marrow edema along with a hypointense low-signal line. The detection of nondisplaced incomplete stress fractures of the femoral neck is important for treatment. Stress fractures of the femoral neck are on the compressive or tensile aspect of the neck. Tensile stress fractures are at greater risk for displacement, and thus are generally recommended for pinning. Compressive stress fractures, seen more often in children, are usually treated nonsurgically, with crutches used to avoid weight bearing.

*Osteonecrosis*

Osteonecrosis is an important cause of hip pain because of the associated morbidities. Osteonecrosis is the death of cellular elements of bone and bone marrow after the interruption of blood flow to that area. This disruption in flow can be a result of trauma, such as from fracture of the femoral neck or dislocation of the hip, or of nontraumatic causes, such as steroid use, alcohol abuse, sickle cell disease, radiation, or pancreatitis. Collapse and secondary degenerative changes are often a result of osteonecrosis that occurs in weight-bearing joints. Patients often present with nonspecific signs and symptoms that include pain in the hip and limitation of motion.

Common methods used in the assessment of osteonecrosis include plain radiographs, radionuclide bone scanning, and MR imaging. The plain radiographic findings of osteonecrosis are less sensitive than those of other modalities in the detection of the early stages of osteonecrosis. The advantage of this method over others is that it is able to detect early changes of subchondral collapse and to evaluate the secondary degenerative changes in the femoral head and acetabulum as a result of the osteonecrosis. The most sensitive tests for the detection of early osteonecrosis are radionuclide bone scanning and MR imaging. Radionuclide bone scanning is used because these patients typically present with increased radionuclide uptake as a result of new bone formation during the reparative phase. MR imaging has an extremely high sensitivity and specificity and is seen as the "gold standard" for the evaluation of osteonecrosis. MR imaging is able to demonstrate marrow-based pathologic findings by indicating fatty marrow and tissue water. In advanced osteonecrosis, subchondral focal lesions of the femoral head, often fractures, are seen on MR imaging as low signal on T1- or T2-weighted images beneath the articular surface.

From a historical standpoint, the classification of osteonecrosis-based on MR imaging findings was proposed by Mitchell and colleagues [14] and correlates the MR imaging appearance with histologic features. More recently, however, this classification system has been questioned, because most AVN lesions have mixed signal and do not adhere to the classifications. Class A lesions have signal characteristics that are isointense to fat on T1- and T2-weighted images. Class B lesions have a signal intensity that is isointense to blood and is thought to be representative of an intermediate stage of osteonecrosis. Class C lesions have a signal characteristic that is isointense to fluid and is also representative of an intermediate stage of osteonecrosis. Class D lesions have signal characteristics of fibrous tissue and low signal on T1- and T2-weighted images. The class D lesion is thought to represent a late stage in the progression of osteonecrosis and is associated with deformity of the femoral head and secondary degenerative changes in the hip joint.

A recent review of eight football players who incurred a traumatic posterior hip subluxation in the National Football League (NFL) reported on its clinical significance and the value of the MR imaging in evaluating this injury [15]. MR imaging was performed in seven of the eight players acutely after injury and was able to determine the presence of an effusion. Because of the traumatic nature of the injury, the effusion was thought to be a hemarthrosis. CT-guided aspiration of the hemarthrosis was subsequently performed for decompression. In addition, MR imaging was able to detect disruption of the iliofemoral ligament. The integrity of the surrounding hip capsule was also apparent by MR imaging as well as bony marrow edema in the region of the posterior acetabular lip (all players had acetabular lip fractures). Finally, no patient had acute osteonecrosis as determined by evaluation of the femoral head. Patients had follow-up MR imaging at 6 to 8 weeks after being injured, with only one patient demonstrating signal changes in the femoral head consistent with early osteonecrosis.

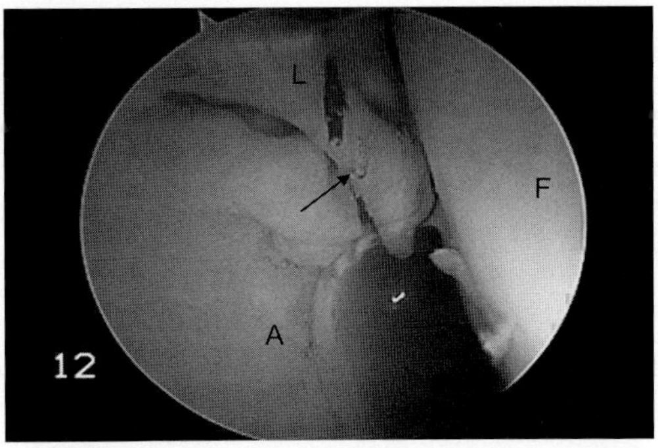


Fig. 3. Arthroscopic view of an anterior labral tear (*arrow* points to tear). A, acetabulum; F, femoral head; L, anterior labrum.

## Hip arthroscopy

With improved techniques and instrumentation, hip arthroscopy has allowed the orthopedic surgeon the means to treat in a minimally invasive manner athletes who present with intra-articular hip loose bodies, labral tears, LT tears, and chondral injuries (Figs. 2 and 3). Of late, hip impingement and hip instability can be further addressed.

After performing a careful history and physical examination, the hip arthroscopist should order hip MR imaging and/or MR arthrography to confirm a clinically suspected diagnosis or to detect other intra-articular pathologic findings. If such findings are not detected, an extra-articular diagnosis must be considered, such as a lumbar or sacral disorder, iliopsoas tendonitis, or piriformis syndrome, to cite just a few differential diagnoses.

An effusion, although nonspecific, would point to an intra-articular process. If the effusion could be better defined by the radiologist, whether it is attributable to a synovial condition (eg, PVNS) or to a chondral injury, this would greatly enhance the preoperative discussion with the patient as to clinical outcome. The presence of a subtle labral tear in the presence or absence of an articular cartilage injury may better prognosticate an athlete's return to play. The ability to determine by MR imaging whether an injury is acute, chronic, traumatic, or insidious in onset may also be helpful for the treating physician.

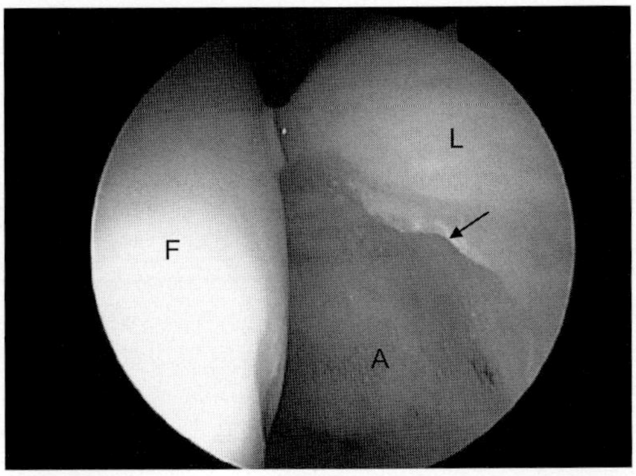


Fig. 2. Arthroscopic view of an anterior labral tear (*arrow* points to tear). A, acetabulum; F, femoral head; L, anterior labrum.

Hip arthroscopy can be performed with the patient in the supine or lateral position, with a fracture table used to allow for gentle traction. Under C-arm fluoroscopic control, proper distraction of the hip joint is confirmed and fluid is injected in the central compartment via the anterolateral portal site. Three portals are used for visualization and instrumentation: anterolateral, posterolateral, and anterior. Two arthroscopes (30° and 70°) are used interchangeably for improved visualization of the femoral head, pulvinar, and labrum. More recently, hip arthroscopy has extended to the peripheral compartment to allow viewing of the anterior neck region and to address femoroacetabular impingement. Blind spots for the arthroscopist still exist, most notably at the posteromedial aspect of the femoral head as well as at the posterior aspect of the femoral neck. Careful evaluation by the radiologist at these zones would be helpful.

## Summary

MR imaging is an invaluable method for the workup of a painful hip. It is showing increased sensitivity and specificity for many of the soft tissue and bony abnormalities of the hip, especially with the addition of intra-articular contrast (MR arthrography). Chondral injuries of the femoral head and acetabulum remain an area in MR imaging that should continue to improve with new gradient protocols.

## References


[1] Byrd JW, Jones KS. Diagnostic accuracy of clinical assessment, magnetic resonance imaging, magnetic resonance arthrography, and intra-articular injection in hip arthroscopy patients. Am J Sports Med 2004;32:1668–74.

[2] Erb RE. Current concepts in imaging the adult hip. Clin Sports Med 2001;20:661–96.

[3] Newberg AH, Newman JS. Imaging the painful hip. Clin Orthop 2003;406:19–28.

[4] Dinauer PA, Murphy KP, Carroll JF. Sublabral sulcus at the posteroinferior acetabulum: a potential pitfall in MR arthrography diagnosis of acetabular labral tears. AJR Am J Roentgenol 2004;183: 1745–53.

[5] Lage LA, Patel JV, Villar RN. The acetabular labral tear: an arthroscopic classification. Arthroscopy 1996;12:269–72.

[6] McCarthy J, Noble P, Aluisio FV, et al. Anatomy, pathologic features, and treatment of acetabular labral tears. Clin Orthop 2003;406:38–47.

[7] Kelly BT, Williams RJ III, Philippon MJ. Hip arthroscopy: current indications, treatment options, and management issues. Am J Sports Med 2003; 31:1020–37.

[8] Gray AJ, Villar RN. The ligamentum teres of the hip: an arthroscopic classification of its pathology. Arthroscopy 1997;13:575–8.

[9] Bencardino J, Kassargian A, Palmer W. Magnetic resonance imaging of the hip: sports related injuries. Top Magn Reson Imaging 2003;14:145–60.

[10] McCarthy J, Noble P, Schuck M, et al. The role of labral lesions to development of early degenerative hip disease. Clin Orthop 2001;393:25–37.

[11] Anderson K, Strickland S, Warren R. Hip and groin injuries in athletes. Am J Sports Med 2001;29: 521–33.

[12] Wahl CJ, Warren RF, Adler RS, et al. Internal coxa saltans (snapping hip) as a result of overtraining: a report of 3 cases in professional athletes with a review of causes and the role of ultrasound in early diagnosis and management. Am J Sports Med 2004; 32:1302–9.

[13] DeAngelis NA, Busconi BD. Assessment and differential diagnosis of the painful hip. Clin Orthop 2003; 406:11–8.

[14] Mitchell DG, Rao VM, Dalinka MK, et al. Femoral head avascular necrosis: correlation of MR imaging, radiographic staging, radionuclide imaging, and clinical findings. Radiology 1987;162: 709–15.

[15] Moorman CT III, Warren RF, Hershman EB, et al. Traumatic posterior hip subluxation in American football. J Bone Joint Surg Am 2003; 85:1190–6.

ELSEVIER
SAUNDERS

Magn Reson Imaging Clin N Am
13 (2005) 641–652

MAGNETIC
RESONANCE
IMAGING CLINICS
of North America

# Imaging of the Acetabular Labrum

Cheryl Petersilge, MD*

*Case Western Reserve University, Cleveland, OH, USA*

The labrum is a critical structure within the hip joint. Its role in the function and pathology of the hip is only currently being fully explored. Over the past 5 years, our understanding of this structure has evolved significantly. Detailed studies of its anatomy have been performed. Many reports have been written regarding its appearance on MR imaging and at MR arthrography and its appearance under direct visualization at arthroscopy and in cadaveric specimens. Labral pathology is currently known to be a significant cause of pain. It is believed that labral pathology is a significant factor in the development and progression of osteoarthritis of the hip, and this role is only beginning to be understood. This association between labral pathology, anatomic variations within the hip joint, and osteoarthritis is one of the driving forces behind the efforts to improve the diagnosis and treatment of labral pathology.

## Anatomy

The labrum is a fibrocartilaginous structure that is firmly attached to the rim of the acetabulum (Fig. 1) [1]. Its junction with the osseous margin is irregular, and there may be extension of bone into the substance of the labrum [1,2]. The labrum is widest anteriorly and superiorly; it is thickest superiorly and posteriorly [1,3,4]. At the margins of the acetabular notch the labrum blends imperceptibly with the transverse ligament. Sulci are formed at the junction of these two structures and should not be confused with labral pathology. The joint capsule attaches to the acetabular rim adjacent to the labrum. At the anterior and posterior margins of the joint the capsule attaches at the base of the labrum, which creates small perilabral or labrocapsular sulci. At the superior aspect of the joint the capsule inserts several millimeters above the labrum, which creates a larger perilabral sulcus or recess.

According to some investigators, the labrum blends imperceptibly with the articular cartilage [1,4]. Other investigators describe a cleft at the junction of the articular cartilage and labrum at the anterosuperior quadrant of the hip joint, however [5,6]. The anatomy of this junction is critical to the interpretation of MR arthrography and is discussed later in this article.

Detailed histologic examination of the labrum has demonstrated that it is composed of fibrocartilaginous tissue and dense connective tissue [5]. Three separate layers have been identified within the labrum. Along the articular surface a randomly oriented fibrillar network is present. Chondrocytes that are present within these collagen fibrils create a fibrocartilaginous layer [5,6]. Next a lamellar layer of collagen fibrils is seen. Along the external surface of the labrum the main substance of the labrum is composed of circumferentially oriented collagen fibrils, which blend with the transverse ligament at the margins of the acetabular notch [5]. These circumferentially oriented fibers are reinforced with perpendicularly oriented collagen fibrils [7].

The blood supply of the labrum is from capsular blood vessels, which are derived from the obturator, superior gluteal, and inferior gluteal arteries [5,8,9]. The blood supply to the labral substance is through small vessels that are located along the capsular side of the labrum [1,5,10]. These vessels do not penetrate deeply, and the articular surface of the labrum is avascular. Vessels also have been identified within the adjacent acetabular rim; however, they do not penetrate into the substance of the labrum [8,10]. The relative

* 7775 Thistle Lane, Novelty, OH 44072.
*E-mail address:* cpetersilge@att.net

1064-9689/05/$ - see front matter 
doi:10.1016/j.mric.2005.08.015

*mri.theclinics.com*

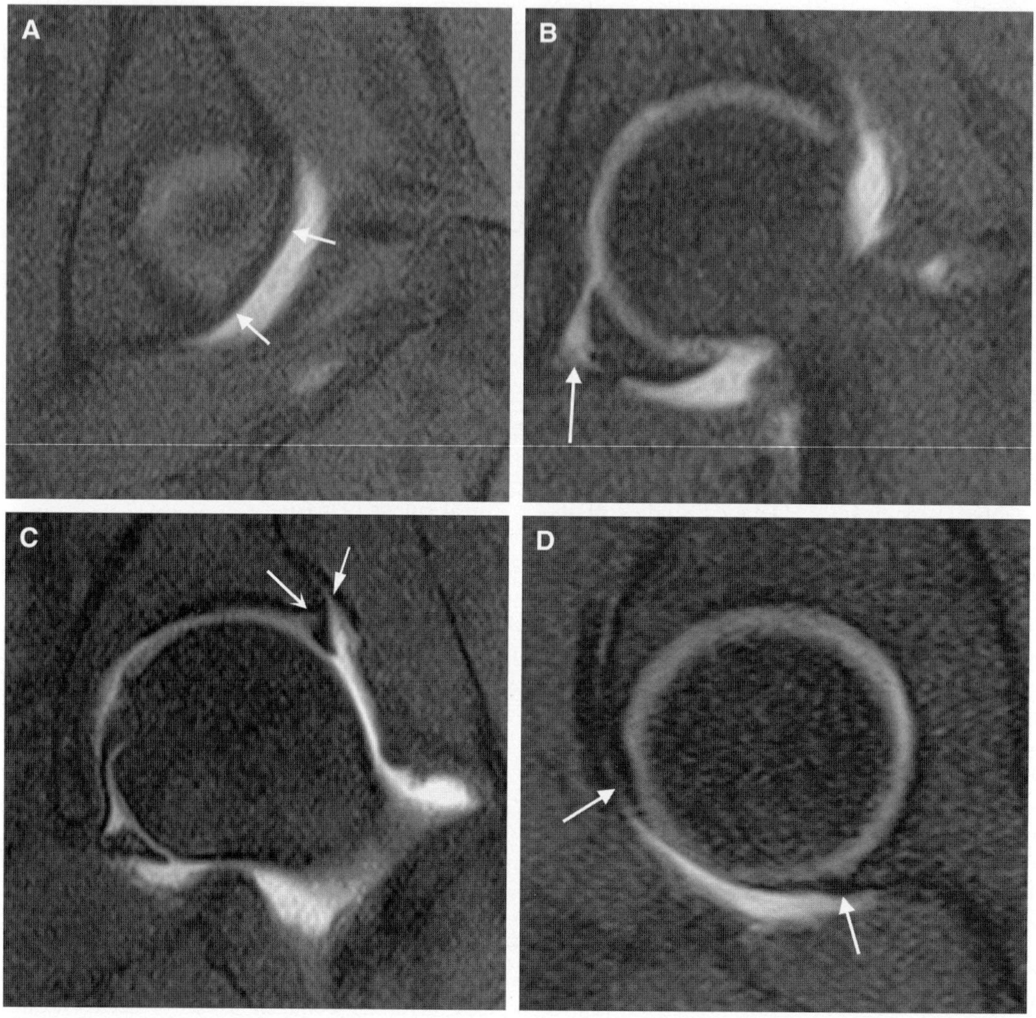


Fig. 1. Normal anatomy with intra-articular gadolinium. Coronal fat saturated T1-weighted images from posterior to anterior (*A–C*) demonstrate the attachment of the labrum along the posterior rim (*A*, *arrows*) and the labroligamentous sulcus at the posteroinferior corner of the joint where labrum and transverse ligament join (*B*, *arrow*). The normal attachment of the superior labrum to the acetabular rim is seen (*C*, *arrow with curved head*) and no separation between the labrum and articular cartilage is evident. The normal perilabral sulci are seen, superiorly where it is larger (*C*, *arrow with straight head*) and posteriorly where it is smaller (*E*, *arrowhead*). On the sagittal fat-saturated T1-weighted image (*D*) the normal labrum blends imperceptibly with the transverse ligament (*arrows*). The posterior perilabral recess is small; the anterior recess (to the left) is barely perceptible. The oblique axial gradient echo image (*E*) also demonstrates the normal labral attachment (*arrow with straight head*). In this image, a portion of the labrum overlies the articular cartilage. Contrast material has entered the iliopsoas bursa medial and lateral to the iliopsoas tendon (*arrows with curved heads*). This communication is normal.

lack of vascularity within the labrum suggests that it has little capacity for repair [10].

Functionally, the role of the labrum is not well understood. It does deepen the socket of the acetabulum, which increases the surface area of the hip [4]. It may play a role in weight bearing [4]. Biomechanical studies have demonstrated that the labrum aids in sealing the hip joint and preventing the expression of fluid when the joint is stressed [11]. By maintaining this seal, forces are distributed within the joint in a manner that protects the articular cartilage [12,13]. The labrum also maintains stability within the joint and prevents lateral subluxation of the femoral head [12]. This

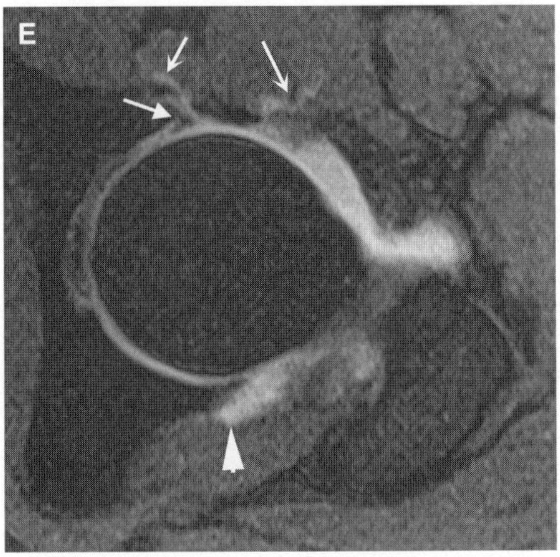


Fig. 1 (*continued*)

function was identified clinically by recognition of the fact that superolateral joint space narrowing on radiographs is an indicator of osteoarthritis secondary to labral pathology [14].

## Clinical background

Initially, identification of labral abnormalities was important because of the role these abnormalities played in the production of hip pain. Treatment was guided by the desire to reduce a patient's pain. Occasionally concerns were raised regarding the relationship between labral pathology and osteoarthritis. Over time our understanding of the association between labral pathology, anatomic variations within the hip joint, and osteoarthritis has evolved [10,14–23]. Currently, labral pathology is believed to be part of a continuum of abnormalities that result in osteoarthritis. Underlying anatomic variations within the hip that lead to labral pathology are recognized.

From his study of 436 patients, McCarthy and associates [10] provided data to support the concept that labral lesions contribute to the development of osteoarthritis. They found a twofold increase in the relative risk of chondral erosion in the presence of labral lesions (Fig. 2) [10]. They proposed the following sequence of events: traction or impingement leads to excessive loading of the labrum at the extremes of joint motion, which leads to fraying along the articular margin of the labrum, which leads to tearing of the articular margin of the labrum, which leads to delamination of the articular cartilage, which produces a cartilage flap adjacent to the labral lesion and eventually more global labral and chondral pathology [9]. Underlying mechanisms of the initial

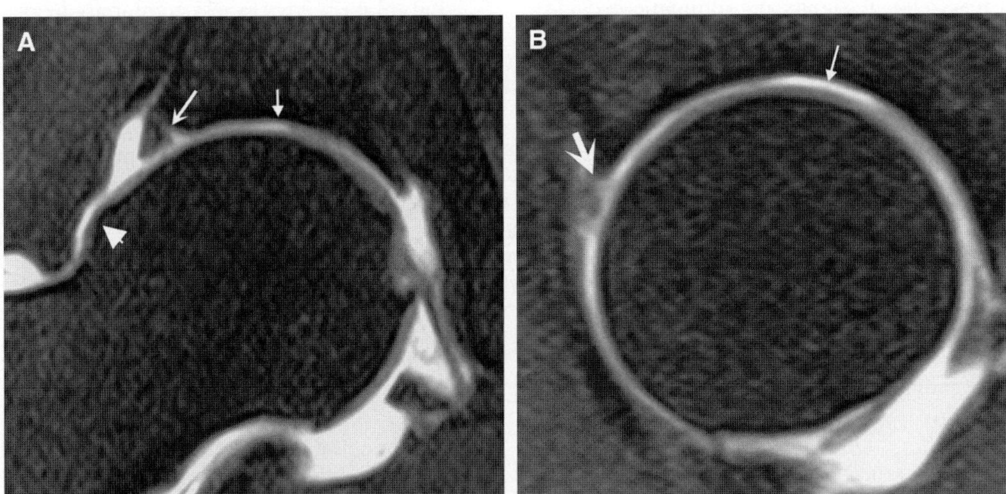


Fig. 2. Fat-saturated T1-weighted coronal (*A*) and sagittal (*B*) images reveal a partial labral detachment with contrast interposed along a portion of the acetabular rim–labral interface (*arrows with curved heads*). Generalized cartilage loss is seen adjacent to the labrum on the sagittal image, and larger defect is noted more centrally within the joint (*A* and *B*, *arrow with straight head*). The changes in this hip are secondary to femoroacetabular impingement as identified by the lateral femoral bump (*arrowhead*).

traction or impingement include developmental dysplasia and femoroacetabular impingement.

Leunig and colleagues [24] explored the cause for peripheral degeneration of the acetabulum in hips of elderly patients. They were driven by the observation that joint degeneration was more commonly found in the periphery rather than a central location, as one would expect if the mechanism of joint wear along the weight-bearing surface were accepted. They found that impingement—and its associated labral pathology—is the most likely reason for this peripheral distribution of degenerative disease.

## Clinical presentation

Patients who have labral pathology may present with pain referable to the hip, groin, pelvis, and even the medial knee. The differential diagnosis in these patients is extensive and includes arthritis, bursitis, infection, stress fracture, musculotendinous injuries, tendon avulsion, and even hernias. Symptoms of mechanical hip pain help to differentiate patients who have labral tears [25]. These mechanical symptoms include pain with range of motion, which may be accompanied by locking, clicking, or catching. A significant correlation between anterior inguinal pain, painful clicking, transient locking, and giving way has been associated with arthroscopically confirmed labral tears [26]. A significant traumatic event is usually not remembered; however, there is an increase in symptoms in young athletic individuals. If any injury is remembered, it is typically a minor twisting injury [9,27]. No female or male predilection is known [10].

Until the introduction of MR arthrography into the arsenal for assessment of the painful hip, these patients often went undiagnosed for many months or years. Because MR arthrography is more widespread, labral pathology is being recognized with greater frequency. As with most soft tissue injuries, radiographs are typically not useful for these patients. The radiographic presence of osteoarthritis is associated with a poor outcome, however [25].

Anatomic variations within the hip joint may predispose patients to the development of labral abnormalities. Patients who have developmental dysplasia of the hip are at increased risk for labral abnormalities, especially superiorly. With the deficient acetabulum superiorly, the labrum is subjected to stresses not present in the normal hip. In patients who have developmental dysplasia, labral pathology should be considered when a patient's pain is out of proportion to radiographic changes. MR arthrography also may be a useful preoperative examination in adolescents and young adults who are considering an osteotomy. In these patients, inspection of the intra-articular structures is not typically performed at the time of surgery, and concomitant labral pathology may not be recognized and treated. Failure to address the associated labral pathology may lead to a poor outcome after osteotomy. Conversely, labral pathology should be considered in patients who have undergone a technically successful osteotomy but continue to have pain.

Femoroacetabular impingement is another form of anatomic variation within the hip joint that is associated with labral pathology. In the Cam type of impingement, an abnormal femoral head neck junction leads to impingement between the abnormal femur and a normal acetabular rim. The first stage of injury occurs within the articular cartilage of the acetabular rim. As the condition progresses, detachment of the labrum may occur. In the Pincer type of impingement, overcoverage of the femoral head by the acetabulum leads to pinching of the labrum between the femur and acetabulum, which leads to labral tear. (See the article by Bredella and Stoller elsewhere in this issue for further discussion of femoroacetabular impingement.)

Labral pathology is less commonly associated with significant injury to the hip. Dislocations of the hip may detach or tear the posterior labrum at the time of dislocation or relocation of the hip. The labral fragment may become trapped between the head and acetabulum and prevent an anatomic reduction [28–31]. Transverse acetabular fractures also may lead to damage of the labrum with avulsion of the labrum from the acetabular rim [32].

## MR imaging of the labrum

### *Technique*

MR imaging is the ideal tool for assessment of the acetabular labrum. As with many other joints, MR arthrography of the hip with its joint distention is the preferred imaging modality for evaluating the labrum. There are reports of the successful assessment of the labrum without joint distention, however [33]. In a study by Czerny and associates [34], the sensitivity and accuracy for nondistended joints were 30% and 36%, respectively, when compared with surgical findings. Sensitivity and accuracy increased to 90% and 91%, respectively, after joint distention [34].

Joint distention for MR arthrography may be achieved by injection of normal saline or a dilute solution of gadolinium. The standard dilution of gadolinium for joint distention is 0.2 mmol/L of gadopentetate dimeglumine. For a single hip this dilution may be achieved by mixing 0.1 mL of gadopentetate dimeglumine in 20 mL of normal saline. By mixing 15 mL of the dilute gadolinium solution with 5 mL of iodinated contrast, an opacified solution can be injected into the joint. The joint capacity is 8 to 20 mL [35,36]. Intra-articular lidocaine injection also may be useful. Pain relief with intra-articular lidocaine further supports an intra-articular source. Failure to produce pain relief, however, does not exclude an intra-articular source.

With the use of intra-articular gadolinium, a combination of T1-weighted images with and without fat saturation may be used. A surface coil should be used with the following imaging parameters: field of view 14 to 16 cm; section thickness 3 to 5 mm for spin echo and 1.5 mm for gradient echo sequences; matrix 192 to 256×256.

Because of the spherical nature of the acetabulum, it is important to use at least three imaging planes to ensure that all portions of the labrum are assessed adequately. This author prefers to use fat-saturated T1-weighted images in the sagittal, coronal, and oblique axial planes and T1-weighted images in the axial plane. The oblique axial plane is oriented along the long axis of the femoral neck on a coronal image (Fig. 3). This plane has the advantage of providing a more thorough examination of the labrum and is useful for assessing the femoral head neck junction in patients suspected of having acetabulofemoral impingement.

Radial imaging also may be used to achieve this goal [37,38]. Radial imaging has the advantage of providing perpendicular images of the labrum at each portion within the joint with a single imaging sequence. Radial images are obtained with the use of gradient echo sequences. Reconstructions are performed at 10° to 15° increments around the joint. Volume artifacts are partially reduced. With their use of radial imaging, Plotz and colleagues [38] demonstrated an increase in sensitivity and accuracy from 60% and 70%, respectively, for oblique axial and coronal image to 80% and 85%, respectively, with radial

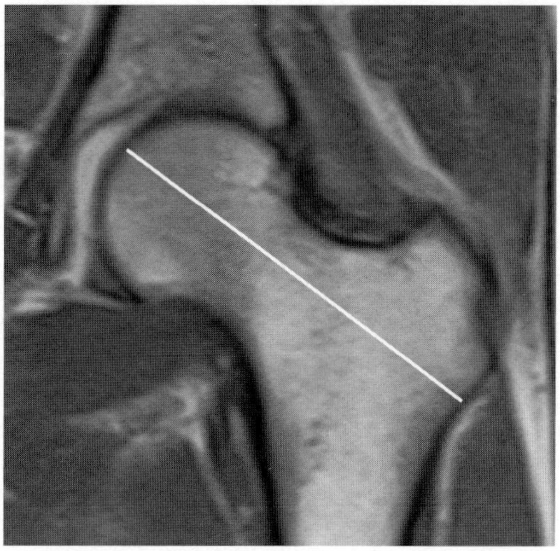

Fig. 3. The axis for the oblique axial/sagittal plane is oriented along the long axis of the femoral neck on a coronal image. Note the difficulty in separating labrum and capsule in this nondistended joint. On this T1-weighted image the labrum has diffuse intermediate signal.

imaging. Specificity was 100% for both techniques. As with every patient who presents with pain referable to the hip or groin, an assessment of the entire pelvis is performed with short tau inversion recovery (STIR) coronal images that include the entire symphysis pubis and the sacrum.

*Normal imaging anatomy*

An understanding of the MR appearance of the normal labrum has been derived from imaging of asymptomatic individuals, assuming that the asymptomatic labrum represents the spectrum of normal. These labra also have been studied without the benefit of joint distention. Unfortunately, it is difficult to know whether these morphologic variations are real or created by the apposition of capsule and the labrum. Significant variations in labral morphology and intrasubstance signal contribute to difficulty in differentiating normal from abnormal labra without the benefit of joint distention.

In studies of asymptomatic individuals, the labrum was triangular in cross-section in 66% to 94% [3,39,40]. Rounded, blunted, and irregular margins have been described. The incidence of triangular labra decreases with increasing age, whereas the incidence of rounded and irregular margins increases with age [39,40]. Absent labra have been noted in 10% to 14% of individuals

[3,39]. A consistent constellation of findings has been associated with the absent labrum [3]. This group of findings includes an absent anterior labrum with a blunted remnant along the anterosuperior and superior portion of the joint. Although those who described this constellation of findings on imaging examination suggested that it represented an anatomic variant of the normal labrum, additional MR arthrographic and arthroscopic studies have not confirmed this impression [1,41].

The labrum is typically of diffuse low signal intensity on all imaging sequences, although in asymptomatic individuals this pattern was only seen in 44%, and the incidence decreased with increasing age [39]. Focal intermediate to slightly high signal intensity may be seen at the labral base [2,3,41]. A wide spectrum of intermediate intrasubstance signal has been reported in asymptomatic labra, and the incidence of intrasubstance signal increases with increasing age [39,40]. Intrasubstance signal is more common in men than women [39]. This intermediate signal is most commonly located within the superior and anterior labrum but may be identified at any point within the joint [3,40].

Globular, linear, or curvilinear intermediate or high signal intensity is seen in 58% of labrum on T1-weighted and proton density–weighted images [3]. This signal may involve the articular surface, making distinction between these labra and labra with tears difficult. Intralabral intermediate signal has been described in 37% of labra on T2-weighted images. Bright signal on T2-weighted images has been reported in 15% (7/47) of labra [3]. The cause of this intrasubstance signal is not clear. Studies have demonstrated poor correlation between histologic changes of degeneration and labral signal [2]. The increasing incidence with age, however, does suggest at least a degenerative component.

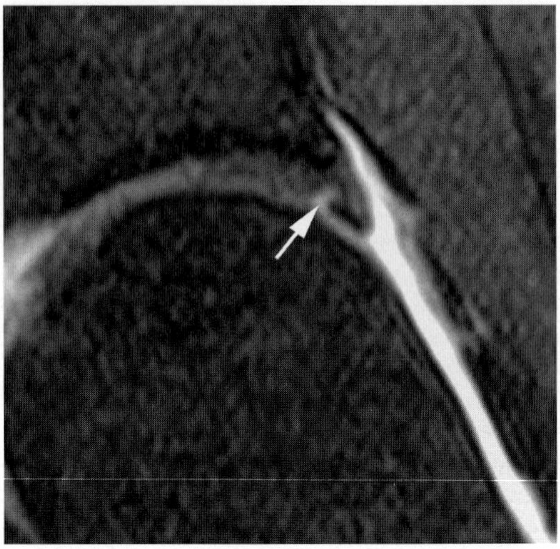

Fig. 4. MR appearance of probable normal labrocartilaginous cleft. On this coronal fat-saturated T1-weighted image with intra-articular gadolinium, contrast material is present between the articular cartilage and the labrum (*arrow*). As opposed to the detachments seen in other figures, this contrast does not extend into the interface between the labrum and the bone.

### *The perilabral sulcus*

Few pitfalls have been recognized in the interpretation of MR arthrography of the hip. The one that continues to plague persons who perform this test is a question about the presence of a normal sulcus at the anterosuperior aspect of the joint (Fig. 4). To date, no conclusive data are available about whether such a sulcus may exist normally. A review of the existing information will help the reader to draw his or her own conclusion.

A discussion of the terminology for all of the sulci of the hip should be the first step in this discussion. First are the perilabral sulci, which are located at the labrocapsular junction on the capsular surface of the labrum. They are normal, although loss of the sulcus can be an indicator of labral disease [34]. To avoid confusion, spaces should be referred to as the perilabral recesses. Next is the sulcus created by the junction of the transverse ligament and the labrum, also a normal finding. This sulcus should be known as the labroligamentous sulcus. Another sulcus is located at the posteroinferior aspect of the joint, and it recently has been described as a normal variant [42]. This sulcus is actually a labrocartilaginous cleft. It was found in 22.6% of the 23 hips examined. The last and most confusing of the sulci is the sublabral sulcus at the anterosuperior margin of the joint. This perilabral sulcus is also actually a labrocartilaginous cleft. Whether this finding is a normal variant or always pathologic is a subject of great debate.

Cadaveric studies of fetal specimens have demonstrated a cleft that was seen only in the anterosuperior portion of the joint [5,6]. This cleft was identified in 4/74 (5%) of specimens [6]. In another study of 25 cadavers (age range 23–77 years), Peterson and associates [5] described a physiologic cleft at the junction of the articular cartilage. The cleft was partial in 6 (24%) and complete in 13 cadavers. Cotten and colleagues [3] identified a possible sublabral sulcus in 3 young volunteers in their study of 46 (6.5%) asymptomatic individuals. At surgery, a cleft between the cartilage and the acetabular labrum is commonly identified (Robert Sterling, MD, personal communication, 2005).

Histologic studies have concluded that the articular cartilage and the labrum blend together seamlessly, which suggests that a separation between the articular cartilage and labrum would be abnormal [1,2,4]. Hodler and associates [2] examined 12 cadaver hips from elderly individuals to make their observations. The conclusions of Seldes and colleagues [1] and Tan and colleagues [4] are drawn from studies of 67 cadaveric specimens with an average age of 78 years.

Seldes and Tan, however, report tears at the anterosuperior margin in 74% of hips, and 89% of these tears were detachments [1,4]. In their study, few normal anterosuperior labral margins were examined. The average age of their specimens was 78 years. Is it possible that this abnormality is similar to the Type I superior labral anterior to posterior tear (SLAP) in the shoulder? The finding is of significance is the younger population but not the older population.

In their study of six cadaveric hips (age range 72–84 years), Czerny and colleagues [41] did not identify any sublabral sulci. Dinauer and colleagues [42] and Petersilge and colleagues [36] in their studies of 23 and 24 hips, respectively, were unable to confirm the presence of a sulcus (labrocartilaginous cleft) at the anterosuperior portion of joint.

In an arthroscopic study of 56 hips, Fitzgerald [27] found 41 tears with separation of the articular cartilage and labrum. Most tears were in the anterior aspect of the hip. Based on visual inspection, they reported that evidence of attempted healing of the defect was usually seen but a residual sulcus could be identified. The sulcus measured 2 to 5 mm in width and 8 to 20 mm in length, which would suggest that the sulcus is abnormal.

This author currently believes that a normal cleft is located between the margin of the articular cartilage and the labrum. The literature suggests that this normal variant has an incidence of 5% to 6%, thus any conclusive evidence would require examination of at least 20 hips to identify one cleft. In this author's experience, the cleft is seen in the anterosuperior aspect of the joint without extension anteriorly or superiorly in a joint that is otherwise normal. The margins of the cartilage edge and the border of the labrum are sharp. In contrast, any extension of contrast into the acetabular (osseous) labrum junction should be considered abnormal. Any irregularity of the margins of the cartilage edge or the adjacent labrum would indicate that the separation between labrum and cartilage is abnormal.

## Labral pathology

A combination of imaging and clinical and laboratory studies has contributed to our overall understanding of labral pathology. Evaluation of the labrum includes an assessment of morphology, distribution of contrast material, and assessment of the perilabral recess [34]. Pathologic changes are most commonly located in the anterosuperior aspect of the hip joint [1,4,10,21,27,34,36,41]. Extension of the abnormalities into other portions of the joint may be seen in 32% of cases (Fig. 5) [1,4,10]. Tears at multiple separate sites are less common and occur in only 6.9% of joints [10]. These multiple tears usually involve the anterior and posterior portions of the joint. The posterior lesion is believed to be a secondary lesion created by instability that results from the anterior lesion [10]. Isolated posterior lesions were most commonly associated with direct trauma to the hip [9,10]. Tears isolated to the posterosuperior aspect of the joint were more common than anterosuperior abnormalities in the Japanese literature on adolescent patient tears [20,43].

Traditionally in the imaging literature the terms "tear" and "detachment" when applied to structures such as the labrum have distinctly different definitions. Detachments are recognized by the interposition of contrast material at the acetabular-labral interface, whereas tears are identified by the presence of contrast material within the substance of the labrum (Figs. 6 and 7) [34,36]. Within the clinical literature, however, the terms tear and detachment are intermingled. Detachments are often reported as one form of tear. In most series, detachments are seen much more commonly than intrasubstance tears, with up to 90% of tears being detachments [1,27,41,44]. These differences in terminology should be noted whenever reviewing this literature.

At arthroscopic and cadaveric inspection, the description of labral pathology varies. Seldes and

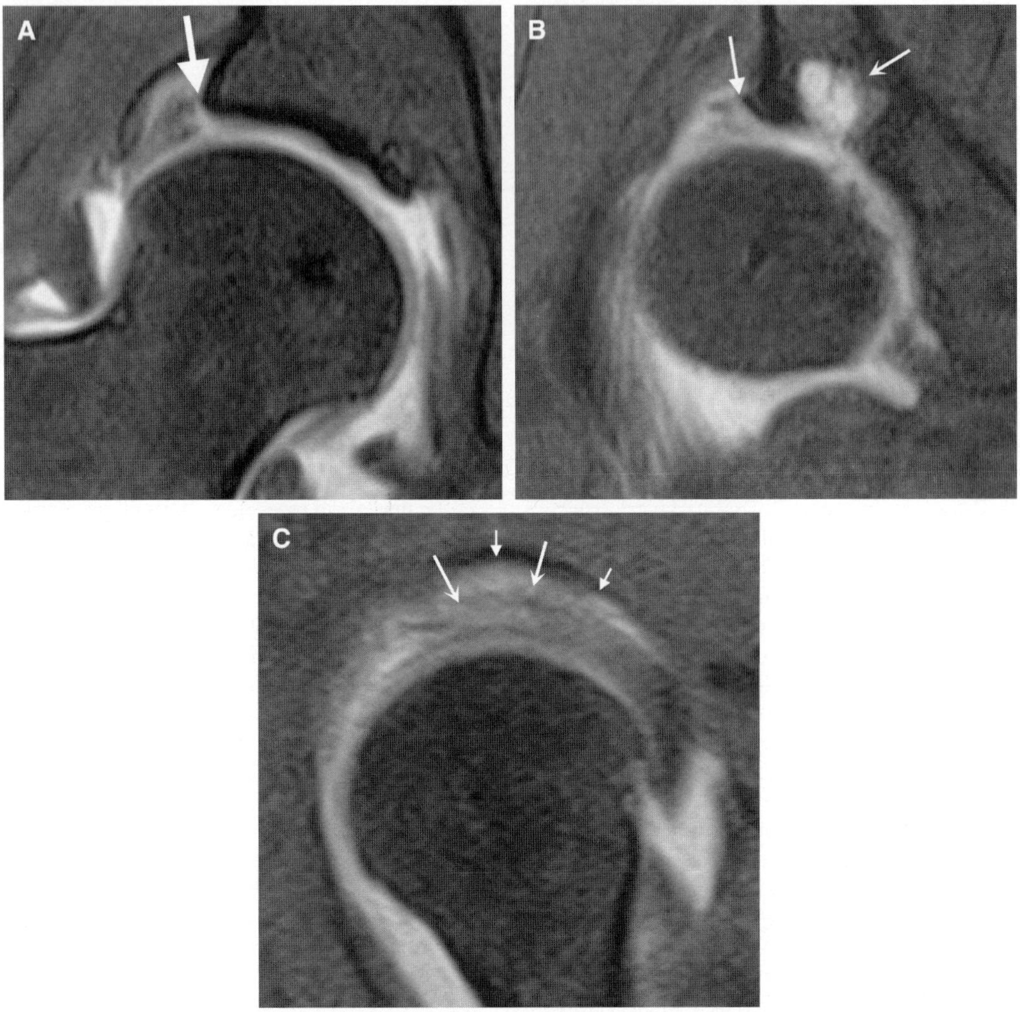


Fig. 5. Fat-suppressed T1-weighted images with intra-articular gadolinium from a patient with developmental dysplasia of the hip. Coronal images from posterior to anterior (*A* and *B*) reveal a labral detachment (*arrows with straight heads*). The labrum is likely degenerative with irregular margins and diffuse intermediate signal. A large subchondral cyst is present (*B*, *arrow with curved head*). Note the disruption of the articular cartilage and subchondral bone at the base of the cyst. On the sagittal image (*C*) the labral detachment is visible (*short arrows*). An intrasubstance tear (*long arrows*) is also seen with significant distortion of the anterior aspect of the labral (on the left). The tear and detachment involve the anterior and superior labrum.

associates [1] reviewed 77 cadaveric hips and described two types of labral tears. Type I tears (detachments) occur between the articular cartilage and the labrum, and type II tears occur within the substance of the labrum [1]. The same definition is used by Leunig and associates [44]. Tears and detachments occur along the articular surface of the labrum [1,10]. Tears occur along the course of the circumferentially oriented fibers of the labrum, which explains the appearance of longitudinal or bucket handle–type tears (Fig. 8).

Lage and associates [21] classified labral tears into four types. Radial flap and radial fibrillated tears occur within the substance of the labrum. Longitudinal peripheral tears occur at the labral base and likely represent what other authors refer to as detachments. Longitudinal peripheral tears (detachments) were not the most common type of tear identified in this study; they accounted for only 16.2% of tears. The last type of tear is the unstable tear, which is identified by subluxing labral fragments.

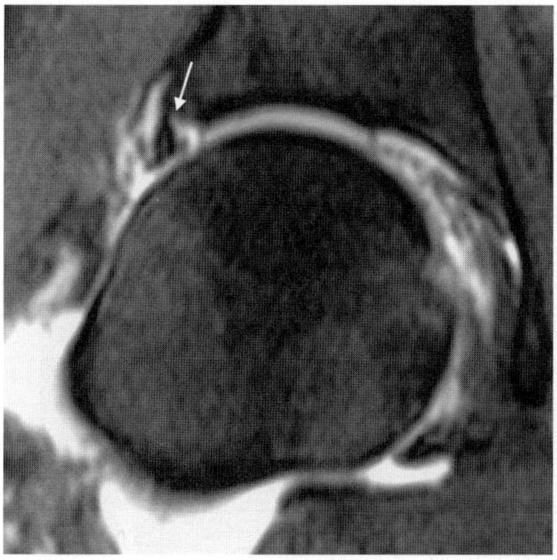

Fig. 6. Coronal fat-saturated T1-weighted image with intra-articular gadolinium demonstrates an extensive partial detachment of the superior labrum. The arrow identifies the point at which the labrum remains attached to the rim.

Based on his study of 436 patients with an average age of 37.4 years, McCarthy and colleagues [10] also described two types of labral pathology, although the types differ from those of Seldes. They described fraying at the labral-cartilage junction and tearing of the labrum with separation from the articular cartilage (chondrolabral separation) [10]. They referred to this chondrolabral separation as the watershed lesion. Fraying occurs at all regions within the hip, whereas 86% of chondrolabral separations are present in the anterior aspect of the joint. Fraying and chondrolabral separation did not occur adjacent to each other. Posterior and lateral fraying was associated with anterior tears, however, which suggested that they may be secondary lesions related to abnormal joint motion caused by the anterior tear.

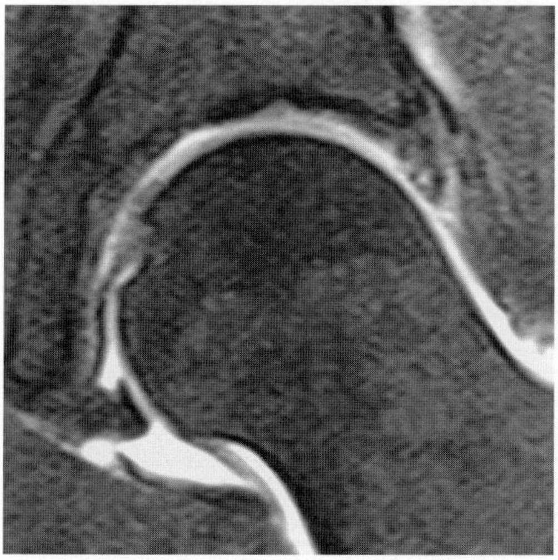

Fig. 7. On this coronal fat-saturated T1-weighted image with intra-articular gadolinium, the superior labrum has diffuse heterogeneous intermediate signal within. A tear is confirmed along the articular surface with the intrasubstance collection of contrast material.

Cartilaginous lesions are frequently associated with labral pathology. Complete assessment of an MR arthrogram includes detailed evaluation of the articular cartilage. Only moderate sensitivity for detection of cartilage lesions has been reported, however [45,46]. This lower sensitivity is partly caused by the thin articular cartilage of the hip. Cartilage flaps are particularly difficult to identify because they often lay within their bed against the subchondral bone. Cartilaginous abnormalities predominate on the acetabular articular surface, especially anterosuperiorly, with few lesions on the femoral head [24,46]. As the severity of labral pathology progresses, the incidence of cartilage lesions increases [1]. The most severe cartilaginous abnormalities are seen when the labrum is completely detached from the margin of the acetabulum [1].

In McCarthy and colleagues' [10] study of 436 patients, 62.6% had cartilaginous lesions. Most lesions were located in the anterior aspect of the joint, and the most severe lesions were seen anteriorly. A statistically significant relationship was identified between the severity of cartilage lesions and the presence of labral lesions. Chondral flaps were most common (present in 62% of hips), whereas localized full-thickness wear was seen in 38% and global degenerative disease with foci of full-thickness loss was seen in 6%. A strong association was seen between labral lesions and cartilaginous lesions, with 73% of labral lesions accompanied by a cartilaginous lesion. Only 6% of cartilaginous lesions did not have associated labral lesions. The strongest association was identified between labral disease (tears and fraying) and the presence of serious articular degeneration. Similar findings also were identified in a study of patients with mild developmental dysplasia of the hip [47]. Labral tears, labral fraying, and cartilage lesions all increase in prevalence with increasing age.

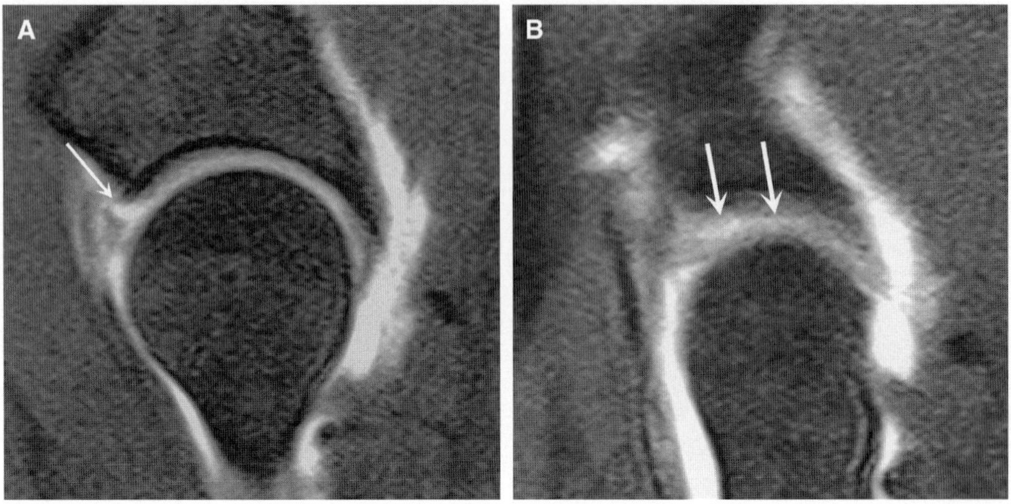

Fig. 8. Sagittal fat-saturated T1-weighted images with intra-articular gadolinium from medial to lateral demonstrate a labral detachment that extends from anterior (*A, arrow*) to superior (*B, arrows*) in the configuration of a longitudinal peripheral tear along the circumferentially oriented fibers of the labrum.

Distinct pathologic changes occur in the labrum and acetabular rim in association with developmental dysplasia of the hip, and the term "acetabular rim syndrome" has been used by Klaue and associates [48] to describe these changes (Fig. 9). These investigators recognize two types of anatomic abnormalities with different pathologic changes within the rim. In type I changes, the acetabulum is shallow and vertical, and the femoral head and acetabulum are incongruent. In this situation the labrum is subject to chronic shear stress because of the increased weight-bearing role. This stress leads to labral hypertrophy and subsequent separation from the

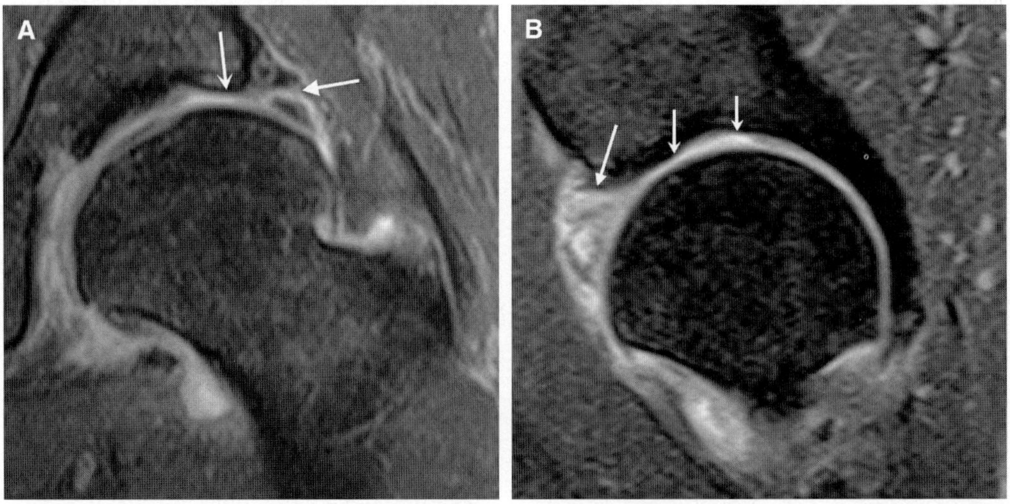

Fig. 9. Coronal and sagittal fat-saturated T1-weighted images with intra-articular gadolinium in a patient with developmental dysplasia. A detachment is present at the base (*A* and *B*, *arrows with straight heads*). A large cartilage defect is present in the acetabular rim adjacent to the labral abnormality (*A* and *B*, *arrows with curved heads*). On the sagittal image, note the hypertrophy of the anterior labrum with a large intrasubstance collection of contrast consistent with tear.

acetabular margin. These findings also have been identified by other investigators [10,49–51]. Soft tissue para-acetabular cysts may form. Identification of periarticular cysts should suggest the possibility of underlying labral tear or detachment [18,52]. Although these cysts are more commonly seen in patients with developmental dysplasia, they are not unique to that patient population [36,42,48,51,53].

With type II changes, the acetabulum and femoral head are congruent and the acetabular roof is short. The acetabular rim is stressed and eventually may fail with a fatigue fracture and os acetabuli formation. Intraosseous cysts may form. McCarthy and Lee [47] hypothesized that with disruption of the chondrolabral interface, joint fluid is driven into the subchondral bone. This fluid leads to undermining of the articular cartilage and creates cartilage flaps, continued subchondral injury, and subchondral cyst formation.

The labrum plays a critical role in producing hip pain and is a key structure in the development of osteoarthritis. Our knowledge of this structure continues to grow, including the spectrum of the normal and the appearance of pathologic changes.

## References


[1] Seldes RM, Tan V, Hunt J, et al. Anatomy, histologic features and vascularity of the adult acetabular labra. Clin Orthop Relat Res 2001;382:232–40.

[2] Hodler J, Yu JS, Goodwin D, et al. MR arthrography of the hip: improved imaging of the acetabular labrum with histologic correlation. AJR Am J Roentgenol 1995;165:887–91.

[3] Cotten A, Boutry N, Demondion X, et al. Acetabular labrum: MRI in asymptomatic volunteers. J Comput Assist Tomogr 1998;22:1–7.

[4] Tan V, Seldes RM, Katz MA, et al. Contribution of acetabular labrum to articulating surface area and femoral head coverage in adult hip joints: an anatomic study in cadavera. Am J Orthop 2001;30: 809–12.

[5] Peterson W, Peterson F, Tillman B. Structure and vascularization of the acetabular labrum with regard to the pathogenesis and healing of labral lesions. Arch Orthop Trauma Surg 2003;123:283–8.

[6] Walker JM. Histological study of the fetal development of the human acetabulum and labrum: significance in congenital hip disease. Yale J Biol Med 1981;54:255–63.

[7] Ito K, Leunig M, Ganz R. Histopathologic features of the acetabular labrum in femoroacetabular impingement. Clin Orthop Relat Res 2004;429:262–71.

[8] Kelly B, Shapiro GS, Digiovanni CW, et al. Vascularity of the hip labrum: a cadaveric investigation. Arthroscopy 2005;21:3–11.

[9] McCarthy J, Noble P, Aluisio FV, et al. Anatomy, pathologic features, and treatment of acetabular labral tears. Clin Orthop Relat Res 2003;406:38–47.

[10] McCarthy JC, Noble PC, Schuck MR, et al. The role labral lesions to development of early degenerative hip disease. Clin Orthop Relat Res 2001; 393:25–37.

[11] Ferguson SJ, Bryant JT, Ganz R, et al. The acetabular labrum seal: a poroelastic finite element model. Clin Biomech (Bristol, Avon) 2000;15:463–8.

[12] Ferguson SJ, Bryant JT, Ganz R, et al. The influence of the acetabular labrum on hip joint cartilage consolidation: a poroelastic finite element model. J Biomech 2000;33:953–60.

[13] Ferguson SJ, Bryant JT, Ganz R, et al. An in vitro investigation of the acetabular labrum seal in hip joint mechanics. J Biomech 2003;36:171–8.

[14] Byrd JW, Jones KS. Osteoarthritis cause by an inverted acetabular labrum: radiographic diagnosis and arthroscopic treatment. Arthroscopy 2002;18: 741–7.

[15] Dorrell JH, Catterall A. The torn acetabular labrum. J Bone Joint Surg Br 1986;68B:400–3.

[16] Altenberg AR. Acetabular labrum tears: a cause of hip pain and degenerative osteoarthritis. South Med J 1977;70:174–5.

[17] Harris WH, Bourne RB, Oh I. Intra-articular acetabular labrum: a possible etiological factor in certain cases of osteoarthritis of the hip. J Bone Joint Surg Am 1979;61A:510–4.

[18] Hase T, Ueo T. Acetabular labral tear: arthroscopic diagnosis and treatment. Arthroscopy 1999;15: 138–41.

[19] Ganz R, Parvizi J, Beck M, et al. Femoroacetabular impingement: a cause for osteoarthritis of the hip. Clin Orthop Relat Res 2003;417:112–20.

[20] Ikeda T, Awaya G, Suzuki S, et al. Torn acetabular labrum in young patients arthroscopic diagnosis and management. J Bone Joint Surg Br 1988;70B:13–6.

[21] Lage LA, Patel JV, Villar RN. The acetabular labral tear: an arthroscopic classification. Arthroscopy 1996;12:269–72.

[22] Ueo T, Suzuki S, Iwasaki R, et al. Rupture of the labra acetabularis as a cause of hip pain detected arthroscopically, and partial limbectomy for successful pain relief. Arthroscopy 1990;6:48–51.

[23] Noguchi Y, Miura H, Takasugi S, et al. Cartilage and labrum degeneration in the dysplastic hip generally originates in the anterosuperior weight-bearing area: an arthroscopic observation. Arthroscopy 1999;15:496–506.

[24] Leunig M, Beck M, Woo A, et al. Acetabular rim degeneration. Clin Orthop Relat Res 2003;413:201–7.

[25] Fargo LA, Glick JM, Sampson TG. Hip arthroscopy for acetabular labral tears. Arthroscopy 1999;15: 132–7.

[26] McCarthy JC. The diagnosis and treatment of labral and chondral lesions. AAOS Instructional Course Lectures 2004;53:573–7.
[27] Fitzgerald RH. Acetabular labrum tears: diagnosis and management. Clin Orthop 1995;311:60–8.
[28] Dameron TB. Bucket-handle tear of acetabular labrum accompanying posterior dislocation of the hip. J Bone Joint Surg Am 1959;41:131–4.
[29] Paterson I. The torn acetabular labrum: a block to reduction of a dislocated hip. J Bone Joint Surg Br 1957;39B:306–9.
[30] Rashleigh-Belcher HJC, Cannon SR. Recurrent dislocation of the hip with a "Bankart-type" lesion. J Bone Joint Surg Br 1986;68B:398–9.
[31] Shea K, Kalamchi A, Thompson GH. Acetabular epiphysis-labrum entrapment following traumatic anterior dislocation of the hip in children. J Pediatr Orthop 1986;6:215–9.
[32] Leunig M, Sledge JB, Gill TJ, et al. Traumatic labral avulsion from the stable rim: a constant pathology in displaced transverse acetabular fractures. Arch Orthop Trauma Surg 2003;123:392–5.
[33] Mintz D, Hooper T, Connell D, et al. Magnetic resonance imaging of the hip: detection of labral and chondral abnormalities using noncontrast imaging. Arthroscopy 2005;21:385–93.
[34] Czerny C, Hofmann S, Neuhold A, et al. Lesions of the acetabular labrum: accuracy of MR imaging and MR arthrography in detection and staging. Radiology 1996;200:225–30.
[35] Edwards DJ, Lomas D, Villar RH. Diagnosis of the painful hip by magnetic resonance imaging and arthroscopy. J Bone Joint Surg Br 1995;77B:374–6.
[36] Petersilge CA, Haque MA, Petersilge WJ, et al. Acetabular labral tears: evaluation with MR arthrography. Radiology 1996;200:231–5.
[37] Kubo T, Horii M, Harada Y, et al. Radial-sequence magnetic resonance imaging in evaluation of acetabular labrum. J Orthop Sci 1999;4:328–32.
[38] Plotz CMJ, Brossmann J, von Knoch M, et al. Magnetic resonance arthrography of the acetabular labrum: value of radial reconstructions. Arch Orthop Trauma Surg 2001;121:450–7.
[39] Lecouvet FE, Vande Berg BC, Malghem J, et al. MR imaging of the acetabular labrum: variations in 200 asymptomatic hips. AJR Am J Roentgenol 1996; 167:1025–8.
[40] Abe I, Harada Y, Oinuma K, et al. Acetabular labrum: abnormal findings at MR imaging in asymptomatic hips. Radiology 2000;216:576–81.
[41] Czerny C, Hofmann S, Urban M, et al. MR arthrography of the adult acetabular-labral complex: correlation with surgery and anatomy. AJR Am J Roentgenol 1999;173:345–9.
[42] Dinauer PA, Murphy KP, Carroll JF. Sublabral sulcus at the posteroinferior acetabulum: a potential pitfall in MR arthrography diagnosis of acetabular labral tears. AJR Am J Roentgenol 2004;183: 1745–53.
[43] Suzuki S, Awaya G, Okada Y, et al. Arthroscopic diagnosis of ruptured acetabular labrum. Acta Orthop Scand 1986;57:513–5.
[44] Leunig M, Werlen S, Ungersbock A, et al. Evaluation of the acetabular labrum by MR arthrography. J Bone Joint Surg Br 1997;79B:230–4.
[45] Knuesel PR, Pfirrmann CW, Noetzli HP, et al. MR arthrography of the hip: diagnostic performance of a dedicated water-excitation 3D double-echo steady-state sequence to detect cartilage lesions. AJR Am J Roentgenol 2004;183:1729–35.
[46] Schmid MR, Notzli HP, Zanetti M, et al. Cartilage lesions in the hip: diagnostic effectiveness of MR arthrography. Radiology 2003;226:382–6.
[47] McCarthy JC, Lee J. Acetabular dysplasia: a paradigm of arthroscopic examination of chondral injuries. Clin Orthop Relat Res 2002;405:122–8.
[48] Klaue K, Durnin CW, Ganz R. The acetabular rim syndrome. J Bone Joint Surg Br 1991;73B:423–9.
[49] Haller J, Resnick D, Greenway G, et al. Juxtaacetabular ganglionic (or synovial) cysts: CT and MR features. J Comput Assist Tomogr 1989;13:976–83.
[50] Horii M, Kubo T, Inoue S, et al. Coverage of the femoral head by the acetabular labrum in dysplastic hips. Acta Orthop Scand 2003;74:287–92.
[51] Leunig M, Podeszwa D, Beck M, et al. Magnetic resonance arthrography of labral disorders in hips with dysplasia and impingement. Clin Orthop 2004;418: 74–80.
[52] Schnarkowski P, Steinbach LS, Tirman PF, et al. Magnetic resonance imaging of labral cysts of the hip. Skeletal Radiol 1996;25:733–7.
[53] Magee T, Hinson G. Association of paralabral cysts with acetabular disorders. AJR Am J Roentgenol 2000;174:1381–4.

ELSEVIER
SAUNDERS

Magn Reson Imaging Clin N Am
13 (2005) 653–664

MAGNETIC
RESONANCE
IMAGING CLINICS
of North America

# MR Imaging of Femoroacetabular Impingement

Miriam A. Bredella, MD[a,*], David W. Stoller, MD, FACR[b]

[a]*Division of Musculoskeletal Radiology, Department of Radiology, Massachusetts General Hospital, 55 Fruit Street, Yawkey Building 6400, Boston, MA 02114, USA*
[b]*California Pacific Medical Center, 3700 California Street, Suite G 350, San Francisco, CA 94188, USA*

Multiple causative factors lead to osteoarthritis (OA) of the hip. In a number of cases, however, no exact mechanism can be determined (idiopathic OA) [1–3]. In recent years, femoroacetabular impingement (FAI) has been found to cause a progressive degenerative process leading to early OA of the hip [4,5]. FAI is a distinct pathologic entity that occurs as a result of abnormal abutment between the proximal femur and acetabular rim because of morphologic abnormalities affecting the proximal femur, acetabulum, or both. Repetitive microtrauma from impingement of the femoral head against the acetabulum, especially during flexion and internal rotation, when the femoral head is in contact with the acetabular rim, which is then subject to abnormal stress, causes degeneration of the acetabular labrum and articular cartilage. Degeneration and tearing of the labrum as well as progressive damage to the adjacent acetabular cartilage are precursors of OA [4–9]. Patients with FAI are usually young and physically active and present with slow onset of hip or groin pain, often after minor trauma or without preceding trauma, restricted flexion and internal rotation, and a positive impingement test (pain with flexion and internal rotation). The pain gradually increases over time and is activity dependent. Sports activities, such as soccer, kickboxing, tennis, baseball, football, or volleyball, that require hip flexion with variable torque or axial loading may aggravate symptoms and are often associated with FAI [4,10–12].

Radiographs in patients with FAI are often read as normal, and no treatment is initiated. On closer review, however, subtle abnormalities may be visible, including bony prominence of the anterolateral femoral head-neck junction; reduced offset of the femoral head-neck junction, synovial herniation pits, and changes of the acetabulum, such as an os acetabuli, ossification of the acetabular rim, or the "crossover" or "posterior wall" signs seen in acetabular retroversion [1,4,6,9,12–14]. MR imaging is often used in the evaluation of young adults with hip and groin pain. MR imaging and MR arthrography are the modalities of choice to evaluate the acetabular labrum and articular cartilage. Low offset of the femoral head, subchondral cysts, and ossification of the acetabular rim as well as labral tears and chondral injuries can be seen on MR imaging in patients with FAI [7,8,11,12,15–17]. Acetabular rim lesions on MR imaging have been shown to correlate with results of the impingement test [18]. The recognition of FAI and its relation to early OA of the hip requires early diagnosis and treatment to prevent or delay degeneration of the hip.

## Pathomechanisms of femoroacetabular impingement

It is thought that OA results from abnormal axial loading exceeding the tolerance level of the articular cartilage and subchondral bone. Joint damage is therefore expected first in the weight-bearing area of the acetabulum, femoral head, or both [15,19]. Several studies have shown damage to the acetabular rim in the anterosuperior quadrant in hips without apparent abnormalities [6,8,15,20], suggesting FAI as the trigger for OA in these hips [18].

* Corresponding author.
*E-mail address:* mbredella@partners.org (M.A. Bredella).

1064-9689/05/$ - see front matter 
doi:10.1016/j.mric.2005.08.001

FAI is well recognized after total hip arthroplasty. It is also known to occur in patients with abnormal hip anatomy, such as developmental hip dysplasia (DDH), slipped capital femoral epiphysis (SCFE), Legg-Calve-Perthes (LCP) disease, or posttraumatic deformity, where a mismatch between the femoral head-neck junction and the acetabulum has occurred [9,15,21–26]. FAI in patients without preexisting hip disease has been recognized in recent years and might be secondary to variations in normal anatomy or unrecognized developmental anomalies. These variations in proximal femoral and acetabular anatomy can lead to FAI [4,5,27]. The anatomic configuration of the femoral head and neck and acetabulum allows joint clearance during hip movement. Loss of the femoral head-neck offset or excessive acetabular coverage results in decreased joint clearance between the femoral neck and acetabulum. As a result, impingement of the femoral neck against the acetabulum and labrum occurs during terminal motion of the hip, leading to lesions of the acetabular labrum or adjacent articular cartilage (Fig. 1) [5,18,20,21]. The detection of subtle anatomic abnormalities of the femoral head-neck junction and acetabulum is important for surgical planning, because arthroscopic labral or chondral debridement alone addresses only the site of secondary damage attributable to FAI and does not alter the underlying cause. This can lead to progression of the early labral and chondral lesions to OA [4,6,9,11,18,20,28,29].

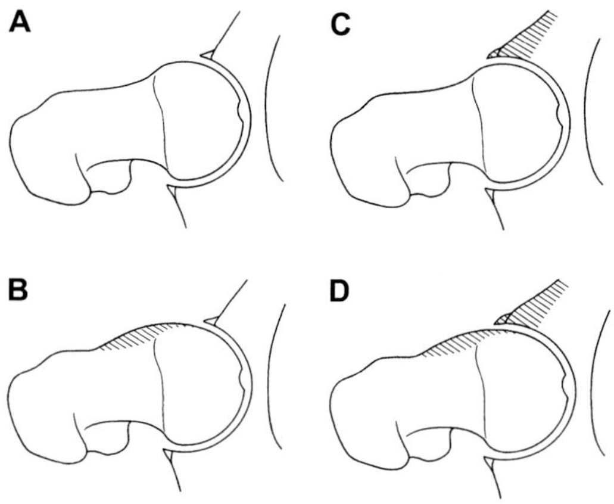


Fig. 1. Pathomechansims of FAI. Reduced clearance during joint motion leads to repetitive abutment between the proximal femur and anterior acetabular rim. Normal clearance of the hip (*A*), reduced femoral head-neck offset (*B*), excessive overcoverage of the femoral head by the acetabulum (*C*), and combination of reduced head-neck offset and excessive anterior overcoverage (*D*) are shown. (*From* Lavigne M, Parvizi J, Beck M, et al. Anterior femoroacetabular impingement. Part 1. Techniques of joint preserving surgery. Clin Orthop Relat Res 2004;418:62; with permission.)

### Types of femoroacetabular impingement

Two types of FAI can be distinguished. Impingement can be attributable to femoral causes (cam impingement) or acetabular causes (pincer impingement). Cam impingement is caused by abutment of an abnormal femoral head against the acetabulum during forceful motion [4,6–9,20]. Pincer impingement is the result of linear contact between the acetabular rim and the femoral neck as a result of acetabular abnormalities, such as acetabular retroversion, leading to anterior overcoverage of the femoral head [4,14,20,30,31].

### Cam impingement

Femoral causes of impingement include insufficient femoral head-neck offset, subtle displacement of the femoral epiphysis, SCFE, or postsurgical or traumatic deformities. [9,15,21–26]. Posterior placement of the femoral head on the femoral neck with inadequate anterior femoral head-neck offset results in contact and impingement between the femoral neck and acetabular rim when the hip is flexed or internally rotated, resulting in abnormal forces on the acetabular cartilage and subchondral bone in the anterosuperior rim area, which leads to damage to the acetabular labrum and articular cartilage [4,5,8–10,21,22,24, 29,32]. Cam impingement is more frequently seen in young athletic men [4,6].

Decreased offset of the femoral head-neck junction can be seen on MR imaging or radiographs as a prominent lateral extension of the femoral head at the step-off to the adjacent femoral neck (Fig. 2) [8,15]. The offset refers to the difference between the widest diameter of the femoral head and the most prominent part of the femoral neck. On cross-table lateral radiographs of the hip, a deficient anterior head-neck offset is present if the anterior head-neck junction extends beyond a circle around the femoral head [6]. Loss of femoral head-neck offset results in decreased clearance between the femoral neck and acetabulum during terminal motion [5]. A congruent but nonspherical head, a short neck, or a small head-to-neck ratio, especially when located

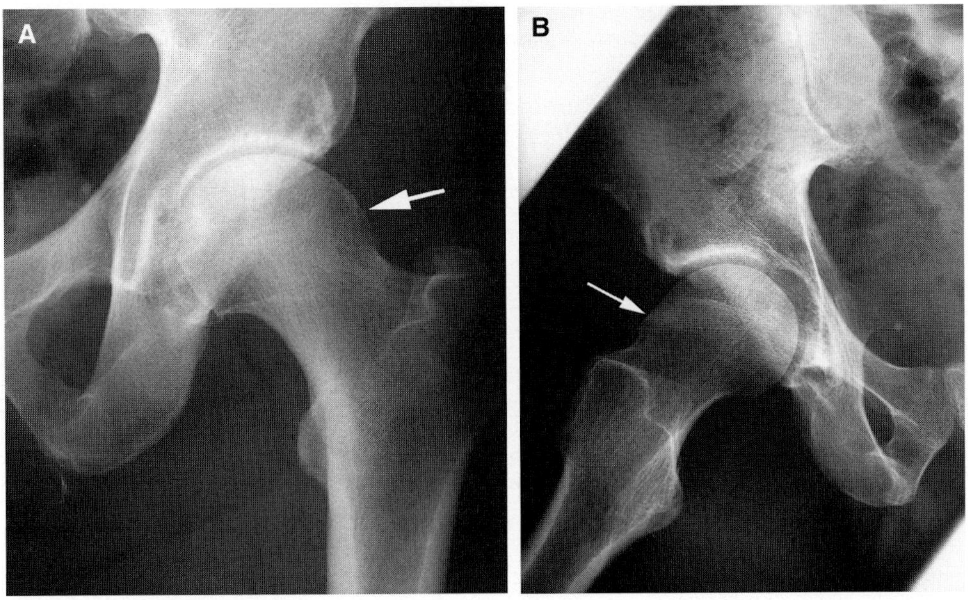


Fig. 2. (*A*) Radiograph demonstrating nonspherical femoral head resulting in decreased femoral head-neck offset (*arrow*). (*B*) Frog-leg lateral radiograph demonstrates decreased femoral head-neck offset and an osseous bump at the femoral head-neck junction (*arrow*). (*B*, Courtesy of Z. Rosenberg, MD, New York, NY.)

anteriorly, is a morphologic feature of FAI that can be detected with MR imaging.

Stuhlberg and colleagues [33] described the presence of a "pistol-grip" deformity in 40% of patients who develop OA of the hip. The term *pistol-grip* deformity refers to a flattened femoral head-neck junction, depicted on radiographs or MR images as flattening of the usually concave surface of the femoral head, a bump on the anterolateral aspect of the femoral neck, or failure of the femoral head to be centered over the femoral neck [5,33]. Jager and coworkers [9] noted an osseous bump at the anterolateral femoral head-neck junction in patients with FAI. Tanzer and Noiseux [5] described a pistol-grip deformity as a cause of FAI in 100% of patients with idiopathic arthritis of the hip. In a study by Leunig and colleagues [15], 80% of hips with FAI had a lack of anterolateral head-neck offset. In a study using MR imaging of the hip, Siebenrock and coworkers [29] described abnormal lateral extension of the femoral head epiphysis in patients with FAI and a decreased head-neck offset. Delayed separation of the common femoral head and greater trochanteric physis or eccentric closure of the femoral head epiphysis usually affects the anterosuperior aspect of the femoral head-neck junction, suggesting an epiphyseal growth abnormality as the underlying cause for decreased femoral head-neck junction [29,34].

Murray [13] calculated the "femoral head ratio" on anteroposterior (AP) radiographs, constructing an axis of the femoral neck by using the midpoint between the trochanters and the narrowest portion of the femoral neck and dividing the width of the femoral head above the axis by that below [11,13].

Notzli and colleagues [11] described a method using MR imaging to quantify the concavity of the femoral head-neck junction. The anterior extent of the concavity of the femoral neck was defined as a point where the distance from the cortex to the center of the femoral head exceeds the radius of the cartilage-covered femoral head. Widening of the femoral neck anterior to this line reduces the concavity of the neck. The angle formed between the axis of the neck and a line connecting the center of the head and neck at its narrowest point (alpha angle) was found to be larger in patients with FAI compared with a control group (Fig. 3). The alpha angle measured 74.0° ± 5.4° in patients with FAI and 42° ± 2.2° in the normal control group [11]. All causes of impingement attributable to the shape of the femoral head-neck junction, such as a wide femoral neck, osteophyte formation, or posterior displacement of the femoral head, result in an increased alpha angle [11]. In the study by Notzli and colleagues [11], all patients with a positive impingement test

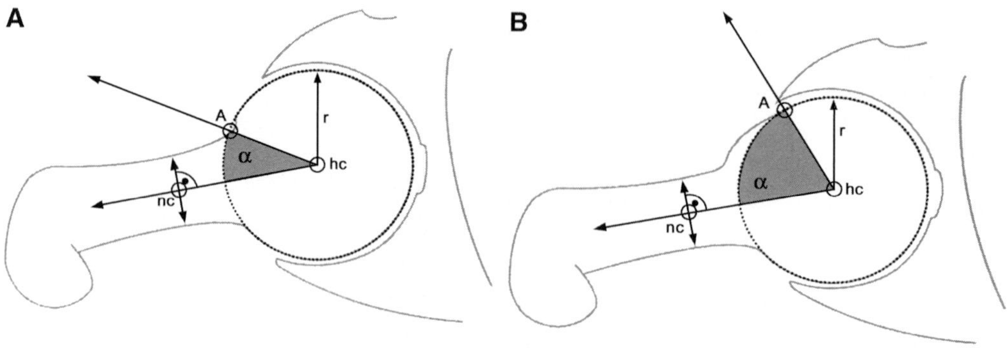


Fig. 3. Construction of the alpha angle to evaluate the femoral head-neck junction. Point A is the anterior point where the distance from the center of the head (hc) exceeds the radius (r) of the subchondral surface of the femoral head. The alpha angle is measured as the angle between A-hc and hc-nc, with nc being the center of the neck at the narrowest point. Hip in a normal subject (*A*) and a typical deformation (*B*). (*From* Noetzli HP, Wyss TF, Stoecklin CH, et al. The contour of the femoral head-neck junction as a predictor for the risk of anterior impingement. J Bone Joint Surg Br 2002;84(4):556–60; with permission.)

result demonstrated abnormalities on MR imaging, such as degeneration of the labrum or labral tears, and in 85% of the patients, there was associated damage to the anterolateral acetabular cartilage.

The goal of surgical treatment of cam impingement is to allow a sufficient impingement-free range of motion during flexion and internal rotation. Surgical treatment includes removal of the nonspherical portions of the femoral head and bony prominence of the extra-articular femoral head, thereby improving the femoral head-neck offset. Surgical treatment also includes arthroscopic debridement of labral tears and removal of loose bodies. Cartilage defects are often not repaired, because it has been shown that cartilage repair procedures, such as microfracture, have a low success rate in the hip [4,6,9,20].

## Pincer impingement

In patients with FAI, the femoral head may have normal morphology and the abnormal abutment between the femoral head and acetabulum is the result of acetabular abnormalities. The acetabular rim syndrome, a precursor of OA, has been described in patients with DDH. In dysplastic hips with a shallow acetabulum and insufficient acetabular coverage of the femoral head, the acetabular surface is reduced, leading to increased load and pressure on the acetabulum (Fig. 4). This leads to labral tears, chondral lesions, intraosseous cysts in the acetabular roof, and bony fragmentation (os acetabuli). Acetabular rim syndrome in DDH is characterized by similar MR imaging findings in an identical location as FAI [23].

Acetabular retroversion, coxa profunda, or protrusio acetabuli results in overcoverage of the femoral head by increasing the relative depth of the acetabulum [4,6,12]. Abutment of the femoral

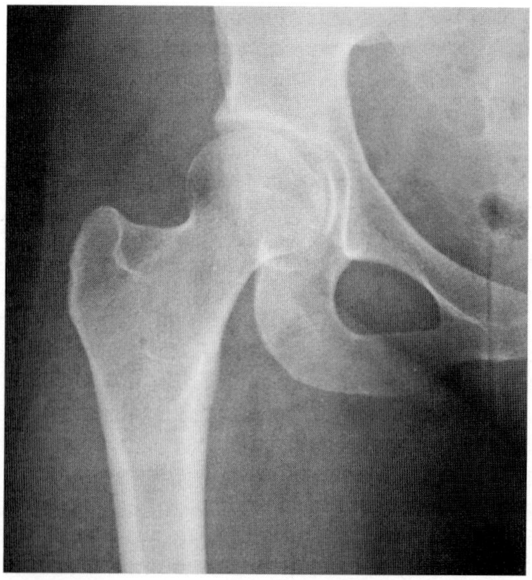

Fig. 4. Radiograph of a patient with developmental hip dysplasia shows a shallow acetabulum with partial uncovering of the femoral head. This leads to increased pressure on the acetabular roof and subsequent labral and chondral lesions and later OA. (Courtesy of Z. Rosenberg, MD, New York, NY.)

head against the acetabulum results in degeneration of the labrum with ganglion formation or ossification of the acetabular rim, which then further deepens the acetabulum, leading to worsening of the overcoverage [4,12,14]. Persistent anterior abutment of the femoral head against the acetabulum can result in chondral injury of the femoral head in the "contre-coup" area of the posteroinferior acetabulum. Chondral lesions are often limited to a small acetabular rim area and are often more benign compared with the deep chondral lesions and extensive labral tears seen in cam impingement [4,6]. Pincer impingement is more frequently seen in middle-aged athletic women [4,6].

In the normal hip, the acetabular opening is anteverted from the sagittal plane. Retroversion of the acetabulum has been described as a posteriorly oriented acetabulum with reference to the sagittal plane [12,14]. Acetabular retroversion can occur as part of a complex acetabular developmental deformity, as result of posttraumatic dysplasia, or as an isolated deformity, which is considered a precursor to OA [12,14,27,35,36]. In retroversion, the anterior acetabular roof edge lies lateral to the posterior edge. As the acetabular opening spirals downward, it becomes more anteverted; however, the anterior edge of the acetabulum is located in a more lateral position compared with normal, and the posterior edge is more medially located (Fig. 5).

Acetabular retroversion can be diagnosed on AP radiographs on the basis of two distinctive features: the crossover or "figure of eight" and posterior wall signs [12,14]. The crossover sign is created by the anterior aspect of the acetabular rim being more laterally located than the posterior aspect of the cranial aspect of the acetabulum. The anterior aspect of the acetabular rim is directed more horizontally and medially, thereby crossing over the more straight and vertical posterior aspect of the acetabular rim (Fig. 6) [12,14]. The posterior wall sign is the outline of the posterior edge of the posterior wall of the acetabulum. In the normal acetabulum, the line descends through the center point of the femoral head or lateral to it. In the retroverted acetabulum, this line is medial to the center point, indicating relatively less posterior coverage [12,14].

A retroverted acetabulum can be seen on axial MR or CT images as increased coverage of the anterior femoral head [14]. The prominent anterolateral edge of the acetabulum predisposes to impingement during flexion and internal rotation, resulting in labral degeneration and/or tears and adjacent cartilage. Labral tears predispose to

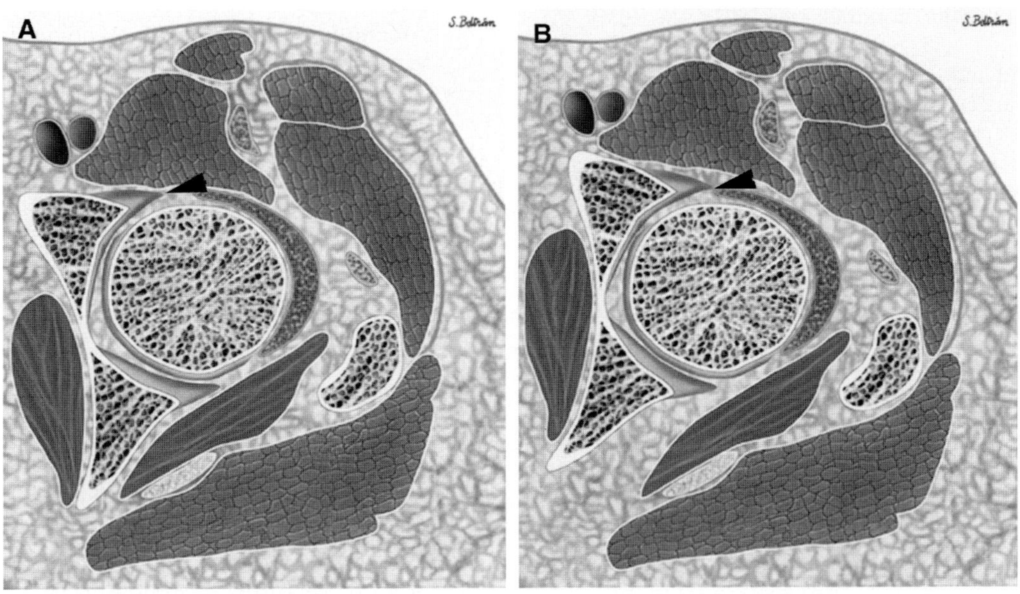


Fig. 5. Acetabular retroversion. (*A*) Normal orientation of the acetabulum. Note normal location of the anterior lip (*arrowhead*). (*B*) Retroversion of the normal acetabulum resulting in anterior overcoverage. The anterior lip (*arrowhead*) extends more laterally compared with normal.

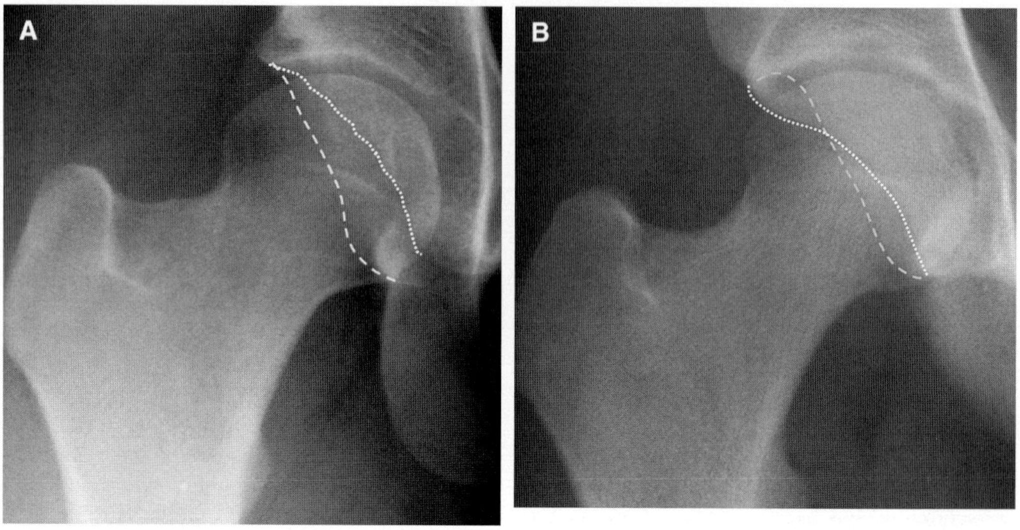



Fig. 6. Radiographs of acetabular retroversion. (*A*) Normal acetabulum. The dotted line represents the anterior acetabular rim, and the broken line represents the posterior acetabular rim. (*B*) Crossover sign in a patient with acetabular retroversion, where the anterior rim (*dotted line*) crosses over the posterior rim (*broken line*). (Courtesy of S. Anderson, MD, and M. Tannast, MD, Bern, Switzerland.)

extraosseous ganglia formation with splitting of the labrum and acetabular cartilage. This allows penetration of synovial fluid into subchondral bone, leading to subchondral cyst formation [12,14]. In later stages of FAI, there may be evidence of damage from impingement and even fragmentation of the bony margin of the prominent anterior acetabular edge. In the study by Reynolds and coworkers [14], retroversion was bilateral and symmetric in all patients.

Surgical treatment of pincer impingement includes arthroscopic debridement of labral lesions and reduction of anterior acetabular overcoverage by excising the bony prominence at the acetabular rim. The goal is to allow sufficient impingement-free range of motion during flexion and internal rotation [6,12,14,20]. Acetabular retroversion has been successfully treated with reverse periacetabular osteotomy [12].

## MR imaging protocol

Our protocol for MR imaging of the hip is designed to image bilateral hips and the unilateral hip in question. We use a phased-array torso coil or body coil on a 1.5-T magnet (General Electric Medical Systems, Milwaukee, Wisconsin). Our protocol includes oblique-coronal (parallel to the axis of the femoral neck) T1-weighted, fast spin-echo (FSE) (repetition time per milliseconds [TR]/echo time per milliseconds [TE] = 650/17);

**Box 1. Summary of MR imaging findings in femoroacetabular impingement**

*Femoral findings*

- Decreased femoral head-neck offset
- Dysplastic femoral bump at physeal scar
- Subchondral edema/cysts at, adjacent to, or remote from femoral bump
- Chondral fissures or defects ± joint space narrowing (advanced stage of FAI)
- Femoral head edema (advanced stage of FAI with worse prognosis)
- Capsular thickening and synovitis
- Thickening of iliofemoral ligament

*Acetabular findings*

- Acetabular retroversion
- Subchondral edema or cysts of the acetabular rim
- Cysts of fluid, synovial, or fat signal depending on stage
- Subchondral sclerosis of the acetabular rim
- Chondral fissures or defect in superior or superior-lateral acetabular rim
- Labral tears
- Paralabral cysts

oblique-coronal axial fat-saturated (FS), proton density (PD), FSE (TR/TE 3000/51); and oblique-coronal short tau inversion recovery (STIR) (TR/TE/inversion time per milliseconds [TI] = 5000/34/150) sequences of both hips, using a large field of view (FOV) of 36 cm. Using a four-channel phased-array cardiac coil, sagittal and oblique-coronal PD FSE (TR/TE = 3000/51), oblique-coronal T2*gradient-recalled echo (GRE) (TR/TE = 500/15, 20° flip angle), and coronal T1 FSE images of the affected hip are performed with a small FOV (16–18 cm). Slice thickness is 4.5 mm, with a 0.4-mm interslice gap and a number of excitations (NEX) of 3 to 4. Imaging time is approximately 35 minutes.

MR arthrography is usually performed to assess the acetabular labrum, because several studies have shown its high accuracy in detecting labral lesions [37–40]. After the intra-articular administration of dilute gadolinium at a dose of 10 to 15 mL, MR imaging of the affected hip is performed. Before MR imaging, the intra-articular

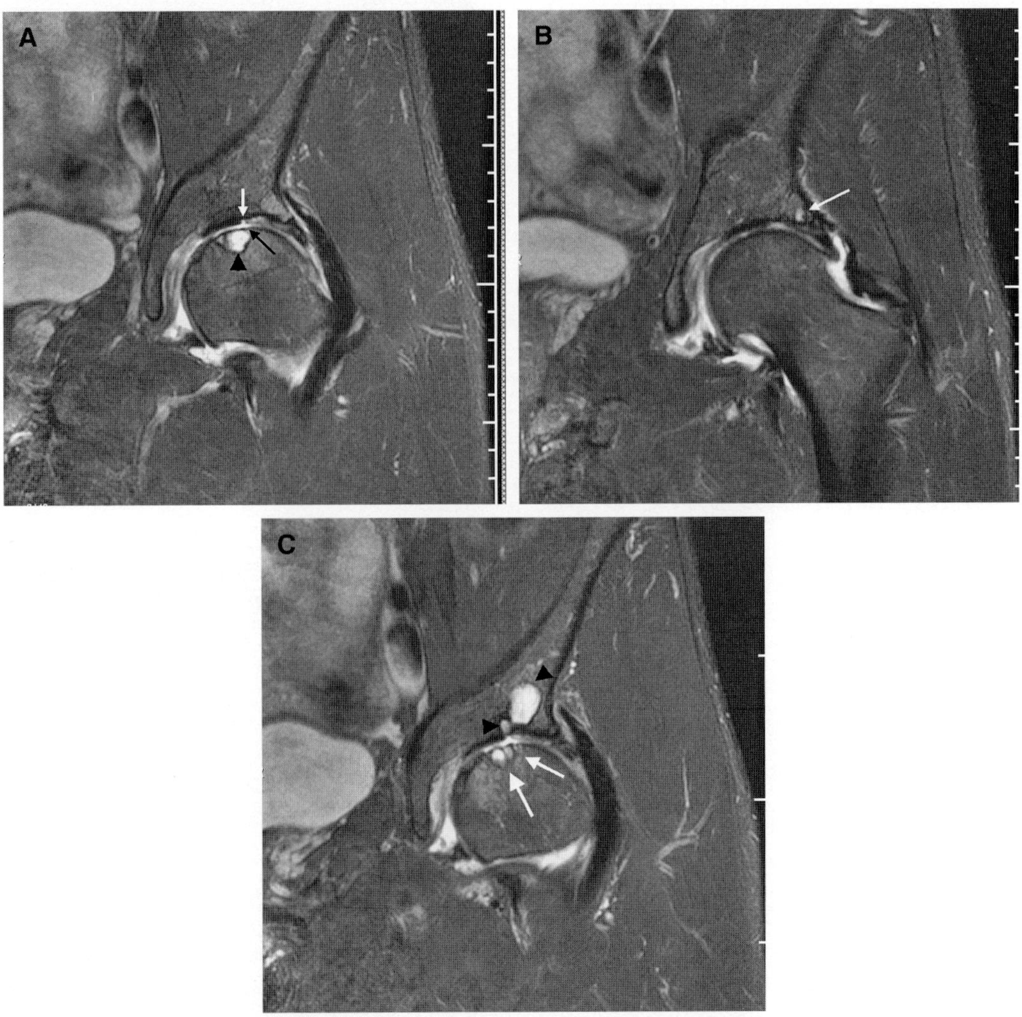


Fig. 7. MR imaging findings in advanced FAI. (*A*) Coronal FS PD FSE MR image in a patient with advanced FAI demonstrates an acetabular cartilage defect (*white arrow*) and a cartilage defect of the femoral head (*black arrow*) with an underlying large subchondral cyst (*black arrowhead*). Joint space narrowing is present. (*B*) Coronal FS PD FSE MR image of the same hip demonstrates a subchondral cyst of the acetabular rim (*arrow*). (*C*) Coronal FS PD FSE MR image shows cartilage loss with a large subchondral cyst of the acetabular rim (*black arrowheads*) and femoral head (*white arrows*). Changes involving the femoral head are seen in a later stage of FAI.

position of the needle is confirmed under fluoroscopic guidance with a small amount of water-soluble iodinated contrast, followed by administration of the dilute gadolinium mixture. The gadolinium mixture is made by injection of gadolinium (0.4 mL) into a 50-mL bag of normal saline. We draw 10 mL of this mixture into a 20-mL syringe, followed by water-soluble iodinated contrast (5 mL; Isovue-M-200) and lidocaine 1% (5 mL). Ten to 15 mL of this mixture is then injected into the hip. After administration of the gadolinium mixture, the patient is brought to the MR imaging unit in a wheelchair to avoid weight bearing, which may cause extravasation of contrast. MR imaging of the affected hip is performed with a small FOV (16–18 cm) using FS. T1-weighted, FSE sequences in all three planes (TR/TE = 650/17) and axial and coronal FS PD FSE (TR/TE = 3000/51).

If the anterior superior quadrant of the acetabular labrum is suspicious for a tear but findings on conventional sequences are indeterminate, radial imaging can be performed. For radial imaging, a plane orthogonal to the acetabular rim and labrum is prescribed off a true sagittal localizer.

The accurate assessment of a reduced femoral head-neck junction may require oblique axial images obtained perpendicular to the femoral neck to visualize the head and neck junction and the femoral bump on a single image.

## MR imaging findings of femoroacetabular impingement

MR imaging findings of FAI (Box 1) include edema and sclerosis of the lateral acetabular rim visualized as hypointense on T1. Subchondral edema is hyperintense on FS PD FSE images. Acute subchondral acetabular cysts are hyperintense on FS PD FSE images (Fig. 7). Intermediate signal intensity synovial or granulation tissue is associated with maturation of subchondral cysts. In the younger patient population, the conversion of the cyst to fat signal intensity indicates an attempt at healing [41].

The articular cartilage is hyperintense in areas of chondral softening. This softening progresses from articular cartilage fissures to frank chondral fragmentation resulting in a full-thickness chondral defect in the superior portion on the acetabular roof (Figs. 8 and 9). Subchondral sclerosis is visualized on coronal and sagittal images and is associated with chondral involvement. Chondral

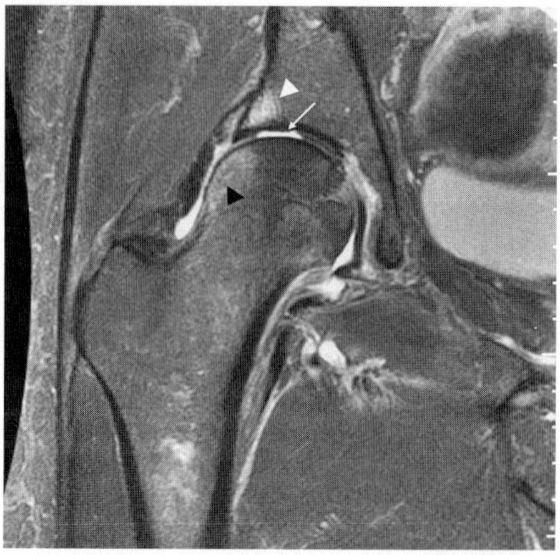

Fig. 8. Coronal FS PD FSE MR image shows bone marrow edema of the acetabular rim (*white arrowhead*), a large chondral defect (*white arrow*), and bone marrow edema in an area of a dysplastic femoral bump adjacent to the physeal scar (*black arrowhead*).

lesions are frequently associated with joint space narrowing and represent a later stage of FAI (see Fig. 7), usually less responsive to impingement surgery [17,41].

On MR imaging, the acetabular labrum appears as a triangular low signal intensity structure

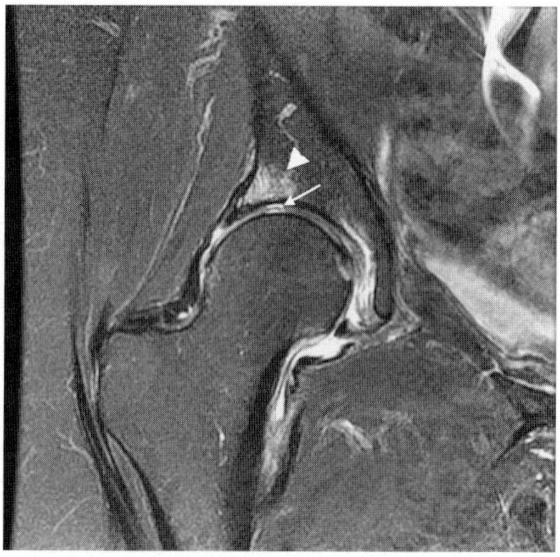

Fig. 9. Coronal FS PD FSE MR image demonstrates changes of FAI with subchondral bone marrow edema of the acetabular rim (*arrowhead*) and an articular cartilage defect (*arrow*). Degenerative changes of the labrum are present.

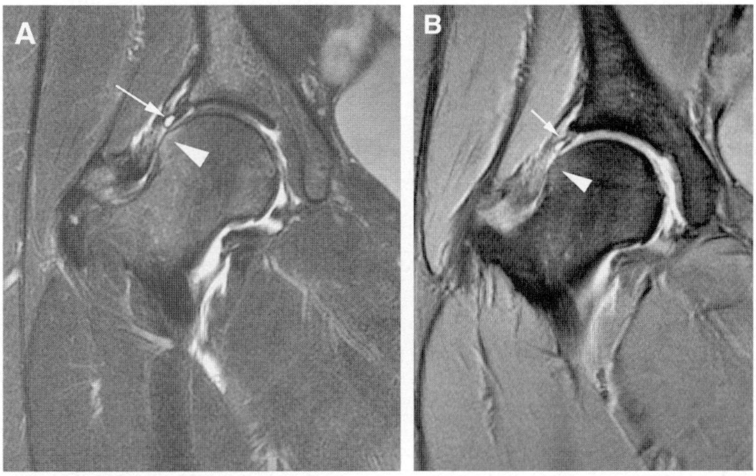


Fig. 10. (*A*) Coronal FS PD FSE MR image demonstrates a labral tear with paralabral cyst (*arrow*). A dysplastic femoral bump lateral to the physeal scar is present (*arrowhead*). (*B*) Coronal GRE image of the same hip demonstrates increased conspicuity of the convex contour of the dysplastic femoral bump (*arrowhead*). Labral tear with a paralabral cyst is identified (*arrow*).

with sharp margins. A recess is seen between the outer margin of the labrum and the joint capsule. With degeneration of the labrum, there is increased signal on FS PD FSE images. Labral tears usually present as a fluid-filled cleft at the base of the labrum adjacent to the acetabular cartilage. Complete detachment of the labrum can be seen in advanced tears. Paralabral cysts that are hyperintense on FS PD FSE images may be present within the adjacent bone or in an extra-articular location (Fig. 10) [18,41,42].

A dysplastic femoral bump is located lateral (directly lateral, superolateral, or inferolateral) to the physeal scar of the femoral head-neck junction (Figs. 11 and 12). This bump exists as a discrete contour convexity that may be associated with subchondral edema (see Fig. 8) and cystic change. The finding of a femoral-sided subchondral cyst

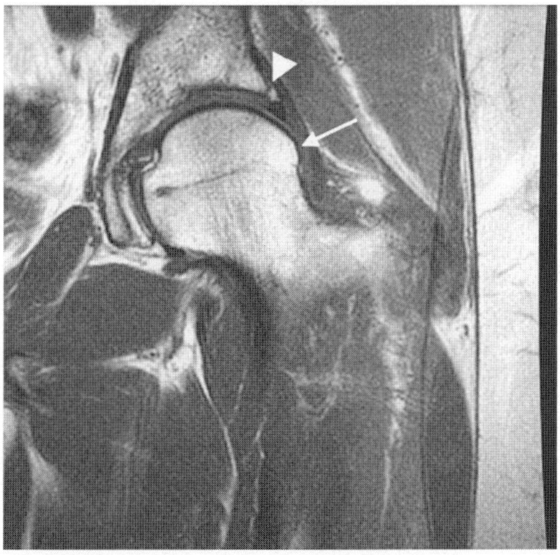

Fig. 11. Coronal T1-weighted MR image demonstrates a decreased femoral head-neck offset with a dysplastic femoral bump (*arrow*). A small os acetabuli is present (*arrowhead*). An os acetabuli is often seen in patients with FAI.

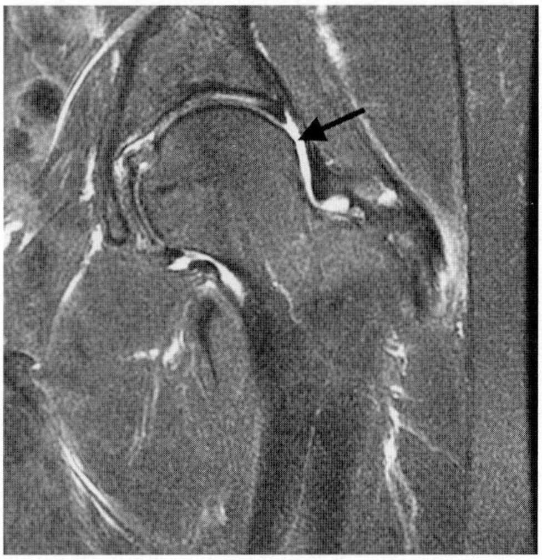

Fig. 12. Coronal FS PD FSE MR image demonstrates the dysplastic femoral bump (*arrow*).

represents the point of impingement on the femur and is not a normal variation of synovial herniation [9,41]. T2* GRE coronal images increase the conspicuity of the convex contour associated with the dysplastic femoral bump at the head-neck junction (see Fig. 10). GRE improves the visualization of altered trabecular bone in the area of impingement because of increased sensitivity to susceptibility of altered trabecular architecture [41]. A reduced femoral head-junction can be assessed on oblique axial images obtained perpendicular to the femoral neck to visualize the head and neck junction and the femoral bump on a single image (Fig. 13).

Thickening of the joint capsule, often with synovitis, and thickening of the iliofemoral ligament laterally are associated with the inflammatory changes in FAI (Fig. 14). The iliofemoral ligament is divided arthroscopically to allow the outflow of small loose bodies, and debris not removed during the initial arthroscopic treatment. Sectioning of this ligament also provides pain relief secondary to capsular contraction [41].

The acetabular contour (slope) as visualized on anterior coronal images represents a sensitive indictor of acetabular dysplasia (DDH). Lateral acetabular rim syndrome as originally described in DDH is characterized by similar MR imaging findings in an identical location as seen in FAI [18]. Leunig and colleagues [18] described hypertrophy of the acetabular labrum and increased incidence of paralabral cysts in patients with DDH compared with patients with FAI. In our experience, however, a hypertrophied labrum or paralabral cysts are frequently seen in patients with FAI without DDH (Fig. 15).

Anterior overcoverage of the acetabulum with a retroverted acetabulum is common in patients

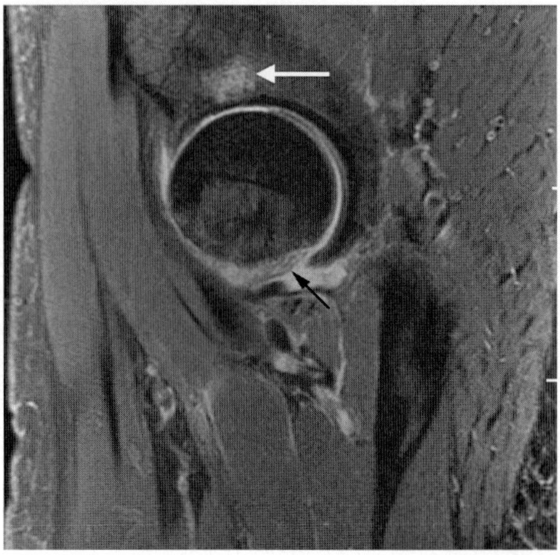

Fig. 14. Sagittal FS PD FSE MR image in a patient with FAI deomonstrates bone marrow edema of the acetabular rim (*white arrow*). Synovitis of the capsule is noted (*black arrow*).

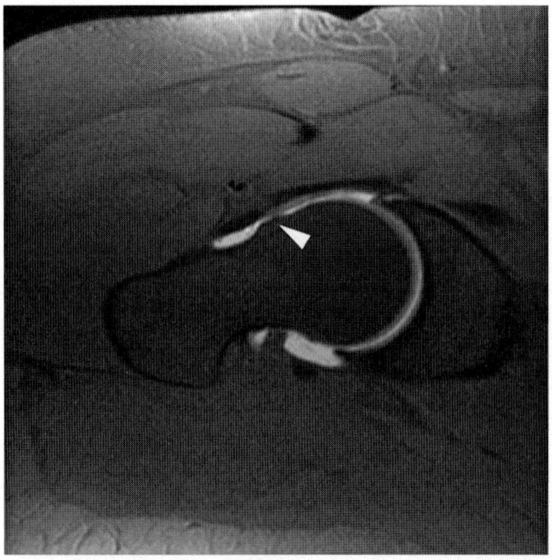

Fig. 13. Oblique axial FS PD FSE MR image obtained perpendicular to the femoral neck demonstrates a decreased femoral head-neck offset with a dysplastic femoral bump (*arrowhead*), resulting in an increased alpha angle in a patient with FAI. (Courtesy of A. Kassarjian, MD, Boston, MA.)

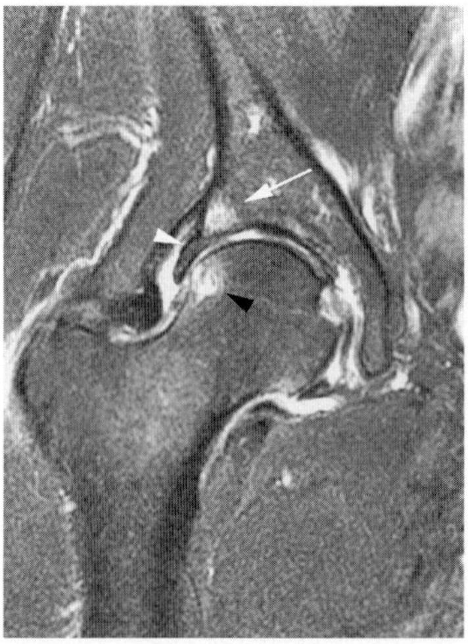

Fig. 15. Coronal FS PD FSE image demonstrates a hypertrophied labrum (*white arrowhead*) and changes from FAI with bone marrow edema of the acetabular rim (*white arrow*) and a dysplastic femoral bump with edema (*black arrowhead*). In this patient, no changes of developmental dysplasia could be identified.

with pincer type FAI [12]. MR imaging has not been used routinely to evaluate acetabular overcoverage and retroversion; however, a retroverted acetabulum can be assessed in the axial plane [12,14].

## Summary

FAI is a common cause of OA of the hip. It can be caused by decreased offset of the femoral head and neck, resulting in abutment of the femoral neck against the acetabular rim (cam impingement) and abutment of this area into the well-constrained socket (pincer impingement) within normal range of motion [15]. This repetitive mechanical trauma to the hip joint causes mechanical wear of the labrum and articular cartilage; left untreated, it causes pain, labral tears, and chondral injuries leading to progressive OA of the hip. The identification of FAI as a cause of OA allows appropriate therapy early and thus delays or prevents end-stage arthritis.

MR imaging and MR arthrography are accurate noninvasive imaging modalities able to demonstrate acetabular labral disease and adjacent cartilage damage as well as the subchondral cysts and synovial herniation pits associated with impingement. In addition, MR imaging is able to detect underlying subtle anatomic variations of the femoral head-neck junction and acetabulum associated with FAI.

## References

[1] Harris WH. Etiology of osteoarthritis of the hip. Clin Orthop Relat Res 1986;213:20–33.
[2] Aronson J. Osteoarthritis of the young adult hip: etiology and treatment. Instr Course Lect 1986;35: 119–28.
[3] Typpo T. Osteoarthritis of the hip. Radiologic findings and etiology. Ann Chir Gynaecol Suppl 1985; 201:1–38.
[4] Ganz R, Parvizi J, Beck M, et al. Femoroacetabular impingement: a cause for osteoarthritis of the hip. Clin Orthop Relat Res 2003;417:112–20.
[5] Tanzer M, Noiseux N. Osseous abnormalities and early osteoarthritis: the role of hip impingement. Clin Orthop Relat Res 2004;429:170–7.
[6] Beck M, Leunig M, Parvizi J, et al. Anterior femoroacetabular impingement: part II. Midterm results of surgical treatment. Clin Orthop Relat Res 2004; 418:67–73.
[7] Ito K, Leunig M, Ganz R. Histopathologic features of the acetabular labrum in femoroacetabular impingement. Clin Orthop Relat Res 2004;429:262–71.
[8] Ito K, Minka MA II, Leunig M, et al. Femoroacetabular impingement and the cam-effect. A MRI-based quantitative anatomical study of the femoral head-neck offset. J Bone Joint Surg Br 2001;83:171–6.
[9] Jager M, Wild A, Westhoff B, et al. Femoroacetabular impingement caused by a femoral osseous head-neck bump deformity: clinical, radiological, and experimental results. J Orthop Sci 2004;9:256–63.
[10] Murphy S, Tannast M, Kim YJ, et al. Debridement of the adult hip for femoroacetabular impingement: indications and preliminary clinical results. Clin Orthop Relat Res 2004;429:178–81.
[11] Notzli HP, Wyss TF, Stoecklin CH, et al. The contour of the femoral head-neck junction as a predictor for the risk of anterior impingement. J Bone Joint Surg Br 2002;84:556–60.
[12] Siebenrock KA, Schoeniger R, Ganz R. Anterior femoro-acetabular impingement due to acetabular retroversion. Treatment with periacetabular osteotomy. J Bone Joint Surg Am 2003;85:278–86.
[13] Murray RO. The aetiology of primary osteoarthritis of the hip. Br J Radiol 1965;38:810–24.
[14] Reynolds D, Lucas J, Klaue K. Retroversion of the acetabulum. A cause of hip pain. J Bone Joint Surg Br 1999;81:281–8.
[15] Leunig M, Beck M, Woo A, et al. Acetabular rim degeneration: a constant finding in the aged hip. Clin Orthop Relat Res 2003;413:201–7.
[16] Leunig M, Werlen S, Ungersbock A, et al. Evaluation of the acetabular labrum by MR arthrography. J Bone Joint Surg Br 1997;79:230–4.
[17] Schmid MR, Notzli HP, Zanetti M, et al. Cartilage lesions in the hip: diagnostic effectiveness of MR arthrography. Radiology 2003;226:382–6.
[18] Leunig M, Podeszwa D, Beck M, et al. Magnetic resonance arthrography of labral disorders in hips with dysplasia and impingement. Clin Orthop Relat Res 2004;418:74–80.
[19] Buckwalter JA, Lohmander S. Operative treatment of osteoarthrosis. Current practice and future development. J Bone Joint Surg Am 1994;76:1405–18.
[20] Lavigne M, Parvizi J, Beck M, et al. Anterior femoroacetabular impingement: part I. Techniques of joint preserving surgery. Clin Orthop Relat Res 2004;418:61–6.
[21] Beck M, Leunig M, Clarke E, et al. Femoroacetabular impingement as a factor in the development of nonunion of the femoral neck: a report of three cases. J Orthop Trauma 2004;18:425–30.
[22] Eijer H, Myers SR, Ganz R. Anterior femoroacetabular impingement after femoral neck fractures. J Orthop Trauma 2001;15:475–81.
[23] Klaue K, Durnin CW, Ganz R. The acetabular rim syndrome. A clinical presentation of dysplasia of the hip. J Bone Joint Surg Br 1991;73:423–9.
[24] Leunig M, Casillas MM, Hamlet M, et al. Slipped capital femoral epiphysis: early mechanical damage to the acetabular cartilage by a prominent femoral metaphysis. Acta Orthop Scand 2000;71:370–5.

[25] Myers SR, Eijer H, Ganz R. Anterior femoroacetabular impingement after periacetabular osteotomy. Clin Orthop Relat Res 1999;363:93–9.
[26] Pitto RP, Klaue K, Ganz R, et al. Acetabular rim pathology secondary to congenital hip dysplasia in the adult. A radiographic study. Chir Organi Mov 1995; 80:361–8.
[27] Tonnis D, Heinecke A. Acetabular and femoral anteversion: relationship with osteoarthritis of the hip. J Bone Joint Surg Am 1999;81:1747–70.
[28] Chell J, Flowers MJ. Is diagnostic arthroscopy of the hip worthwhile? J Bone Joint Surg Br 2000; 82:306.
[29] Siebenrock KA, Wahab KH, Werlen S, et al. Abnormal extension of the femoral head epiphysis as a cause of cam impingement. Clin Orthop Relat Res 2004;418:54–60.
[30] Ferguson SJ, Bryant JT, Ganz R, et al. The acetabular labrum seal: a poroelastic finite element model. Clin Biomech (Bristol, Avon) 2000;15:463–8.
[31] Ferguson SJ, Bryant JT, Ganz R, et al. An in vitro investigation of the acetabular labral seal in hip joint mechanics. J Biomech 2003;36:171–8.
[32] Crowninshield RD, Maloney WJ, Wentz DH, et al. Biomechanics of large femoral heads: what they do and don't do. Clin Orthop Relat Res 2004;429: 102–7.
[33] Stuhlberg SD, Cordell L, Harris WH, et al. Unrecognized childhood hip disease: a major cause of idiopathic osteoarthritis of the hip. St. Louis (MO): CV Mosby; 1975.
[34] Morgan JD, Somerville EW. Normal and abnormal growth at the upper end of the femur. J Bone Joint Surg Br 1960;42:264–72.
[35] Dora C, Zurbach J, Hersche O, et al. Pathomorphologic characteristics of posttraumatic acetabular dysplasia. J Orthop Trauma 2000;14:483–9.
[36] Murphy SB, Kijewski PK, Millis MB, et al. Acetabular dysplasia in the adolescent and young adult. Clin Orthop Relat Res 1990;261:214–23.
[37] Czerny C, Hofmann S, Neuhold A, et al. Lesions of the acetabular labrum: accuracy of MR imaging and MR arthrography in detection and staging. Radiology 1996;200:225–30.
[38] Czerny C, Hofmann S, Urban M, et al. MR arthrography of the adult acetabular capsular-labral complex: correlation with surgery and anatomy. AJR Am J Roentgenol 1999;173:345–9.
[39] Hodler J, Yu JS, Goodwin D, et al. MR arthrography of the hip: improved imaging of the acetabular labrum with histologic correlation in cadavers. AJR Am J Roentgenol 1995;165:887–91.
[40] Petersilge CA, Haque MA, Petersilge WJ, et al. Acetabular labral tears: evaluation with MR arthrography. Radiology 1996;200:231–5.
[41] Stoller DW, Tirman PFJ, Bredella MA. Femoroacetabular impingement. In: Stoller, Tirman, Bredella, editors. Diagnostic imaging: orthopaedics. Salt Lake City (UT): Amirsys; 2004. p. 82–5.
[42] Sadro C. Current concepts in magnetic resonance imaging of the adult hip and pelvis. Semin Roentgenol 2000;35:231–48.

ELSEVIER
SAUNDERS

Magn Reson Imaging Clin N Am
13 (2005) 665–676

MAGNETIC
RESONANCE
IMAGING CLINICS
of North America

# MR Imaging of the Hip: Osseous Lesions

Javier Beltran, MD*, Oleg Opsha, MD

*Department of Radiology, Maimonides Medical Center, 4802 Tenth Avenue, Brooklyn, NY 11219, USA*

Recent technologic advances in gradient strength, pulse sequence, and surface coil design allow for unprecedented soft tissue resolution. The hip joint is only one of the areas in which MR imaging has become the modality of choice for evaluation of bone and soft tissue pathologic findings. The hip is one of the frequent indications for MR imaging in patients presenting with symptoms in which the diagnosis is not resolved with plain films. In this article, the imaging techniques and MR imaging manifestations of the osseous entities are discussed, including trauma (insufficiency and stress fractures, subchondral fractures, and osteochondritis dissecans [OCD]), osteonecrosis, transient osteoporosis, bone marrow edema syndrome, and bone tumors that have a predilection for the hip area. Because of space constrains, only the adult hip is discussed.

## Technical notes

The first decision to make with hip MR imaging is whether to image both hips simultaneously or only the symptomatic hip. It is an important decision because it influences other decisions, such as coil and pulse sequence selection as well as whether or not to inject contrast material intra-articularly or intravenously. This decision is compounded by the common situation in which no pertinent clinical information is provided. As a general guideline, imaging of both hips simultaneously may be appropriate if one is looking for osteonecrosis (given the frequency of bilateral involvement) or metastasis. In most other clinical situations, single hip imaging provides better spatial and contrast resolution, because a dedicated surface coil can be used.

When bilateral hip imaging is chosen, the body coil, preferably phase array, is used [1]. The following set of pulse sequences is recommended: T1-weighted coronal and fast spin echo (FSE) T2-weighted or short tau inversion recovery (STIR) axial. If there are positive findings, one may choose to stop at this time or to switch to single hip imaging using a dedicated surface coil, such as a flexible coil, for better anatomic resolution of small structures, such as the acetabular labrum, or for better evaluation of the articular surfaces or subchondral area of the femoral head.

When single hip imaging is indicated, the following pulse sequences are recommended: coronal T1-weighted high-resolution with a 512 matrix, axial T2-weighted FSE or STIR, sagittal two-dimensional (2D) or three-dimensional (3D) gradient recalled echo (GRE; fast low-angle shot [FLASH], spoiled gradient recalled [SPGR]), or T2-weighted or STIR sequences.

Intravenous contrast material may be useful to assess tissue viability in osteonecrosis and in cases of suspected infection or bone or soft tissue tumors. T1-weighted high-resolution images with fat saturation in the axial sagittal and coronal planes are recommended when using intravenous contrast material. The most recent innovation is the so-called "indirect" MR arthrogram, replacing the intra-articular or "direct" MR arthrogram. Indirect MR arthrography is performed injecting a standard dose of gadolinium chelate (1 mmol/kg) intravenously, followed by 10 to 15 minutes of gentle exercise before imaging using T1-weighted fat-saturated images with high resolution in all three orthogonal planes in addition to a T2-weighted sequence, preferably in the axial plane. This technique provides enough diffusion of contrast material through the synovium to outline the articular surfaces and produce some distention of the capsule and its recesses. An added advantage of

* Corresponding author.
*E-mail address:* jbeltran46@msn.com (J. Beltran).

1064-9689/05/$ - see front matter 
doi:10.1016/j.mric.2005.08.011

indirect MR arthrography is that it produces enhancement of hyperemic tissues. Furthermore, if a preexisting joint effusion is present, the injected contrast material mixes with the joint fluid, giving an excellent arthrographic effect with high resolution provided by the use of the T1-weighted fat-saturated images with a 512 matrix.

Intra-articular direct MR arthrography entails the placement of a needle into the hip joint, generally using fluoroscopic guidance, and injecting a dilution (10–15 mL) of gadolinium chelate (0.1 mL) and saline (20 mL). The patient is then taken immediately into the MR imaging suite, and the same pulse sequences as described for indirect MR arthrography are used. The main advantage of direct MR arthrography over indirect MR arthrography is the full distention of the joint capsule and its recesses. The disadvantages, however, are significant: it requires additional scheduling for fluoroscopy, and it is an invasive procedure with added morbidity.

The indications for indirect or direct MR arthrography include assessment of the articular surfaces when studying OCD and assessment of the acetabular labrum.

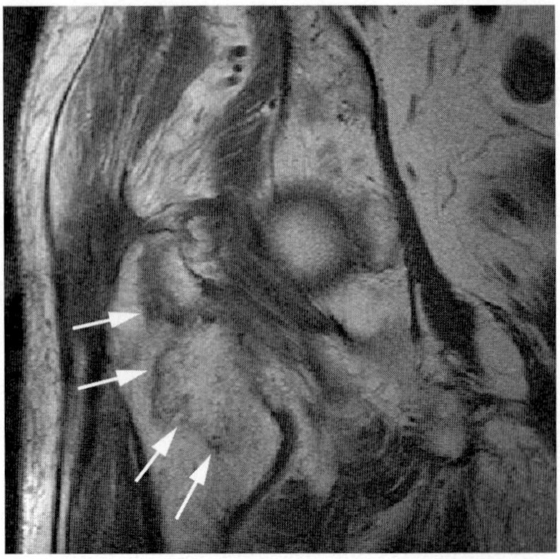

Fig. 1. Occult intertrochanteric fracture in an elderly woman with hip pain after a fall. Radiographs (not shown) were negative. A coronal T1-weighted image demonstrates the irregular fracture line in the intertrochanteric region (*arrows*).

## Trauma

### *Pelvic and hip fractures*

Fractures involving the pelvis and hip can be divided into acute posttraumatic fractures, stress fractures, and insufficiency fractures. Occult posttraumatic fractures in the elderly are a frequent indication for MR imaging of the hip (Fig. 1), and they can occur in the femoral neck, greater trochanter, acetabulum, or parasymphyseal or ischial bone. Insufficiency fractures of the femoral neck, sacrum, pubic bones, and acetabulum may also occur. In these generally osteoporotic patients, plain films may not demonstrate the fracture line and bone scintigraphy may demonstrate increased uptake only several days after the trauma. MR imaging is highly sensitive for detecting the fracture and the surrounding edema immediately after the traumatic event [2–4]. In some cases, CT with multiplanar and surface reconstructions may be helpful to confirm the presence of a fracture extending to the cortical bone; however, in many cases, CT may not add significant information. CT has a definite role in the preoperative evaluation of major pelvic and acetabular fractures, but this topic is beyond the scope of this article.

Verbeeten and colleagues [3] recently evaluated the accuracy of MR imaging in the evaluation of occult hip fracture and its economic impact in a series of 33 patients. They concluded that the accuracy of MR imaging was 100% and that the financial impact was significant, by shortening the time to diagnosis, permitting superior visualization of the bone and soft tissue injuries, and preventing unnecessary hospitalization and delays in definitive treatment. Given the high accuracy of MR imaging for the diagnosis of occult fractures, some authors have proposed the use of a "limited" low-cost study of the hips using a T1-weighted coronal sequence [5]. Some investigators believe that the added value of T2-weighted sequences is significant, however, because they allow one to distinguish bone sclerosis from edema [6].

In a recent study of 73 patients examined with MR imaging (total of 76 MR imaging studies) for possible hip fractures, Oka and Monu [6] found the following distribution of fractures: greater trochanter, 4 fractures; intertrochanteric, 5 fractures; femoral neck, 8 fractures; acetabular, 5 fractures; and obturator ring, 13 fractures. On two occasions, they found bone marrow edema without cortical disruption. Associated muscular injuries (eg, edema, hematoma, hemorrhage) were present in 66% of their cases. In retrospective analysis of the plain radiographs, these authors found an incidence of 46% occult fractures not seen on radiographs.

Based on the MR imaging assessment of hip fractures, the concept of an "incomplete" femoral

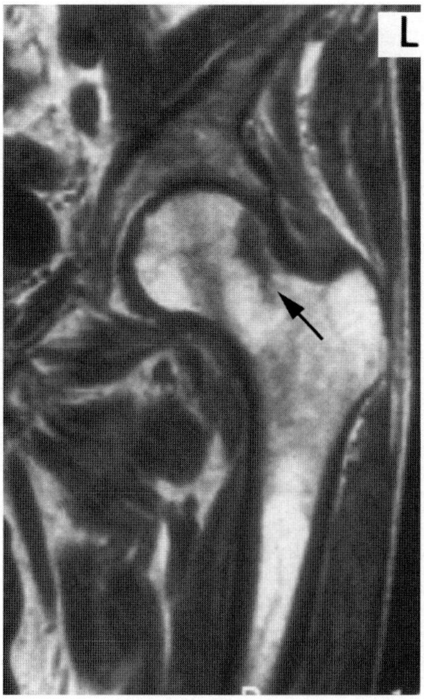


Fig. 2. Incomplete femoral neck fracture in an elderly man with left hip pain after a fall. A coronal T1-weighted image demonstrates a vertically oriented fracture of the left femoral neck (*arrow*). The fracture line stops in the midportion of the neck.

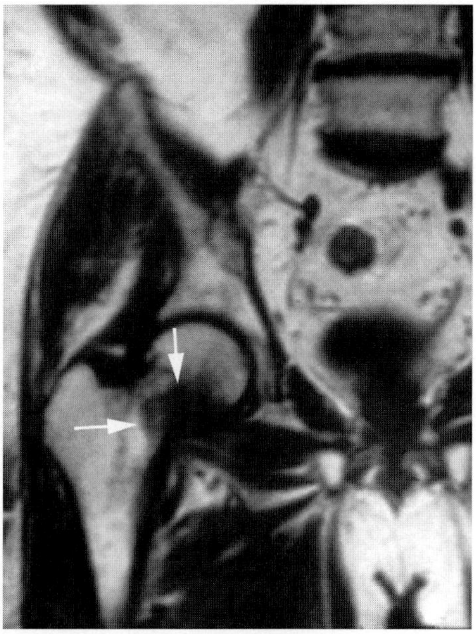

Fig. 3. Insufficiency fracture in an active elderly woman with right hip pain without a history of trauma. A coronal T1-weighted image shows a focal area of abnormal signal intensity in the medial aspect of the femoral neck (*arrows*). Plain films (not shown) demonstrated an irregular sclerotic band in the same area corresponding to incomplete healing of an insufficiency fracture.

neck fracture has emerged. These fractures are normally not evident on plain films, and they are often seen extending vertically from the lateral greater trochanter but not reaching the contralateral cortex (Fig. 2). The significance of this finding is important, because incomplete fractures can evolve into complete and displaced fractures if the patient continues weight bearing.

Another type of hip lesion related to stress or insufficiency is a fracture that occurs at the level of the internal aspect of the femoral neck, where the primary compression trabeculae are confluent toward the calcar. These fractures are most often incomplete and are seen on MR imaging as a low signal intensity area or band in the inner aspect of the femoral neck with or without a fracture line (Figs. 3 and 4). A similar insufficiency fracture can be seen in the supra-acetabular area (Fig. 5).

Parasymphyseal insufficiency fractures of the os pubis are frequently encountered in the paramenopausal female and elderly populations. They may show misleading radiographic signs suggesting malignancy on plain films, and MR imaging has been shown to be helpful not only in establishing the diagnosis but in determining the benign nature of the fracture [7]. Hyperintense mass lesions on T2-weighted images, with hypointensity on T1-weighted images and peripheral and septal enhancement after intravenous administration of contrast material, have been described as characteristic findings in this type of fracture [7]. Similarly, Seo and coworkers [8] found that healing or nonunited insufficiency fractures involving the ischiopubic bones in the elderly population may pose a question about the possibility of an underlying metastatic process on conventional radiographs because of lysis and callus formation at the fracture site. In these cases, these authors [8] proposed the use of contrast-enhanced MR imaging to exclude a pathologic fracture demonstrating a cleft-like elongated area of high signal intensity, excluding a metastatic lesion.

Pathologic fractures of the femoral neck are relatively frequent, and one manifestation in the region of the hip is an avulsion of the lesser trochanter. MR imaging may be helpful to determine the malignant nature of the fracture (Fig. 6).

Sacral insufficiency fractures are well described in the literature [9–12]. MR imaging has been

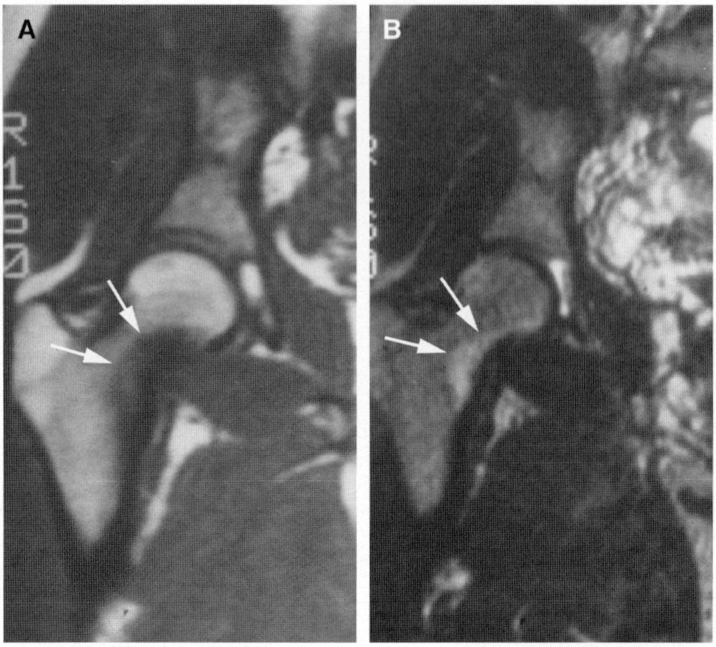


Fig. 4. Stress-related edema in a young marathon runner with severe right hip pain. Plain films (not shown) were normal. A bone scan (not shown) demonstrated increased uptake in the right femoral neck. T1-weighted (*A*) and T2-weighted (*B*) coronal images depict a focal area of edema in the inner aspect of the femoral neck (*arrows*) in the area of the confluence of the primary compressive trabeculae. The patient was treated conservatively with rest and began her training again several months later. Follow-up MR imaging revealed no residual abnormality. The lesion would have probably progressed to a full-blown stress fracture if the patient had continued her strenuous physical activity.

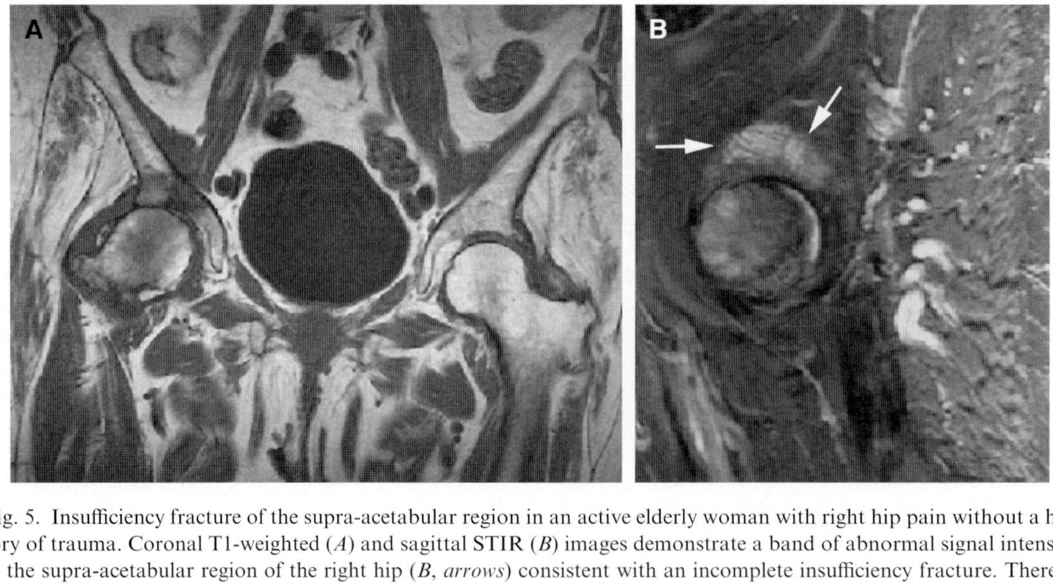


Fig. 5. Insufficiency fracture of the supra-acetabular region in an active elderly woman with right hip pain without a history of trauma. Coronal T1-weighted (*A*) and sagittal STIR (*B*) images demonstrate a band of abnormal signal intensity in the supra-acetabular region of the right hip (*B*, *arrows*) consistent with an incomplete insufficiency fracture. There is degenerative disease of the right hip, with reactive bone marrow edema in the femoral head.

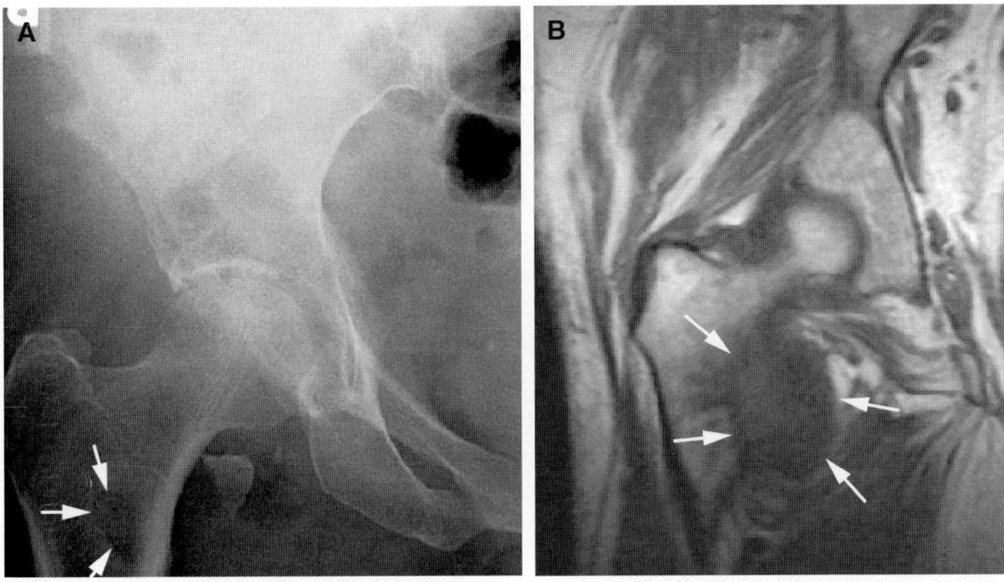


Fig. 6. Pathologic fracture of the lesser trochanter. (*A*) Plain film demonstrates an avulsion fracture of the lesser trochanter associated with a lytic area in the proximal femur (*arrows*). (*B*) Coronal T1-weighted image shows a proximal femoral mass with extraosseous extension (*arrows*), which corresponded to a metastatic lesion.

found to demonstrate early edema along the sacral ala, parallel to the sacroiliac joints, unilaterally or bilaterally, sometimes associated with transverse sacra fractures. The recognition of these fractures is also important because it explains the acute onset of low back pain in the elderly population and helps in excluding a primary bone tumor or metastatic disease.

The signal intensity changes observed with MR imaging in patients with traumatic, insufficiency, or stress fractures is best detected with STIR pulse sequences because of their high sensitivity for even small amounts of free water in the tissues, which appear immediately after the fracture takes place. Resolution of the bone marrow edema may take a long time, however. Slocum and colleagues [13] studied the time to resolution of bone marrow edema in 10 patients with these types of fractures. They found that 90% of the patients showed resolution of the bone marrow edema within 6 months of the initial diagnosis of the fracture (7 patients within 3 months, 2 patients within 6 months, and 1 patient within 12 months).

### *Subchondral fractures*

Subchondral fractures of the femoral head are now a well-recognized entity that may lead to extensive bone marrow edema and eventual collapse of the femoral head, with subsequent bone resorption and rapid development of osteoarthritis. Subchondral fractures are mostly occult on plain films and may be related to stress in the young population or may represent insufficiency fractures caused by osteoporosis in the elderly population or in patients with other causes of osteoporosis [4,14] rather than to direct trauma [14]. This entity may be misdiagnosed as osteonecrosis [15] or transient osteoporosis of the hip (TOH) because of the extensive bone marrow edema that is seen during the first few months. In fact, TOH and subchondral fracture may be the same condition. Another disease that may be linked to subchondral fracture of the femoral head is rapidly destructive osteoarthritis or Postel's disease. MR imaging demonstrates bone marrow edema, joint effusion, and a faintly seen subchondral hypointense line that represents the fracture as discussed elsewhere in this article. This line is better seen once the bone marrow edema subsides (Fig. 7) [16].

### *Osteochondritis dissecans*

OCD or osteochondral fractures are relatively rare in the femoral head. When they occur, the radiographic findings may be subtle [17] or absent [18]. OCD is mostly related to an acute injury, with shearing forces causing the osteochondral

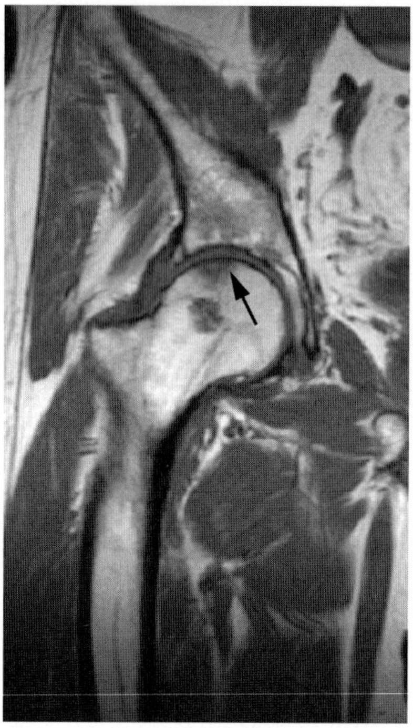

Fig. 7. Subchondral fracture in an active elderly man with acute onset of right hip pain after a tennis game. MR imaging of the right hip (not shown) demonstrated diffuse edema of the femoral head and neck, and a diagnosis of TOH versus osteonecrosis was made. The patient was treated conservatively with rest. Coronal T1-weighted follow-up MR imaging obtained 4 months later demonstrates no residual edema and a subchondral nondepressed fracture (*arrow*). The subchondral bone plate is preserved. There is an incidental enchondroma in the femoral head-neck junction.

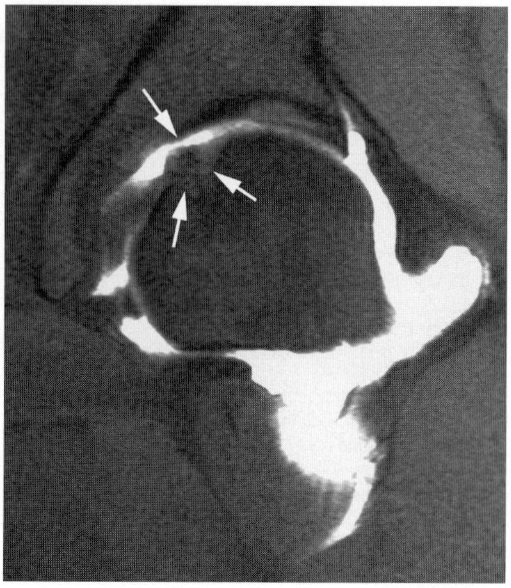

Fig. 8. OCD (osteochondral fracture) in a young female patient with severe hip pain after a fall from a horse. Plain films (not shown) demonstrated a focal irregularity in the femoral head, suspicious for OCD. The patient was treated conservatively. An MR arthrogram was obtained several months later to assess the degree of healing and congruency of the articular surface, because the patient continued to have pain. A T1-weighted fat-saturated image after intra-articular injection of contrast material demonstrates a slightly displaced osteochondral fragment (*arrows*). There is no dissection of contrast material between the fragment and the donor site, indicating some degree of healing. The articular surface is irregular and incongruent, however. A follow-up MR arthrogram was performed 1 year later, as shown in Fig. 9.

fracture. MR imaging manifestations of OCD in the hip include a crater and a fragment of cartilage and bone, generally located in the weight-bearing portion of the femoral head (Fig. 8). The fragment may be in situ or absent, fragmented, or healing in place (Fig. 9). The value of MR imaging is in the assessment of important data, such as size, location, stability, joint surface congruity, and viability of the fragment. All these findings may influence therapeutic planning. Viability of the fragment is established by the signal intensity of the bone fragment. Isointensity of the fragment with the surrounding bone marrow indicates a viable bone, whereas a hypointense fragment on T1- or T2-weighted pulse sequences indicates necrotic bone. Lack of enhancement of the bone fragment after intravenous injection of contrast material also is an indication of nonviable bone. Native fluid or injected contrast material in the interface between a fragment and a donor site indicates an unstable nonhealing lesion. Articular surface smoothness and joint congruity can be assessed with conventional nonenhanced images, although direct MR arthrography is highly accurate for determining minor surface cartilage irregularities (see Fig. 8).

## Nontraumatic bone marrow lesions

Osteonecrosis or avascular necrosis (AVN) of the femoral head is one of the most frequent indications for MR imaging of the hip. MR imaging has been proven highly sensitive and accurate for the detection of this condition. The findings include an irregular low signal intensity line that demarcates the peripheral aspect of the necrotic segment, which histologically correlates

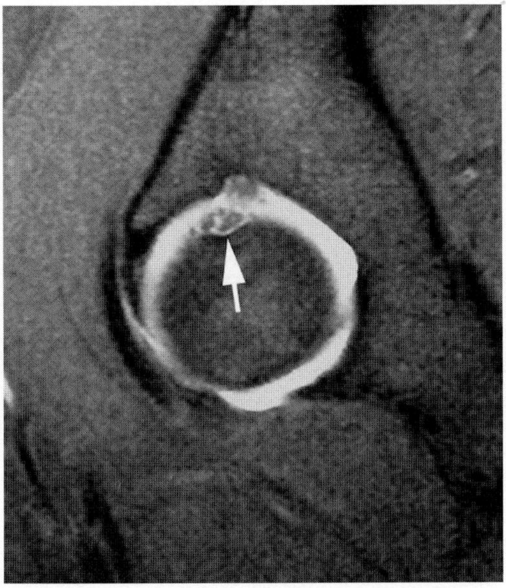

Fig. 9. OCD (osteochondral fracture) in the same patient as in Fig. 8. Sagittal T1-weighted fat-saturated images after intra-articular injection of contrast material demonstrate fragmentation of the osteochondral fragment, persistent incongruity of the articular surface, and dissection of contrast material between the fragments and the donor site (*arrow*), consistent with a nonviable and probably necrotic fragment. The patient was lost to follow-up.

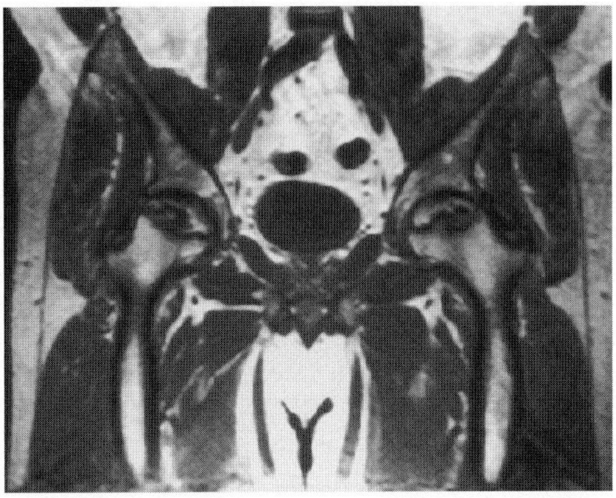

Fig. 10. Bilateral osteonecrosis. A coronal T1-weighted image demonstrates focal areas of bilateral osteonecrosis with a double-line sign. The osteonecrosis involves 100% of the weight-bearing portion of both femoral heads. There is no femoral head collapse or secondary osteoarthritis.

with the reactive interface. Histologically, the reactive interface between viable bone and necrotic bone is composed of two main layers: an external layer with osteoblastic activity and a hyperemic layer with granulation tissue. These two layers are shown on MR imaging as a high-intensity line paralleling a hypointense line. This finding has been termed the *double-line sign*, which is quite characteristic of AVN (Fig. 10). Some investigators, however, claim that the double-line sign may be related to chemical shift artifact [18–20]. Independent of its histopathologic correlation, the presence of a double-line sign is highly suggestive of osteonecrosis. The low signal intensity band corresponds quite closely to the sclerotic margin of osteonecrosis seen on plain films [21], and it is seen in all pulse sequences. The hyperintense line is seen on proton density– and T2-weighted pulse sequences.

Bone marrow edema and joint effusions are additional but nonspecific findings in AVN of the femoral head. Huang and coworkers [22] evaluated 110 hips in 71 patients with surgically proven AVN of the femoral head in search of the incidence and timing of bone marrow edema and joint effusion. These authors found that the peak incidence of bone marrow edema and joint effusion occurred in the advanced stage of the disease and that bone marrow edema had a stronger association with pain than joint effusion. Another recent study by Chan and colleagues [23] in 40 documented cases of AVN of the femoral head indicates that the amount of joint fluid does not correlate with an increase in the intramedullary pressure or the amount of bone marrow edema.

The integrity of the physeal scar has been used a predictor of risk for AVN. In a population with high risk for osteonecrosis, Jiang and Shih [24] found a higher incidence of AVN in patients with a sealed-off physeal scar, suggesting that this finding indicates a more tenuous blood supply to the femoral head, hence increasing the risk for AVN. This observation has not been reproduced at other institutions, however.

In recent years, emphasis has been placed on the assessment of the size of the lesion as compared with the size of the weight-bearing portion of the femoral head [21]. This measurement allows one to determine the potential outcome if minimally invasive treatment, such as core decompression, is considered. Large areas of AVN do not respond to core decompression, and the femoral head eventually collapses, leading to osteoarthritis and a subsequent need for joint replacement. Small lesions (less than 25% of the weight-bearing portion of the femoral head) have a better chance to remain stable without collapse after core decompression [21,25]. A recent review in a group of 39 hips in 35 patients with stage I or II AVN of the femoral head revealed that the index of necrotic extent and the estimation of the percentage involvement of the femoral head are reproducible and reliable methods for quantitatively evaluating the extent of osteonecrosis of the femoral head [25].

The location of focal osteonecrosis involving less than 50% of the weight-bearing portion of the femoral head is also an important predictor of the outcome of the disease. It has been shown that medially or centrally located lesions have a better prognosis than those located laterally [26]. Yoshida and coworkers [27] studied a group of 24 patients with systemic lupus erythematosus with clinically silent AVN of the femoral head, obtaining follow-up MR imaging examinations between 12 and 95 months (mean = 51 months) after the MR imaging diagnosis of AVN was established. They evaluated the percentage of involvement of the femoral head and the medial, central, or lateral location of the process. No surgical intervention was performed in these patients. The authors observed that 15 femoral heads improved (with more than a 15% reduction in the size of their lesions), 5 showed no change, and 4 became worse. All lesions smaller that 25% of the weight-bearing portion of the femoral head improved, and all but two medial or central lesions improved, whereas none of the lateral lesions improved. This study underscores not only the significance of the size and location of the AVN lesion but the potential reversibility of small focal areas of AVN.

Intravenous contrast material in osteonecrosis of the hip has been used in the past for the assessment of the amount of viable bone and to plan minimally invasive procedures, including revascularization and core decompression (Fig. 11) [28].

The MR imaging differential diagnosis of osteonecrosis of the femoral head includes a variety of lesions originating in the bone marrow or the articular surface. The most frequent causes of confusion are transient osteoporosis (discussed in the next section) and subchondral and osteochondral fractures (OCD), as discussed previously. Other lesions that may occasionally produce a similar MR imaging appearance are osteoarthritis or its aggressive manifestation, rapidly destructive osteoarthritis [29]. The usual degenerative disease of the hip manifests itself in the early phases as joint space narrowing attributable to articular cartilage loss, whereas in osteonecrosis, articular cartilage loss is a late manifestation actually representing secondary osteoarthritis attributable to articular surface collapse and joint incongruity. Rapidly destructive osteoarthritis is a relatively rare form of osteoarthritis that is more often seen in elderly women. It is characterized by radiographic findings of typical osteoarthritis progressing to bone resorption and joint collapse with destruction in a short period [29]. This entity may be linked to subchondral fracture or secondary osteonecrosis. Occasionally, a metastatic lesion may

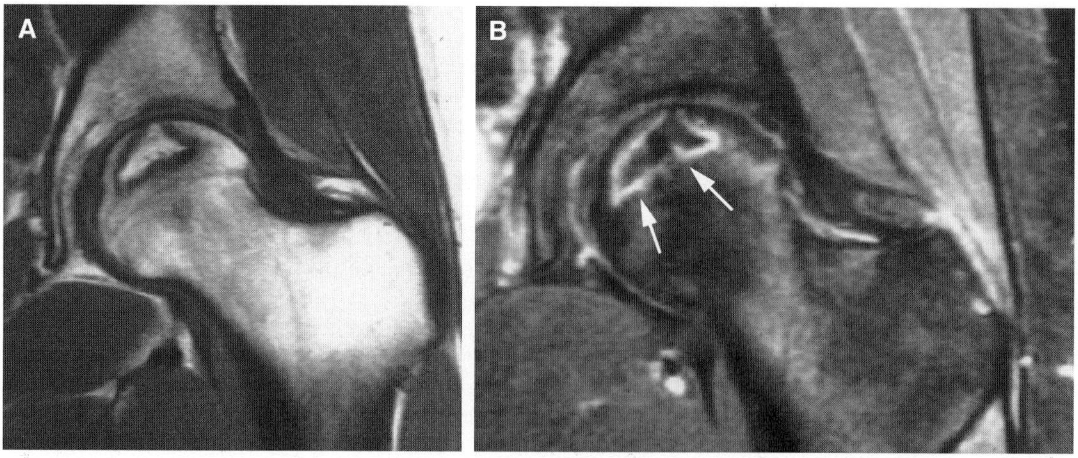


Fig. 11. Osteonecrosis in a young female patient with systemic lupus erythematosus who presented with left hip pain. (*A*) Coronal T1-weighted image demonstrates a triangular-shaped area of osteonecrosis involving a significant portion of the femoral head. Because of her young age, a conservative approach was considered, and a repeat study with intravenous injection of contrast material was performed. (*B*) Coronal T1-weighted fat-saturated image demonstrates rim enhancement of the granulation tissue of the reactive interface (*arrows*), but no contrast material is present within the lesion, indicating nonviable tissue.

simulate a focal lesion of osteonecrosis of the femoral head (Fig. 12).

Acetabular osteonecrosis is a rare accompaniment to aseptic necrosis of the femoral head. In a review of 179 patients with nontraumatic AVN of the femoral head, Fink and colleagues [30] found an incidence of 9.5% of associated AVN of the acetabulum. The criteria for the diagnosis of acetabular osteonecrosis included heterogeneous morphology and irregular contours of the lesion, typical demarcation lines of osteonecrosis, and deficient accumulation of intravenously injected contrast material in the affected regions. The authors concluded that this finding may be significant in the development of early loosening of the acetabular component of total hip replacement.

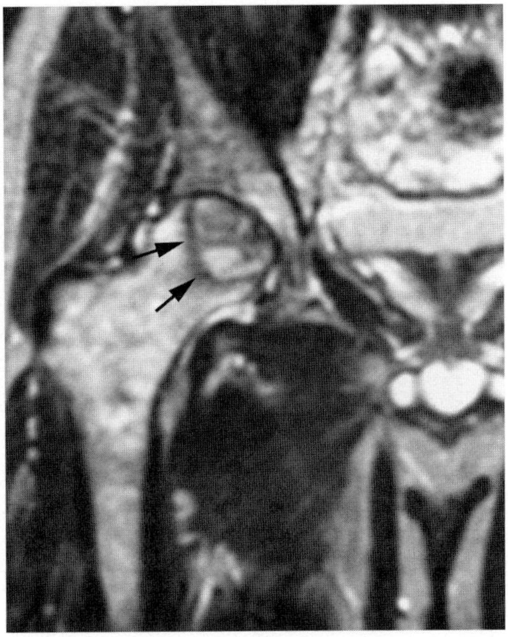

Fig. 12. Metastatic melanoma simulating osteonecrosis in an elderly man with chronic right hip pain. A coronal T2-weighted image demonstrates a focal area of abnormal signal intensity in the femoral head, surrounded by a low signal intensity rim and a questionable double-line sign (*arrows*). There is some bone marrow edema in the femoral neck. The diagnosis of osteonecrosis was made, and given the size of the lesion and continued symptoms, a total hip replacement was planned. At surgery, a tumor was found, which turned out to be metastatic melanoma on histologic examination.

### *Transient osteoporosis of the hip*

TOH, also known as "bone marrow edema syndrome" [31], is another relatively frequent bone marrow condition seen on MR imaging. The entity was described in pregnant women during the third trimester of pregnancy but is now recognized to be more frequent in overweight middle-aged men. The MR imaging findings include extensive bone marrow edema of the femoral head and neck, frequently associated with a joint effusion (Fig. 13). The condition is generally self-limited, with clearing of the clinical symptoms and MR imaging changes in 6 to 8 months.

Some cases of TOH may demonstrate a focal lesion in the subchondral area of the femoral head once the bone marrow edema is cleared, with a hypointense line or band in T1- and T2-weighted pulse sequences. Turner and colleagues [32] suggested that TOH may be a precursor of AVN, based on a small series of 6 cases with findings of TOH that were followed up with MR imaging and developed focal lesions consistent with osteonecrosis. Three of these patients underwent biopsy and confirmed the presence of osteonecrosis. It remains unclear, however, if TOH evolves into osteonecrosis or if it is a manifestation of a subchondral stress or insufficiency fracture or of stress-related edema. Some authors have described similar findings with extensive bone marrow edema involving the head and neck that evolved into focal areas of decreased signal intensity on T1- and T2-weighted pulse sequences and were histologically proved to represent subchondral fractures [33]. These findings suggest that TOH and stress-related edema or stress or insufficiency subchondral fractures may be the same entity. This theory is further supported by the fact that excessive weight is a common denominator in these patients [31,34,35].

Yamamoto and coworkers [36] studied the histologic findings of three patients with clinical and MR imaging evidence of TOH and found focal areas of thin and disconnected bone trabeculae covered by osteoid seams and active osteoblasts. The surrounding bone marrow tissue showed edematous changes and mild fibrosis, but no osteonecrosis was observed in the trabeculae or bone marrow tissue. All three patients improved clinically, and in 3.5 to 9 years of follow-up, there was no evidence of AVN. The authors concluded that their study supports the concept that TOH is not a manifestation of an early reversible phase of osteonecrosis.

Independent of the pathophysiologic mechanisms taking place in these patients, it is clear that in untreated patients with TOH, a subchondral

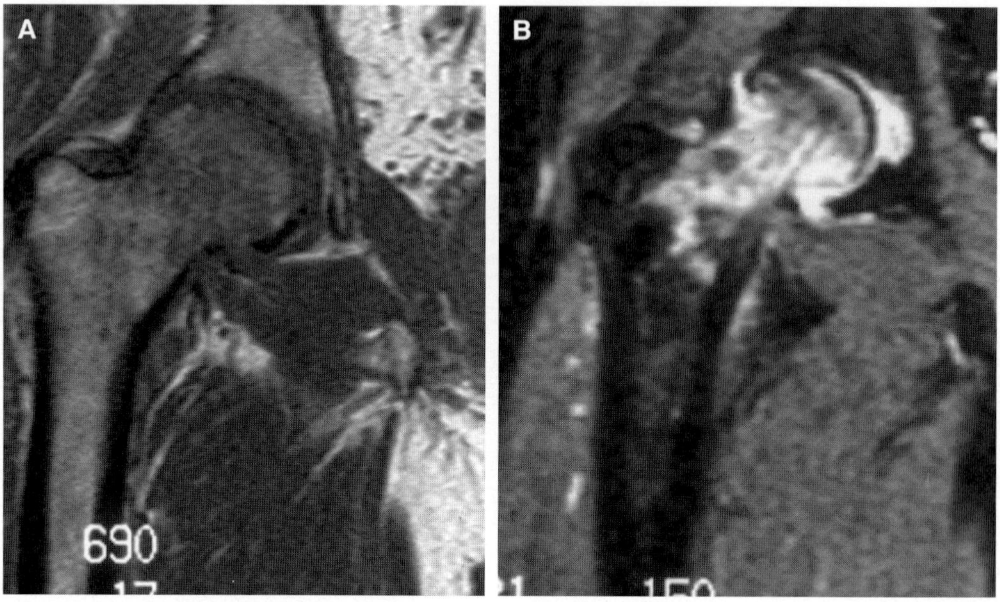


Fig. 13. TOH in a middle-aged overweight man with severe hip pain, without a history of trauma. Coronal T1-weighted (*A*) and STIR (*B*) images demonstrate extensive bone marrow edema in the right femoral head, extending into the neck. Note the presence of a small joint effusion in *B*. No fracture lines are noted.

fracture can develop with persistent weight bearing, leading to femoral head collapse and irreversible secondary degenerative disease requiring hip replacement. It is recommended that careful monitoring of these patients with MR imaging be undertaken during conservative treatment with pain medication and protected weight bearing of the involved hip for a period of 4 to 6 months until the edema is resolved and the clinical symptoms subside. Some investigators recommended core decompression in patients with TOH [37] to decrease pain and shorten the evolution of the process. This procedure is based on the assumption that bone marrow edema is a manifestation of increased intramedullary pressure and is the cause of hip pain. The potential complication of inducing a fracture in an already osteoporotic femoral neck by drilling a tunnel and further weakening the bone is a deterrent of such a procedure, however.

The term *bone marrow edema* syndrome or pattern has been used widely in the recent literature [22,38–41]. This terminology is confusing, because bone marrow edema, as seen on MR imaging, is a nonspecific finding related to a response to any injury or stress to the bone. It is seen in acute fractures, transient osteoporosis, AVN, stress-related injury after continued exercise, stress in an osteoporotic bone, reactive edema in degenerative disease, infection, and tumors, among other conditions. The word "transient" only implies that the edema, the MR imaging signal characteristics, or the bone scan findings are temporary in nature and that some of the listed causes are also temporary. The confusing use of these terms is also compounded by the fact that some cases of TOH have evolved in findings consistent with AVN [39] or subchondral fractures [41]. Because several of the causes of bone marrow edema patterns can be established on the basis of the original or follow-up MR imaging examination (eg, AVN, subchondral fracture, osteochondral lesion or tumor), it is recommended that this nonspecific terminology be avoided.

## Bone and soft tissue tumors

### *Bone tumors*

In general, the primary diagnostic approach to bone tumors is made by their radiographic characteristics, and MR imaging is used for the evaluation of their intramedullary and soft tissue extension, articular extension, and neurovascular bundle involvement. CT is used for assessment of cortical and periosteal extension and for detection of subtle matrix calcifications not seen on plain films. Some tumors, tumor-like conditions, and miscellaneous conditions have a special predilection for the proximal femur. Frequent proximal

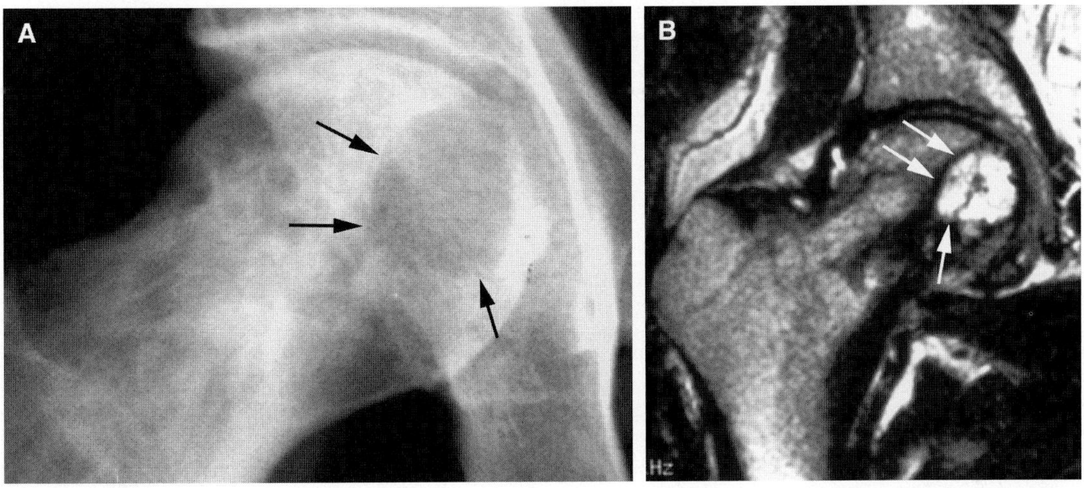


Fig. 14. Clear cell chondrosarcoma in a young man with chronic right hip pain. (*A*) Plain film demonstrates a lytic area in the femoral head (*arrows*), surrounded by irregular sclerosis and focal lucencies. (*B*) Coronal T2-weighted image demonstrates a multilobular hyperintense lesion with a low signal intensity rim (*arrows*). Biopsy of the lesion demonstrated clear cell chondrosarcoma.

femoral tumors include osteoid osteoma, osteoblastoma, chondroblastoma, and chondrosarcoma (including clear cell chondrosarcoma) (Fig. 14).

Special mention is made of osteoid osteomas, which are relatively frequent around the hip. Osteoid osteomas are benign bone-forming tumors that characteristically demonstrate cortical thickening surrounding a nidus. These lesions are better evaluated with plain films and CT than with MR imaging, because the purpose of imaging is to locate the small nidus before surgical removal or percutaneous ablation. Occasionally, however, MR imaging may be used if the plain radiographs do not demonstrate the lesion. Unfortunately, MR imaging findings may be misleading, because these tumors produce extensive bone marrow and soft tissue edema to the point that the edema may obscure the nidus [42].

## References


[1] Kier R, Wain S, Troiano R. Fast spin-echo MR imaging of the pelvis obtained with a phased-array coil: value in localizing and staging prostatic carcinoma. AJR Am J Roentgenol 1993;161:601–6.

[2] Rizzo PF, Gould ES, Lyden JP, et al. Diagnosis of occult fractures about the hip. Magnetic resonance imaging compared to bone scanning. J Bone Joint Surg Am 1993;75:395–401.

[3] Verbeeten KM, Hermann KL, Hasselqvist M, et al. The advantages of MRI in the detection of occult hip fracture. Eur Radiol 2005;15:165–9.

[4] Legroux Gerot I, Demondion X, Louville AB, et al. Subchondral fractures of the femoral head: a review of seven cases. Joint Bone Spine 2004;71:131–5.

[5] Mlinek EJ, Clark KC, Walker CW. Limited magnetic resonance imaging in the diagnosis of occult hip fractures. Am J Emerg Med 1998;16:390–2.

[6] Oka M, Monu JU. Prevalence and patterns of occult hip fractures and mimics revealed by MRI. AJR Am J Roentgenol 2004;182:283–8.

[7] Hosono M, Kobayashi H, Fujimoto R, et al. MR appearance of parasymphyseal insufficiency fractures of the os pubis. Skeletal Radiol 1997;26:525–8.

[8] Seo GS, Aoki J, Karakida O, et al. Ischiopubic insufficiency fractures: MRI appearance. Skeletal Radiol 1997;26:705–10.

[9] Grainger C, Garcia J, Howart NR, et al. Role of MRI in the diagnosis of insufficiency fractures of the sacrum and acetabular roof. Skeletal Radiol 1997;26:517–24.

[10] Resnick D. Osteoporosis. In: Resnick D, editor. Diagnosis of bone and joint disorders. 3rd edition. Philadelphia: WB Saunders; 1995. p. 1783–853.

[11] Blomlie V, Lien HH, Iversen T, et al. Radiation-induced insufficiency fractures of the sacrum: evaluation with MR imaging. Radiology 1993;188:241–4.

[12] Brahme SK, Cervilla V, Vint V, et al. Magnetic resonance appearance of sacral insufficiency fractures. Skeletal Radiol 1990;19:489–93.

[13] Slocum KA, Gorman JD, Puckett ML, et al. Resolution of abnormal MR signal intensity in patients with stress fractures of the femoral neck. AJR Am J Roentgenol 1997;168:1295–9.

[14] Song WS, Yoo JJ, Koo KH, et al. Subchondral fatigue fracture of the femoral head in military recruits. J Bone Joint Surg Am 2004;86:1917–24.

[15] Davies M, Cassar-Pullicino VN, Darby AJ. Subchondral insufficiency fractures of the femoral head. Eur Radiol 2004;14:201–7.

[16] Yamamoto T, Schneider R, Bullough PG. Subchondral insufficiency fracture of the femoral head: histopathologic correlation with MRI. Skeletal Radiol 2001;30:247–54.

[17] Linden B, Jonsson K, Redlund-Johnell I. Osteochondritis dissecans of the hip. Acta Radiol 2003; 44:67–71.

[18] Weaver CJ, Major NM, Garrett WE, et al. Femoral head osteochondral lesions in painful hips of athletes: MR imaging findings. AJR Am J Roentgenol 2002;178:973–7.

[19] Coleman BG, Kressel HY, Dalinka MK, et al. Radiographically negative avascular necrosis: detection with MR imaging. Radiology 1988;168:525–8.

[20] Mitchell DG, Rao VJ, Dalinka M, et al. Hematopoietic and fatty bone marrow distribution in the normal and ischemic hip: new observations with 1.5T MR imaging. Radiology 1986;161:199–202.

[21] Beltran J, Knight CT, Zuelzer WA, et al. Core decompression for avascular necrosis of the femoral head: correlation between long term results and preoperative MR staging. Radiology 1990;175:533–6.

[22] Huang GS, Chan WP, Chang YC, et al. MR imaging of bone marrow edema and joint effusion in patients with osteonecrosis of the femoral head: relationship to pain. AJR Am J Roentgenol 2003;181:545–9.

[23] Chan WP, Liu YJ, Huang GS, et al. MRI of joint fluid in femoral head osteonecrosis. Skeletal Radiol 2002;31:624–30.

[24] Jiang CC, Shih TT. Epiphyseal scar of the femoral head: risk factor of osteonecrosis. Radiology 1994; 191:409–12.

[25] Cherian SF, Laorr A, Saleh KJ, et al. Quantifying the extent of femoral head involvement in osteonecrosis. J Bone Joint Surg Am 2003;85:309–15.

[26] Mont MA, Hungerford DS. Non-traumatic avascular necrosis of the femoral head. J Bone Joint Surg Am 1995;77:459–74.

[27] Yoshida T, Kanayama Y, Okamura M, et al. Long-term observation of avascular necrosis of the femoral head in systemic lupus erythematosus: an MRI study. Clin Exp Rheumatol 2002;20:525–30.

[28] Leung PC. Femoral head reconstruction and revascularization. Treatment for ischemic necrosis. Clin Orthop 1996;323:139–45.

[29] Rosenberg ZS, Shankman S, Steiner GC, et al. Rapid destructive osteoarthritis: clinical, radiographic, and pathologic features. Radiology 1992;182:213–6.

[30] Fink B, Assheuer J, Enderle A, et al. Avascular osteonecrosis of the acetabulum. Skeletal Radiol 1997;26:509–16.

[31] Watson RM, Roach NA, Dalinka MK. Avascular necrosis and bone marrow edema syndrome. Radiol Clin North Am 2004;42:207–19.

[32] Turner DA, Templeton AC, Selzer PM, et al. Femoral capital osteonecrosis: MR finding of diffuse marrow abnormalities without focal lesions. Radiology 1989;171:135–40.

[33] Rafii M, Mitnick H, Klug J, et al. Insufficiency fracture of the femoral head: MR imaging in three patients. AJR Am J Roentgenol 1997;168:159–63.

[34] Guerra JJ, Steinberg ME. Current concepts review—distinguishing transient osteoporosis from avascular necrosis of the hip. J Bone Joint Surg Am 1995;77:616–24.

[35] Hayes CW, Conway WF, Daniel WW. MR imaging of bone marrow edema pattern: transient osteoporosis, transient bone marrow edema syndrome, or osteonecrosis. Radiographics 1993;13:1001–11.

[36] Yamamoto T, Kubo T, Hirasawa Y, et al. A clinicopathologic study of transient osteoporosis of the hip. Skeletal Radiol 1999;28:621–7.

[37] Radke S, Rader C, Kenn W, et al. Transient marrow edema syndrome of the hip: results after core decompression. A prospective MRI-controlled study in 22 patients. Arch Orthop Trauma Surg 2003;123: 223–7.

[38] Radke S, Kirschner S, Seipel V, et al. Magnetic resonance imaging criteria of successful core decompression in avascular necrosis of the hip. Skeletal Radiol 2004;33:519–23.

[39] Radke S, Kenn W, Eulert J. Transient bone marrow edema syndrome progressing to avascular necrosis of the hip—a case report and review of the literature. Clin Rheumatol 2004;23:83–8.

[40] Koo KH, Ahn IO, Song HR, et al. Increased perfusion of the femoral head in transient bone marrow edema syndrome. Clin Orthop 2002;402:171–5.

[41] Miyanishi K, Yamamoto T, Nakashima Y, et al. Subchondral changes in transient osteoporosis of the hip. Skeletal Radiol 2001;30:255–61.

[42] Kransdorf MJ, Stull MA, Gilkey FW, et al. Osteoid osteoma. Radiographics 1991;11:671–96.

ELSEVIER
SAUNDERS

Magn Reson Imaging Clin N Am
13 (2005) 677–690

MAGNETIC
RESONANCE
IMAGING CLINICS
of North America

# Hamstring Injuries of the Hip

Jenny T. Bencardino, MD[a,*], José M. Mellado, MD[b]

[a]*Medical Arts Radiology Group, PC, and Department of Radiology, Huntington Hospital, North Shore Long Island Jewish Health System, 270 Park Avenue, Huntington, NY 11743, USA*

[b]*Institut de Diagnostic per la Imatge, Hospital Universitari de Tarragona Joan XXIII, Carrer Doctor Mallafrè Guasch, 4, 43007 Tarragona, Spain*

Musculotendinous injuries are the most common form of sports-related injury to the hip and pelvis. Hamstring strains account for more than 50% of strain injuries in sprinters [1]. Furthermore, hamstring strains result in the highest number of days lost to play in Australian football players [2]. In fact, at 34%, hamstring strains have the highest recurrence rate of all injuries in the Australian Football League [2].

Hamstring injuries can be classified with regard to the site of involvement. Traumatic disorders at the proximal bone-tendon origin are best defined as avulsion injuries, such as ischial tuberosity fractures and hamstring tendon tears. Musculotendinous lesions include muscle strains and muscle contusions. Strains typically involve the musculotendinous junction, whether proximal, intramuscular, or distal. Conversely, muscle contusions usually affect the deep muscle fibers. Most hamstring injuries occur after indirect trauma from excessive stretching or forceful contraction, leading to avulsion injuries or muscle strains and tears. Insufficient warm-up, lack of flexibility, inadequate muscle strength and endurance, or abnormal contraction and running may predispose to such injuries. In the event of blunt direct trauma, a muscle contusion, intramuscular hematoma, myositis ossificans, or compartment syndrome may develop.

## Anatomic and functional considerations

The hamstrings consist of three muscles that run along the back of the thigh. They include the semitendinosus, the semimembranosus, and the biceps femoris. The hamstring muscles contract to flex the knee and extend the hip. The hamstrings span two joints and are therefore subject to stretching at more than one point. Additional risk factors include composition by fast-contracting type II fibers, eccentric action, and fusiform shape [3–5]. All the hamstring muscles have a complete or near-complete intramuscular tendon extending down the entire length of the muscle belly [6].

The hamstring muscles take their origin from the ischial tuberosity of the pelvis, except for the short head of the biceps femoris [7]. The latter arises from the lower lateral aspect of the linea aspera, with its origin roughly at the midfemoral shaft level. The two heads of the biceps femoris are inserted into the head of the fibula by a common tendon. The semitendinosus and the long head of the biceps femoris have a conjoint origin from the posteromedial aspect of the ischial tuberosity, in close relation to a portion of the adductor magnus that arises from the ischial tuberosity (Fig. 1). The semitendinosus muscle belly is located in the posteromedial aspect of the thigh just off the midline. Distally, the semitendinosus tendon passes behind the medial femoral condyle to insert in the upper medial surface of the tibia, along with the gracilis and sartorius, as the pes anserinus complex [7]. The semimembranosus arises from a long flat tendon at the posterolateral aspect of the ischial tuberosity, lateral to the conjoint tendon of the biceps

* Corresponding author.

*E-mail address:* jbencardino@yahoo.com (J.T. Bencardino).


doi:10.1016/j.mric.2005.08.002

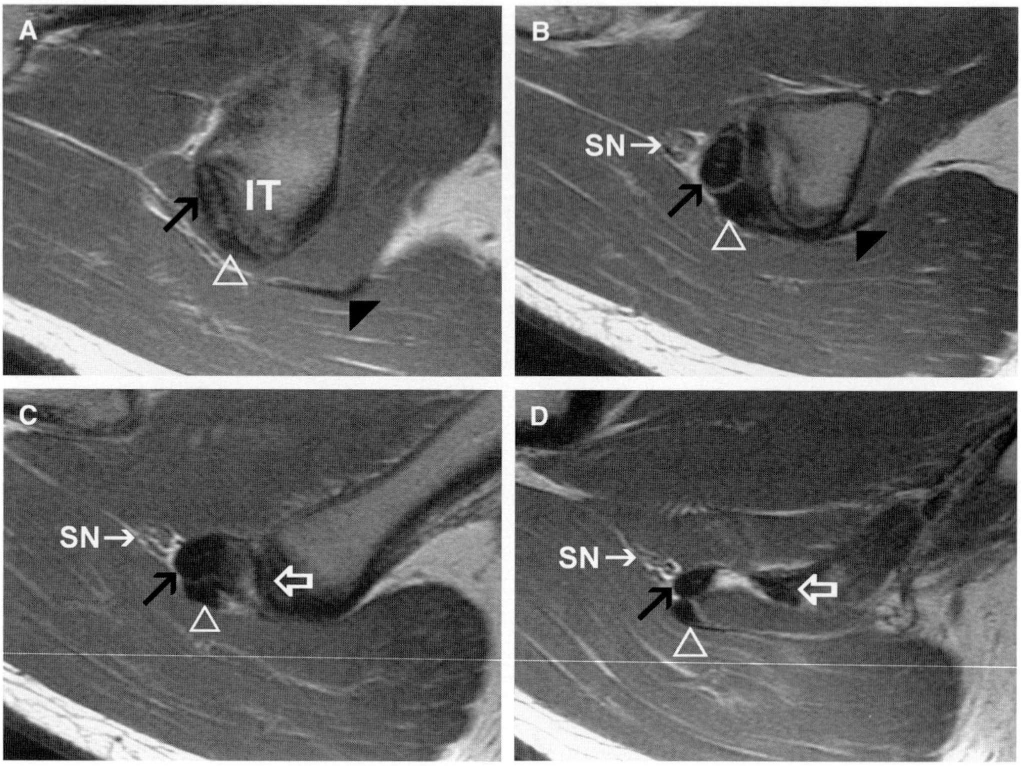


Fig. 1. MR imaging anatomy of the origin of the hamstrings. (*A*) Axial fast spin-echo proton density image through the ischial tuberosity (IT) demonstrates the proximal tendon of the semimembranosus just lateral and anterior to the conjoint tendon of the biceps femoris and semitendinosus. At this level, the sacrotuberous ligament is identified. (*B*) Slightly distal to *A*, the sciatic nerve is identified lateral to the semimembranosus tendon and conjoint biceps femoris–semitendinosus tendon. (*C*) Slightly distal to *B*, the origin of the adductor magnus tendon from the ischial tuberosity is demonstrated. (*D*) Slightly distal to *C*, the proximal tendons of the semimembranosus, conjoint biceps femoris–semitendinosus, and adductor magnus are visualized. The semimembranosus tendon (*black arrow*), conjoint biceps femoris–semitendinosus tendon (*open arrowhead*), adductor magnus tendon (*open arrow*), and sacrotuberous ligament (*black arrowhead*) are shown. SN, sciatic nerve.

femoris and semitendinosus (Fig. 2). The semimembranosus has multiple insertion sites, the primary of which is to the posteromedial aspect of the upper tibia just below the knee.

High-resolution MR images obtained at the level of the ischial tuberosity in the axial plane demonstrate the origin of the hamstring muscle complex in great detail (see Fig. 1). The semimembranosus tendon arises from a flat superolateral oblique facet located in the posterior aspect of the greater tuberosity [8], roughly at the same level of insertion of the sacrotuberous ligament (see Fig. 1). On coronal and sagittal images, the relation between the semimembranosus tendon and the conjoint biceps femoris–semitendinosus tendon can be clearly visualized, because the former travels immediately anterior to the latter (see Fig. 2C). Also, the semimembranosus has a greater length of "bare" tendon as opposed to the most proximal convergence of the conjoint biceps femoris–semitendinosus tendon with its muscle fibers (see Fig. 2C). On axial images through the proximal thigh, the semimembranosus tendon acquires a flat or crescentic configuration traversing a soft tissue plane created by the adductor magnus muscle anteriorly and the biceps femoris–semitendinosus musculotendinous complex posteriorly (Fig. 3A). Once the tendon blends with the most proximal muscle fibers, its crescentic configuration is further augmented as it continues down the posteromedial thigh (see Fig. 3B, C). The biceps femoris–semitendinosus conjoint tendon emanates from an inferomedial transverse facet in the most posterior aspect of the ischial tuberosity (see Figs. 1 and 2) [8]. The conjoint tendon travels slightly posterior and lateral to the semimembranosus tendon in the

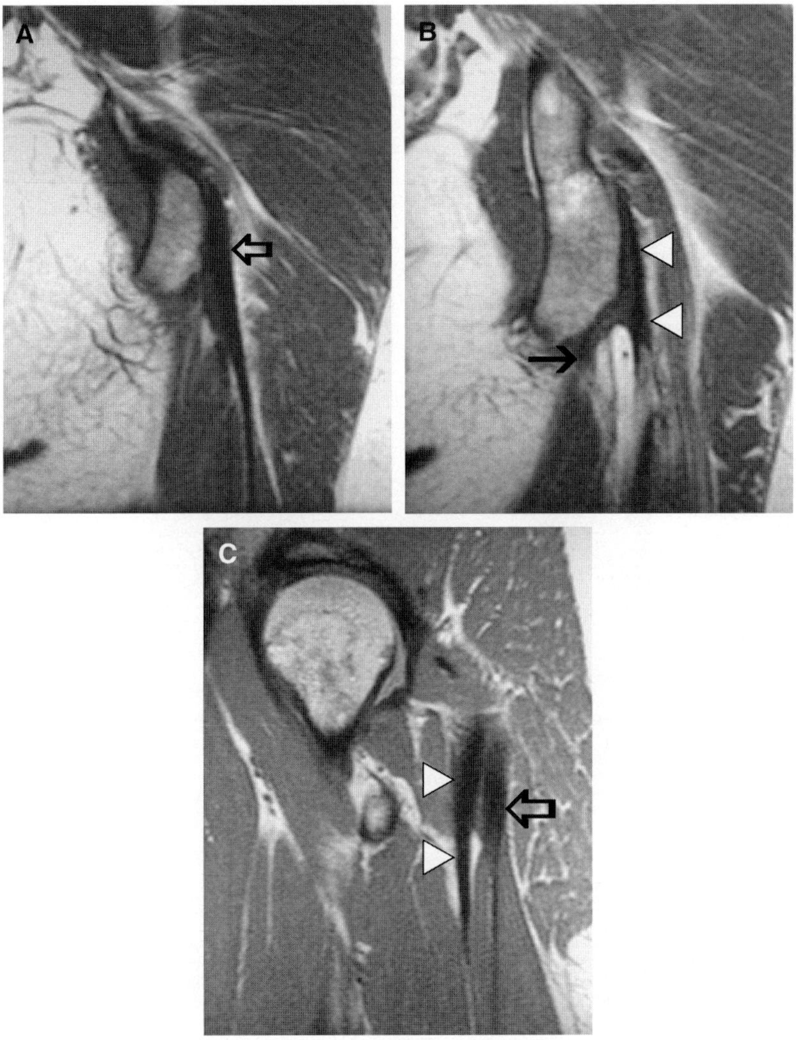


Fig. 2. MR imaging anatomy of the origin of the hamstrings. (*A*) Coronal T1-weighted image through the most posterior aspect of the ischial tuberosity demonstrates the origin of the conjoint biceps femoris–semitendinosus tendon (*open arrow*). (*B*) Coronal T1-weighted image anterior to *A* shows the origin of the semimembranosus tendon (*arrowheads*). Also noted is the oblique course of the "hamstring head" of the adductor magnus tendon (*black arrow*). (*C*) Sagittal fast spin-echo proton density image through the origin of the hamstrings depicts the conjoint biceps femoris–semitendinosus tendon (*open arrow*) arising posterior to the semimembranosus tendon (*arrowheads*) from the ischial tuberosity. Also note the greater length of the "bare" semimembranosus tendon as opposed to the most proximal convergence of the conjoint biceps femoris–semitendinosus tendon with its muscle fibers.

proximal thigh (see Fig. 3A). The "hamstring head" of the adductor magnus tendon arises from the ischial tuberosity just below the level of the hamstring muscle complex, extending in a medial oblique fashion as depicted on axial and coronal images (see Figs. 1C, D and 2B).

The proximal hamstring tendons are in close proximity to the sciatic nerve (see Fig. 1B). The latter travels lateral to the origin of the hamstring tendons, deep to the gluteus maximus muscle, and superficial to the quadratus femoris muscle at the level of the ischial tuberosity. The tibial portion of the sciatic nerve innervates the semimembranosus and the semitendinosus. The biceps femoris has a dual innervation. The long head is supplied by the tibial side of the sciatic nerve, and the short head is supplied by the peroneal side of the sciatic nerve.

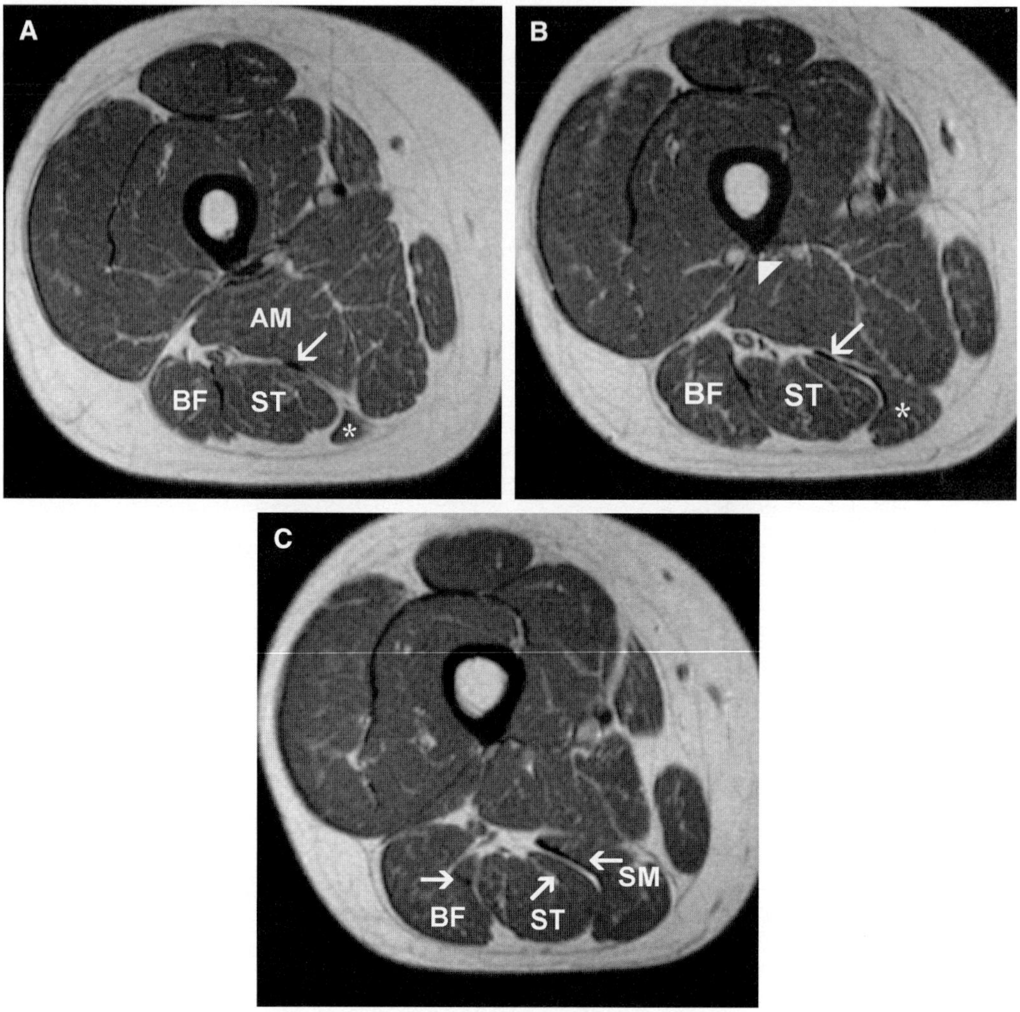


Fig. 3. MR imaging anatomy of the hamstrings in the proximal thigh. (*A*) Axial T1-weighted image demonstrates the semimembranosus tendon as a flat structure wedged between the adductor magnus (AM) and semitendinosus muscle (ST). The most proximal muscle fibers of the semimembranosus (SM) are seen at this level (*). (*B*) Semimembranosus tendon (*white arrow*) acquires a "boomerang" configuration in the middle portion of the thigh. The origin of the short head of the biceps is visualized off the linea aspera (*arrowhead*). (*C*) Individual tendons of the SM, ST, and biceps femoris (BF) are identified.

During walking and running, the hamstrings function primarily to decelerate the extended knee before foot strike and to assist with hip extension after foot strike. In the first half of the swing phase of the running cycle, the hip rapidly flexes. Knee flexion is passive during this period and results from the rapid forward acceleration of the thigh during hip flexion. Midway through the swing phase, however, although hip flexion continues, the knee begins to extend rapidly. During the latter part of the swing phase of gait or float phase of running, the hamstring muscles decelerate the forward swing of the tibia, thus opposing the action of the quadriceps.

## MR imaging strategies

Although clinical assessment may be sufficient for diagnosis and management of muscle injuries, it is currently accepted that MR imaging may provide accurate information with regard to the site, grade, and prognosis of lesions, particularly in the competitive athlete.

Ultrasound has proved to be sensitive and cost-effective in the early detection and grading of muscle injuries and is widely used in this regard. Conventional radiographs or CT may be useful in specific types of injuries, such as avulsion fractures and myositis ossificans. The exquisite soft tissue contrast resolution of MR imaging has been found to be optimal for depiction of most traumatic musculotendinous abnormalities, however.

MR imaging optimally assesses damage to all the components of the musculotendinous unit, including the tendinous origin and insertion sites, the myotendinous junction, and the muscle belly [4,9–11]. MR imaging is also useful for demonstrating occult muscular trauma [12]. The site, extent, and degree of musculotendinous injuries are examined using axial, coronal, and sagittal images oriented along the longitudinal and short axis of the involved musculotendinous unit [9]. The technologist should be instructed to place a capsule over the patient's point of maximal tenderness or above and below the area of concern in the case of a palpable abnormality. In our experience, comparison with the contralateral thigh is helpful to assess the area of signal abnormality at the injured site and to evaluate subtle differences in muscle development better.

Alterations in water content in the affected musculotendinous units are common to all forms of acute traumatic injuries [4,9,11]. T1-weighted images are relatively insensitive to these changes; however, they provide information regarding the presence of methemoglobin (characteristic of subacute hemorrhage) or muscle fatty infiltration [9]. Short tau inversion recovery (STIR) or fat-suppressed T2-weighted sequences enable detection of edematous changes in the musculotendinous unit and are of paramount importance in diagnosing these injuries [4,11]. Detection of intramuscular hemorrhage can be enhanced by the use of gradient-echo T2*-weighted sequences delineating areas of blooming artifact related to the presence of blood products within the muscle. The use of gadolinium-enhanced MR imaging has been suggested as an alternative method for detecting subtle musculotendinous injuries that may otherwise remain undetected [13].

## Proximal bone-tendon disorders

### *Avulsion injuries*

Avulsion injuries at the origin of the hamstrings results from forceful eccentric muscle contraction or excessive passive lengthening [14]. This occurs with the hip flexed and the knee in extension. Pain is typically referred to the buttock region and may be associated with gait disturbances. Loss of function and severe tenderness are frequently the presenting symptoms in this condition, which may manifest as an avulsion fracture or avulsion injury of the proximal hamstring tendons.

Avulsion fractures at the ischial tuberosity are relatively rare injuries typically seen in adolescent athletes before closure of the apophysis [15]. For this reason, comparison with the contralateral side is important to distinguish fracture from unfused apophysis (Fig. 4). Avulsion fractures of the ischial tuberosity are almost exclusively treated conservatively, with an overall good prognosis for spontaneous healing. Bed rest, restricted activity, and return to full athletic performance over the 6 to 12 weeks after the injury are generally adequate for nondisplaced fractures [14]. Surgical repair may be indicated when there is greater than 2 cm displacement of the avulsed fracture fragment. Sciatic nerve involvement has been described as a potential complication secondary to direct compression by abundant callous or avulsed fragment [16]. Furthermore, in some patients, a large hematoma may develop in the posterior thigh as a result of hamstring avulsion injury, which may play a part in the development of posttraumatic sciatic neuropathy [17].

Avulsion fractures are generally diagnosed by radiography [5,18]. In the acute setting, the fracture appears as a crescentic and sharply marginated bone fragment adjacent to the ischial tuberosity (Fig. 5A). In chronic cases, extensive periosteal reaction, callus formation, and lysis at the fracture site may give a more aggressive appearance to the lesion, requiring further investigation with cross-sectional imaging and, eventually, biopsy (see Fig. 5B). On MR imaging, cortical fracture fragments that do not contain bone marrow can be missed. Acute avulsion injury manifests on MR imaging by a hematoma and periosteal stripping at the tendinous attachment site. Waviness and retraction of the torn end of the tendon with or without a fragment of bone may also be present.

Avulsion injuries of the hamstring tendons at the ischial tuberosity are relatively common in adult football players, runners, water skiers, cheerleaders, gymnasts, and dancers. The avulsion injury most frequently involves the conjoint biceps femoris-semitendinosus tendon and

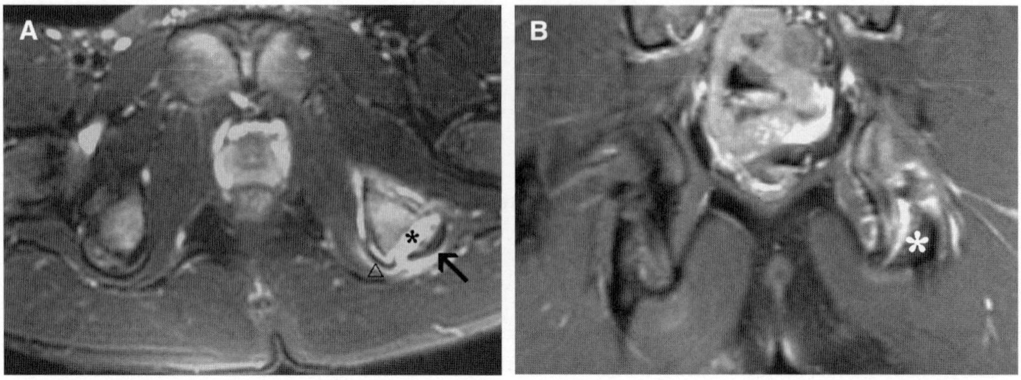


Fig. 4. Avulsion fracture of the ischial tuberosity in a 14-year-old football player. (*A*) Axial fat-suppressed, fast spin-echo, T2-weighted image demonstrates cortical disruption at the attachment of the semimembranosus tendon with a mildly displaced osseous fragment (*arrow*). Fluid outlines the gap between the donor site and the fragment (*). The biceps femoris–semitendinosus tendon origin is preserved (*open arrowhead*). (*B*) Coronal fat-suppressed, fast spin-echo, T2-weighted image shows the displaced fragment (*) as compared with the right ischial tuberosity open growth plate. Incidentally noted is contralateral hamstring tendinosis.

semimembranosus tendons at the ischial tuberosity (Fig. 6). In some patients, however, preservation of the semimembranosus tendon and, less often, of the semitendinosus tendon (anatomic variant) can be observed (Fig. 7) [19]. MR imaging is highly sensitive and specific for the diagnosis of hamstring avulsion injuries as compared with sonography [19]. MR imaging correctly assesses the amount of tendon retraction and the tendon edge morphology, which are important features for preoperative planning.

Acute traumatic hamstring avulsion injury in athletes requires immediate surgical intervention with refixation of the ruptured tendon in anatomic position using a suture anchor system [20].

*Hamstring tendinosis*

In addition to complete tears, partial tears and tendinosis at the origin of the hamstrings have also been reported. Hamstring tendinosis may express itself clinically by gluteal pain and point tenderness while sitting. This condition is more prevalent in young athletes involved in sports that require bursts of speed and repetitive hip stretch, such as football, soccer, basketball, sprinting,

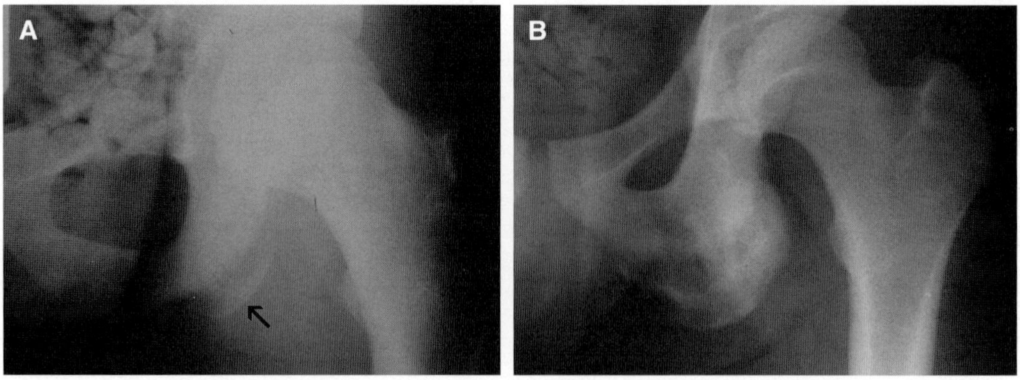


Fig. 5. Ischial tuberosity avulsion. (*A*) Anteroposterior radiograph of the left hip demonstrates a crescentic and sharply marginated bone fragment (*arrow*) adjacent to the ischial tuberosity. (*B*) Follow-up anteroposterior radiograph demonstrates a markedly enlarged ischial tuberosity secondary to exuberant callus formation after avulsion injury. The patient was referred for biopsy to rule out a neoplasm.

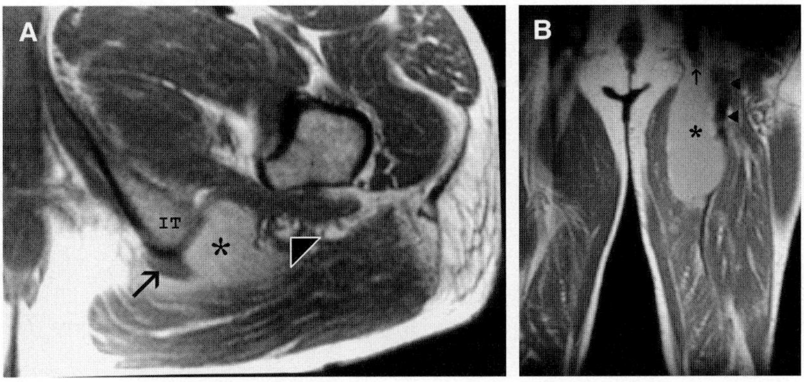


Fig. 6. Hamstring tendon avulsion. (*A*) Axial fast spin-echo proton density image through the left ischial tuberosity (IT) demonstrates complete avulsion of the hamstring tendons outlined by a large hematoma (*). A small proximal tendon stump is identified at the origin of the biceps femoris–semitendinosus tendon (*arrow*). The sciatic nerve (*arrowhead*) is markedly swollen and edematous, explaining patient's neuropathic symptoms. (*B*) Coronal T1-weighted image better demonstrates the amount of retraction of the torn hamstring tendons (*arrowheads*) as well as the size of the associated hematoma (*). Again noted is the small tendon stump at the origin of the conjoint tendon (*arrow*).

rowing, and kickboxing. It may result from chronic repetitive microtrauma leading to intrasubstance degeneration. Hamstring tendinosis may also be secondary to weakening of the tendon by other underlying conditions (gout, diabetes, hyperparathyroidism, and collagen vascular diseases).

On MR imaging, proximal hamstring tendinosis results in increased tendon girth and

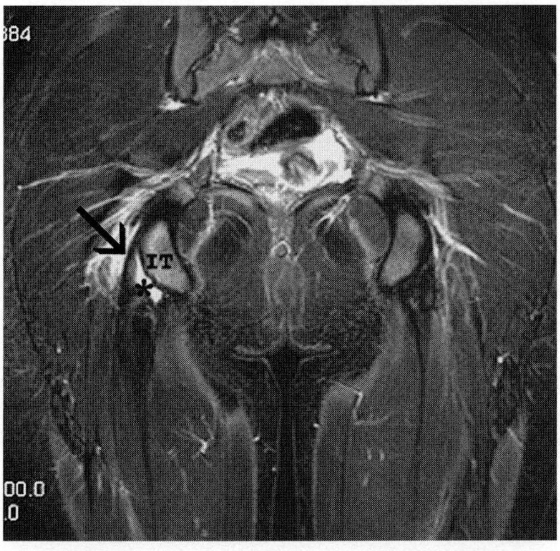


Fig. 7. Partial hamstring tendon avulsion. Preservation of the fibers of the origin of the semimembranosus tendon (*arrow*) is noted in this runner. A small fluid-filled gap is identified interposed between the ischial tuberosity (IT) and the avulsed conjoint tendon (*). Contralateral hamstring tendinosis is noted.

intrasubstance signal heterogeneity. Reactive edema of the ischial tuberosity and, occasionally, a cortical defect can be seen (Fig. 8). Asymmetric involvement of hamstring tendons is a common finding. Advanced tendinosis may lead to hamstring tendon tears. MR imaging features of preexisting hamstring enthesopathy were noted in three of five patients with a partial tear of the hamstring origin [19]. The conjoint tendon was affected in all cases, with preservation of the semimembranosus tendon. Partial tears are characterized by fluid-filled cleavage planes disrupting the homogeneous signal of the hamstring tendons on fat-suppressed, fast spin-echo, proton density or T2-weighted or STIR MR images.

The medical treatment for tendinosis includes rest, anti-inflammatory medication, and a gradually progressive muscle strength and stretching program. Surgery has a limited role in the management of tendinosis unless there is associated proximal hamstring tendon avulsion requiring surgical repair.

Snapping hip syndrome encompasses a variety of intra-articular and extra-articular causes that result in hip pain associated with an audible snapping sound during motion of the hip. "Snapping bottom," subluxation of the tendon of the origin of the long head of the biceps femoris, is a rare condition likely related to degeneration of the tendinous attachment of the muscle at the ischial tuberosity [21]. Long-standing wear and tear secondary to hip hyperflexion is a proposed causative factor. The differential diagnosis includes

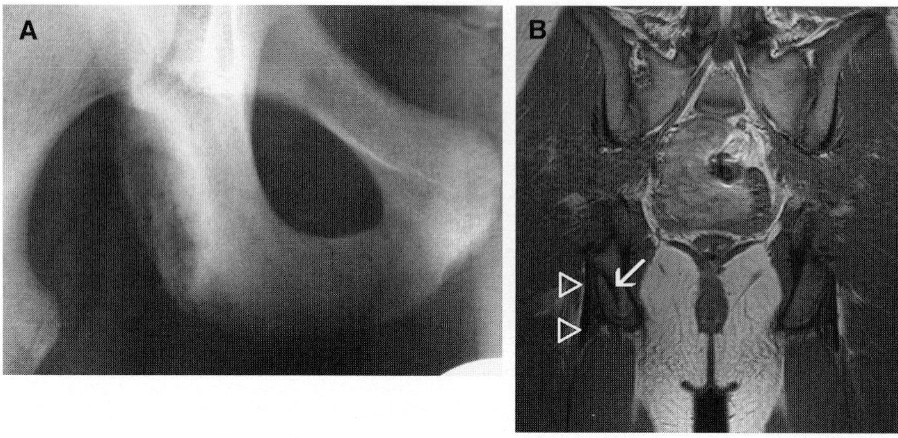


Fig. 8. Hamstring tendinosis. (*A*) Radiograph of the right ischial tuberosity demonstrates a large cortical defect at the site of the origin of the hamstring tendons in this hurdler teenager. (*B*) Coronal T1-weighted image nicely depicts right hamstring tendinosis (*arrowheads*) manifested by thickening and heterogeneous intrasubstance signal associated with a large cortical defect in the right ischial tuberosity (*arrow*). (Courtesy of Z.S. Rosenberg, MD, New York, NY.)

other extra-articular causes of snapping hip syndrome, such as friction of the iliotibial band or gluteus maximus over the greater trochanter, of the iliopsoas tendon over the iliopectineal eminence, and of the iliofemoral ligament over the anterior portion of the hip capsule. Ischiogluteal bursitis, or "weaver's bottom," can also result in pain and swelling of the buttock [22]. In the older nonathletic patient, if conservative measures fail, the treatment of choice for snapping bottom is simple tenotomy.

## Muscle injuries

### *Muscle strain*

Myotendinous strains are induced by indirect trauma from excessive stretch or tension. Eccentric exercise, where the contracting muscle is lengthened, produces microscopic damage in muscle fibers and may result in sensations of stiffness and soreness for the next few days (Fig. 9). Because strain injuries are known to occur during eccentric contraction, it is hypothesized that the microscopic damage from eccentric exercise can progress to muscle strain [23]. The athletes most at risk of hamstring strain are older, with a previous history of such injuries [24,25]. Studies using isokinetic dynamometry have shown that previously injured muscles have a shortened optimum angle of peak torque, making them more prone to damage by eccentric exercise [23,26,27]. The shorter optimum angle may reflect the muscle's preinjury state or be a consequence of the healing process [23]. This knowledge has led to the design of preseason strength training programs emphasizing eccentric overloading as a preventive measure for hamstring strains [28].

Strain injuries most frequently affect the proximal, intramuscular, or distal musculotendinous junction, the weakest point of the musculotendinous unit [11,29]. It is important to keep in mind that the musculotendinous junction of the hamstrings extends completely or almost completely down the length of the muscle belly [6]. Muscle strains are clinically classified as first degree (stretch injury), second degree (partial tear), and third degree (complete rupture) based on absent, mild, or complete loss of muscle function, respectively.

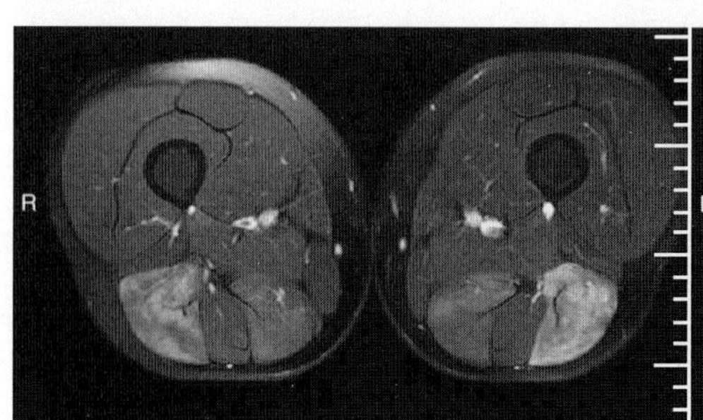


Fig. 9. Delayed-onset muscle soreness. An axial fast spin-echo STIR image demonstrates diffuse interstitial edema of the biceps femoris and semimembranosus muscles bilaterally in a runner athlete.

Muscle strain can be classified on MR imaging based on the extent of disruption present [4,11,30]. First-degree strains imply a minor degree of fiber disruption with fluid leaking through the endomysium. The latter is a thin layer of connective tissue surrounding individual muscle fibers. There is interstitial edema and hemorrhage at the musculotendinous junction, which can extend into the adjacent muscle fascicles because of disruption of the perimysium. This produces a feathery MR imaging pattern (Fig. 10) [11,12]. Second-degree injuries are characterized by a partial tear without retraction. A hematoma at the musculotendinous junction is frequently observed as well as intramuscular and extramuscular laminar fluid collections (Figs. 11 and 12). Extramuscular fluid indicates the presence of a tear of the epimysium, the connective tissue sheath that surrounds a muscle. If skin discoloration and bruising are identified on physical examination, disruption of the deep and superficial fascia should be suspected. Third-degree strain refers to complete rupture of the musculotendinous unit. This diagnosis is usually made on clinical grounds. MR imaging is useful when preoperative assessment of the extent of retraction is needed. In some cases, MR imaging can also pinpoint hematoma, which may require percutaneous drainage [12]. In our experience, not infrequently, patients with grade II to III injuries may present with transient sciatica, which may be attributed to compressive sciatic neuropathy by large gluteal or posterior thigh hematoma.

The most frequently strained hamstring muscle is the biceps femoris, whether as the only site of injury (isolated) or as the primary muscle of involvement [6,19,31–36]. The predominance of the biceps femoris as the site of injury may be attributable to the limited extensibility of the muscle, which originates from the femur and the ischial tuberosity [37]. Multiple hamstring muscle strain injury seems to be a common presentation, with a reported prevalence of 33% to 60% [31,35], although in a recent series by Connell and coworkers [36], only in 4.8% of cases were more than one hamstring muscle involved. Dual injuries of the biceps femoris and semitendinosus have been noted to be the most common concomitant hamstring injury [6,19,31,35].

There is disagreement in the published radiologic literature as to whether the semitendinosus muscle [6,31,35] or the semimembranosus muscle [19,33,34,36] represents the second most common isolated or primary site of hamstring strain. De Smet and Best [35] postulated that differences in the frequency of injuries may reflect the statistical variation within small series or the different injury patterns occurring in various sports. These authors noticed that all the athletes in their series with isolated semitendinosus injury were track and field jumpers.

De Smet and Best [35] were the first investigators to report the geographic distribution of hamstring strain within the musculotendinous unit based on eight potential injury sites, including the origin, proximal tendon, proximal musculotendinous junction, proximal intramuscular musculotendinous junction, distal intramuscular musculotendinous junction, distal musculotendinous junction, distal tendon, and insertion. Injuries of the intramuscular musculotendinous junction were classified as proximal or distal on the basis of their relation to the image that first showed the origin of the short head of the biceps femoris. The short head begins approximately at

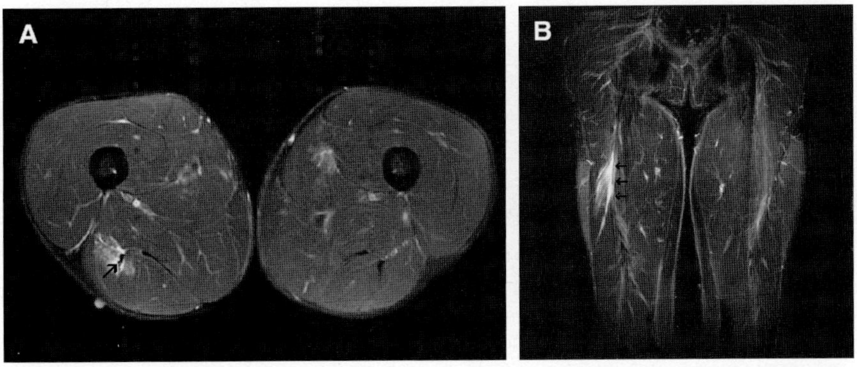


Fig. 10. Grade I biceps femoris muscle strain. Axial (*A*) and coronal (*B*) fat-suppressed, fast spin-echo, T2-weighted images depict a feathery-like edema pattern radiating from the intramuscular tendon of the biceps femoris (*arrows*).

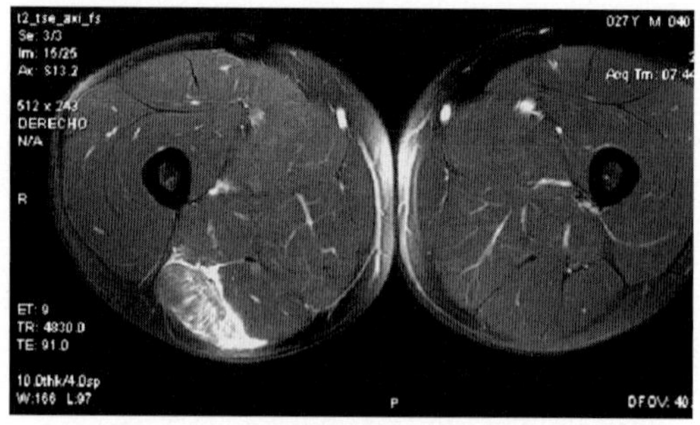


Fig. 11. Grade II biceps femoris muscle strain. Axial fat-suppressed, fast spin-echo, T2-weighted image demonstrates more severe injury exhibiting intramuscular and extramuscular laminar fluid collections. A discrete hematoma at the musculotendinous junction was not identified.

the midfemoral shaft and thus serves as a reproducible landmark for the midpoint of the thigh [38]. In this study, all injuries were located adjacent to the musculotendinous junction. There was a slight predominance of proximal over distal injuries (60%). Although other investigators have concurred with this finding [19], this has not always been observed [31,34]. Despite the concept that proximal hamstring musculotendinous strain tends to have a shorter convalescence interval, Slavotinek and colleagues [31] did not find a statistically significant association between proximal muscle injury and time lost from competition.

In more recent series [19,36], injuries to the epimysial covering have been shown to comprise a significant proportion of biceps femoris muscle strains, up to 35% of the total [19,36]. Epimysial strain is typically located at the boundary of the long head of the biceps with the short head of the biceps (Fig. 13). Slavotinek and colleagues [31] noted linear T2 hyperintensity between muscles in 68% of 37 patients with hamstring muscle strain. These authors postulated that intermuscular laminar collections might represent extension of intramuscular fluid through an epimysial tear, and thus could be considered an indicator of the degree of intramuscular injury. A weak association ($P = .04$) between the presence of focal intermuscular T2 hyperintensity and the number of days lost from competition was noted in this study. Connell and coworkers [36] reported no significant difference in the time it took players with musculotendinous junction tears to return to play compared with players who sustained a myofascial injury, however.

In 1993, Pomeranz and Heidt [34] reported longer convalescence times in 14 athletes with hamstring injury when associated with complete muscle transection, ganglion-like fluid collections, hemorrhage-like signal intensity, distal musculotendinous injury, and greater than 50% cross-sectional muscle involvement. Later research in larger series has validated some of these parameters. In the series by Slavotinek and colleagues [31], measurements of the percentage of abnormal cross-sectional area and approximate volume of abnormal muscle showed a significant association

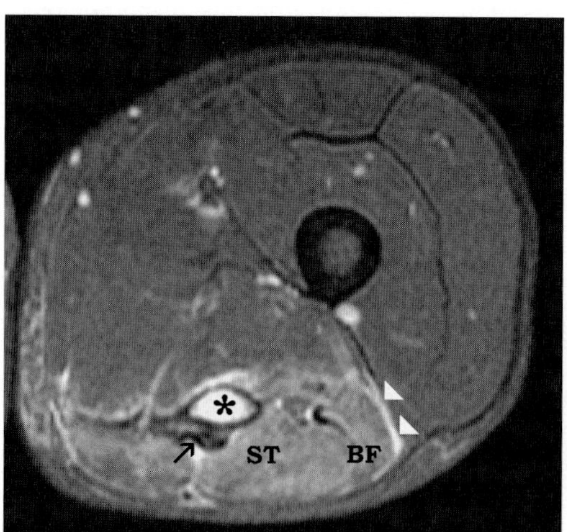


Fig. 12. Grade II hamstring strain. Axial fat-suppressed, fast spin-echo, T2-weighted image shows a focal hematoma (*) adjacent to the semimembranosus intramuscular tendon (*arrow*). Note the diffuse interstitial edema affecting the semimembranosus, semitendinosus (ST), and biceps femoris (BF). A small extramuscular laminar fluid collection is identified (*arrowheads*).

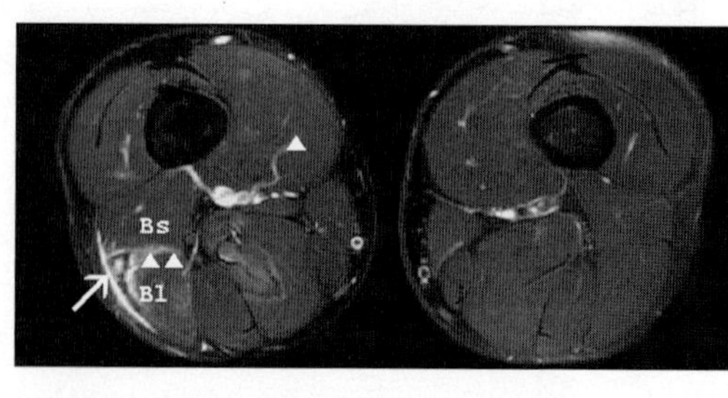


Fig. 13. Epimysial strain of the biceps femoris. Axial fat-suppressed, fast spin-echo, T2-weighted image depicts a small well-defined hematoma located at the boundary of the long head of the biceps (Bl) with the short head of the biceps (Bs). Note the intermuscular (*arrowheads*) and extramuscular (*arrow*) fluid collections.

with subjective pain score, although only an abnormal cross-sectional area greater than 50% was associated with a longer rehabilitation time. No association was found between the location of the injury, whether proximal or distal, and time lost from competition.

In a more recent study, Connell and coworkers [36] showed that the presence of an injury to the biceps femoris, the cross-sectional injury area (as a percentage score), the length of the injury, and injury outside the musculotendinous junction were associated with increased recovery time ($P < .05$). The median duration until return to play for this study population was 21 days. Persistent MR imaging abnormalities were noted in up to 35% of players at 6-week follow-ups in this series, although all but one player were symptom-free and had already returned to competition. This supports the concept that the healing process takes weeks to months to complete histopathologically and may explain the high reinjury rate of greater than 30% among professional football players in Australia [2,24,25].

### *Muscle contusion*

Muscle contusions are secondary to direct trauma, usually by a blunt object. They often occur deep in the muscle belly and thus tend to be less symptomatic than strains, because the latter are commonly localized in the superficial muscle layers [3]. Muscle contusions can be found on MR imaging examinations of patients with high clinical suspicion of hip fracture despite negative radiographs [39].

The MR imaging appearance of muscle contusions varies according to the severity of the lesion. Diffuse edematous changes of the muscle are manifested by a feathery MR imaging appearance on STIR and T2-weighted sequences [12]. Architectural changes other than increased muscle girth are absent. Intramuscular hematoma can develop with more severe trauma. The MR imaging characteristics of an intramuscular hematoma may be affected by its age, state of hemoglobin oxidation, and field strength of the MR imaging system. Acute hematomas are often isointense and hypointense to skeletal muscle on T1 and T2 or STIR images, respectively. Low central T2 signal seen in acute hematomas is probably attributable to the presence of deoxyhemoglobin within intact red blood cells. Subacute hematomas demonstrate increased T1 signal and heterogeneous signal on T2-weighted images because of the presence of extracellular methemoglobin. As the lesion ages, the wall of the hematoma may become hypointense from hemosiderin deposition and fibrosis [10]. Nevertheless, intramuscular or intermuscular hematomas often present as heterogeneous collections on T1- and T2-weighted sequences and do

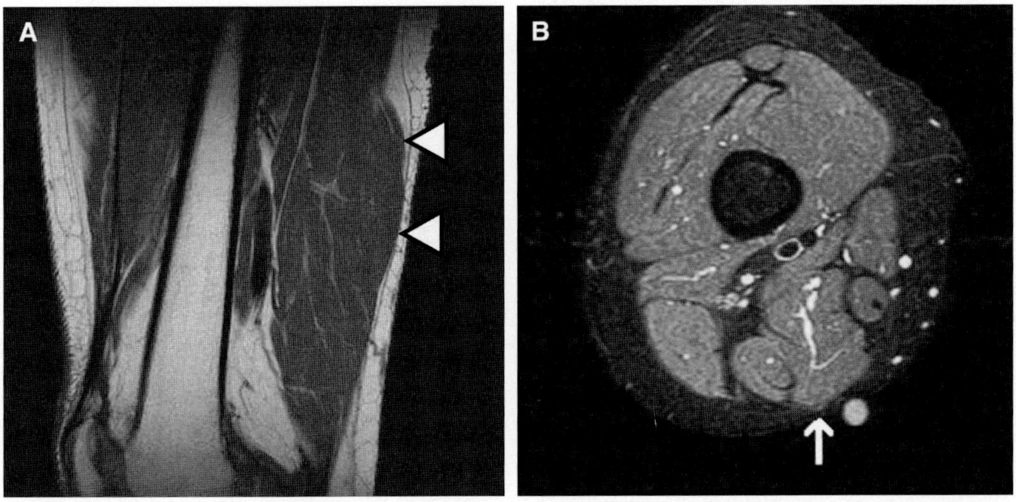


Fig. 14. Semimembranosus muscle hernia. (*A*) Sagittal T1-weighted image of the midthigh demonstrates focal protrusion of the semimembranosus muscle along the posterior thigh fascia (*arrowheads*) in this athlete with clinical symptoms of a painless and hard soft tissue mass. (*B*) Axial fat-suppressed, fast spin-echo, T2-weighted image shows the site of the palpable abnormality (vitamin E capsule), focal discontinuity, and subtle edema of the posterior thigh fascia (*arrow*).

not follow a predictable change in signal over time as opposed to their counterparts in the central nervous system.

### *Myositis ossificans*

Myositis ossificans is a common complication of muscle contusion associated with myonecrosis and hematoma formation [5]. It has been postulated that development of myositis ossificans requires a trauma sufficient to cause proliferative repair with activation of the perimysial tissue–inducible osteoprogenitor cells (IOPCs) [40]. The proliferation typically begins in the periphery and progresses in a centripetal fashion. On microscopic evaluation, three zones can be distinguished in the early phases of myositis ossificans traumatica. An intermediate zone of osteoblasts and immature osteoid surrounds a core of central necrosis and hemorrhage. In the periphery, a shell of mature bone can be identified. A pathologic specimen obtained from the central two zones only may be misinterpreted as osteosarcoma. Identification of the typical peripheral rim of calcification on radiographs or CT in association with a history of previous trauma can help to distinguish myositis ossificans from a soft tissue sarcoma. On MR imaging, however, the signal intensity is often nonspecific and the typical peripheral calcification may be difficult to visualize. The diagnostic performance of MR imaging in the setting of myositis ossificans has not yet been established. Treatment of myositis ossificans includes conservative measures and surgery. Conservative therapy is aimed to prevent further formation of extraosseous ossification. Surgical resection of large lesions may be indicated [41].

### *Compartment syndrome*

Posterior thigh compartment syndrome is an uncommon condition. It has been reported as an unusual complication after spinal surgery in the knee-chest position as well as after craniotomy in the sitting position [42,43]. Presenting clinical symptoms include sciatic neuropathy, systemic manifestations of crush syndrome, acute renal failure, and altered mental status. Increased intracompartmental pressure can be measured by the use of a catheter, which is useful for establishing the diagnosis and monitoring the evolution. Prompt longitudinal fasciotomy is indicated.

### *Muscle hernia*

A muscle hernia is a focal protrusion of muscle tissue through a fascial defect. It is a common disorder in the leg, especially involving the middle and lower thirds. The tibialis anterior hernia was the first such hernia to be described [44] and is said to be the most frequent, although involvement of the extensor digitorum longus, peroneus longus, peroneus brevis, and gastrocnemius has also been reported [45–47]. Muscle hernias usually present in athletes, soldiers, and persons in professions requiring great strain on the legs. Hernias may be multiple and bilateral. Muscle hernias are usually asymptomatic, although they may present with cramping or pain after prolonged activity [45,46,48]. Muscle hernias in the thigh are much more infrequent than in the lower leg, but they may also occur (Fig. 14). To the best of our knowledge, the MR imaging depiction of hamstring muscles hernias has not been reported.

The use of MR imaging when a muscle hernia is suspected may help to clarify the diagnosis and exclude other potential soft tissue masses [48]. An often subtle bulge of the muscle belly is usually noted. Demonstration of the fascial rent (which typically occurs where vessels traverse the fascia) may be extremely difficult, however. The use of fast dynamic imaging during active contraction of the involved muscles allows evaluation of the changes of size and shape of the muscle hernia and may potentially enhance the conspicuity of the fascial tear.

## References

[1] Agre JC. Hamstring injuries. Proposed aetiological factors, prevention, and treatment. Sports Med 1985;2:21–33.

[2] Orchard J, Seward H. Epidemiology of injuries in the Australian Football League, seasons 1997–2000. Br J Sports Med 2002;36:39–44.

[3] Mallone TR. Basic science of musculotendinous structure. In: Garrett WE Jr, Duncan PW, Mallone TR, editors. Muscle injury and rehabilitation. Baltimore (MD): Williams & Wilkins; 1988. p. 1–42.

[4] Palmer WE, Kuong SJ, Elmadbouh HM. MR imaging of myotendinous strain. AJR Am J Roentgenol 1999;173:703–9.

[5] Kneeland JB. MR imaging of sports injuries of the hip. Magn Reson Imaging Clin N Am 1999;7: 105–15.

[6] Garrett WE, Rich FR, Nikolaou PK, et al. Computed tomography of hamstring muscle strains. Med Sci Sports Exerc 1989;21:506–14.

[7] Agur AMR, Dalley AF. Grant's atlas of anatomy. 11th edition. Baltimore (MD): Williams & Wilkins; 2005. p. 366–75.
[8] Ragheb DM, Pathria M, Trudell D, et al. Proximal hamstring attachment complex (PHAC): anatomic and MRI imaging correlation of its attachment sites to the ischial tuberosity in four cadaveric thighs with clinical study of MRI imaging spectrum of commonly encountered pathology [abstract]. AJR Am J Roentgenol 2005;184:26.
[9] Shellock FG, Mink J, Deutsch AL. MR imaging of muscle injuries. Appl Radiol 1994;(February): 11–8.
[10] De Smet AA. Magnetic resonance findings in skeletal muscle tears. Skeletal Radiol 1993;22:479–84.
[11] Steinbach LS, Fleckenstein JL, Mink JH. Magnetic resonance imaging of muscle injuries. Orthopedics 1994;17:991–9.
[12] McNamara MT, Greco A. Miscellaneous muscle lesions. In: Fleckenstein JL, Crues JV III, Reimers CD, editors. Muscle imaging in health and disease. New York: Springer-Verlag; 1996. p. 425–49.
[13] El-Noueam KI, Schweitzer ME, Bhatia M, et al. The utility of contrast-enhanced MRI in diagnosis of muscle injuries occult to conventional MRI. J Comput Assist Tomogr 1997;21:965–8.
[14] Stevens MA, El Khoury GY, Kathol MH, et al. Imaging features of avulsion injuries. Radiographics 1999;19:655–72.
[15] Paletta GA Jr, Andrish JT. Injuries about the hip and pelvis in the young athlete. Clin Sports Med 1995;14:591–628.
[16] Spinner RJ, Atkinsons JL, Wenger DE, et al. Tardy sciatic nerve palsy following apophyseal avulsion fracture of the ischial tuberosity. Case report. J Neurosurg 1998;89:819–21.
[17] Takami H, Takahashi S, Ando M. Late sciatic nerve palsy following avulsion of the biceps femoris muscle from the ischial tuberosity. Arch Orthop Trauma Surg 2000;120:352–4.
[18] Manaster BJ. From the RSNA refresher courses, Radiological Society of North America. Adult chronic hip pain: radiographic evaluation. Radiographics 2000;20(Spec No):S3–25.
[19] Kolouris G, Connell D. Evaluation of the hamstring muscle complex following acute injury. Skeletal Radiol 2003;32:582–9.
[20] Brucker PU, Imhoff AB. Functional assessment after acute and chronic complete ruptures of the proximal hamstring tendons. Knee Surg Sports Traumatol Arthrosc 2005;13(5):411–8.
[21] Rask MR. "Snapping bottom": subluxation of the tendon of the long head of the biceps femoris muscle. Muscle Nerve 1980;3:250–1.
[22] Van Mieghem IM, Boets A, Sciot R, et al. Ischiogluteal bursitis: an uncommon type of bursitis. Skeletal Radiol 2004;33:413–6.
[23] Brockett CL, Morgan DL, Proske U. Predicting hamstring strain injury in elite athletes. Med Sci Sports Exerc 2004;36:379–87.
[24] Verrall GM, Slavotinek JP, Barnes PG, et al. Clinical risk factors for hamstring muscle strain injury: a prospective study with correlation of injury by magnetic resonance imaging. Br J Sport Med 2001; 35:435–40.
[25] Orchard JW. Intrinsic and extrinsic risk factors for muscle strains in Australian football. Am J Sports Med 2001;29:300–3.
[26] Proske U, Morgan DL, Brockett CL, et al. Identifying athletes at risk of hamstring strains and how to protect them. Clin Exp Pharmacol Physiol 2004;31: 546–50.
[27] Jonhagen S, Nemeth G, Erickson E. Hamstring injuries in sprinters. The role of concentric and eccentric hamstring muscle strength and flexibility. Am J Sports Med 1994;22:262–6.
[28] Askling C, Karlsson J, Throstensson A. Hamstring injury occurrence in elite soccer players after preseason strength training with eccentric overload. Scand J Med Sci Ports 2003;13:244–50.
[29] Brandser EA, el-Khoury GY, Kathol MH, et al. Hamstring injuries: radiographic, conventional tomographic, CT, and MR imaging characteristics. Radiology 1995;197:257–62.
[30] Blankenbaker DG, De Smet AA. MR imaging of muscle injuries. Appl Radiol 2004;33:14–26.
[31] Slavotinek JP, Verral GM, Fon GT. Hamstring injury in athletes: using MR imaging measurements to compare extent of muscle injury with amount of time lost from competition. AJR Am J Roentgenol 2002;179:1621–8.
[32] Garrett WE. Muscle strain injuries. Am J Sports Med 1996;24(Suppl):S2–8.
[33] Speer KP, Lohnes J, Garrett WE. Radiographic imaging of muscle strain injury. Am J Sports Med 1993; 21:89–95.
[34] Pomeranz SJ, Heidt RS. MR imaging in the prognostication of hamstring injury. Radiology 1993; 189:897–900.
[35] De Smet AA, Best TM. MRI imaging of the distribution and location of acute hamstring injuries in athletes. AJR Am J Roentgenol 2000;174: 393–9.
[36] Connell DA, Schneider-Kolsky ME, Hoving JL, et al. Longitudinal study comparing sonographic and MRI assessments of acute and healing hamstring injuries. AJR Am J Roentgenol 2004;183: 975–84.
[37] Oakes BW. Hamstring muscle injuries. Aust Fam Physician 1984;13:587–91.
[38] Kujala UM, Orava S, Jarvinen M. Hamstring injuries: current trends in treatment and prevention. Sports Med 1997;23:397–404.
[39] Bogost GA, Lizerbram EK, Crues JV III. MR imaging in evaluation of suspected hip fracture:

frequency of unsuspected of bone and soft-tissue injury. Radiology 1995;197:263–7.
[40] Friedenstein AY. Osteogenic stem cells in the bone marrow. In: Heersche JNM, Kanis JA, editors. Bone and mineral research. Amsterdam: Elsevier Science Publishers; 1990. p. 243–72.
[41] Lipscomb AB, Thomas ED, Johnston RK. Treatment of myositis ossificans traumatica in athletes. Am J Sports Med 1976;4:111–20.
[42] Sancineto C, Monzon DG. Compartment syndrome in the thigh: an unusual complication after spinal surgery. J Spinal Disord Tech 2004;17:335–8.
[43] Poppi M, Giuliani G, Gambari PI, et al. A hazard of craniotomy in the sitting position: the posterior compartment syndrome of the thigh. Case report. J Neurosurg 1989;71:618–9.
[44] Zeiss J, Ebraheim NA, Woldenberg LS. Magnetic resonance imaging in the diagnosis of anterior tibialis muscle herniation. Clin Orthop 1989;244: 249–53.
[45] Braunstein JT, Crues JV. Magnetic resonance imaging of hereditary hernias of the peroneus longus muscle. Skeletal Radiol 1995;24:601–4.
[46] Sherry RH. Herniation of peroneus brevis muscle: report of a case. Bull Hosp Dis 1942;3:69–72.
[47] Alhadeff J, Lee CK. Gastrocnemius muscle herniation at the knee causing peroneal nerve compression resembling sciatica. Spine 1995;20(5): 612–614.
[48] Mellado JM, Pérez del Palomar L. Muscle hernias of the lower leg: MRI findings. Skeletal Radiol 1999; 28(8):465–9.

ELSEVIER
SAUNDERS

Magn Reson Imaging Clin N Am
13 (2005) 691–704

MAGNETIC
RESONANCE
IMAGING CLINICS
of North America

# MR Imaging of the Hip Abductors: Normal Anatomy and Commonly Encountered Pathology at the Greater Trochanter

Jerry Dwek, MD[a,b], Christian Pfirrmann, MD[c], Anthony Stanley, MD[d], Mini Pathria, MD[b], Christine B. Chung, MD[b,*]

[a]*Department of Radiology, Children's Hospital, 3020 Children's Way, San Diego, CA 92123, USA*
[b]*Department of Radiology, University of California—San Diego and Veterans Affairs Health Care System, 3350 La Jolla Village Drive, La Jolla, CA 92161, USA*
[c]*Department of Radiology, University Hospital Balgrist, Forchstrasse 340, CH-8008 Zurich, Switzerland*
[d]*Department of Diagnostic Imaging, National University Hospital, 5 Lower Kent Road, Singapore 119074*

Lateral hip pain, referred to as the greater trochanteric pain syndrome, is a common regional pain syndrome that can prove to be a diagnostic dilemma for the clinician. Historically, lateral hip pain has been routinely attributed to trochanteric bursitis. With the advent of MR imaging as well as a greater appreciation of the spectrum of disease that can affect this region, however, many other considerations for the clinical presentation of lateral hip pain have emerged in the literature [1–13]. Among these are processes affecting the osseous components of the articulation, the joint proper, and the periarticular soft tissues.

Emphasizing the concept that an intimate and detailed knowledge of anatomy affords a more precise and detailed MR imaging interpretation, this article reviews the osseous and soft tissue MR imaging anatomy about the greater trochanter of the hip. The primary focus is on the anatomy and commonly encountered pathologic findings of the abductors of the hip and their attachments to the greater trochanter and intervening bursae.

## Greater trochanteric facet anatomy

Recurring themes are often encountered in the anatomy and pathologic findings of the musculoskeletal system. One such theme is that changes in osseous contour often represent the site of soft tissue attachments. This is the case in the greater tuberosity of the humerus as well as in the greater trochanter of the hip. Just as the rotator cuff muscles wrap around the greater tuberosity of the humerus, the gluteal muscles wrap around the greater trochanter of the hip. The attachment sites of the gluteus medius and minimus are reported to have a common attachment to the greater trochanter in the form of a broad musculotendinous sheet [14]. Although tendon attachment sites can have varying degrees of conspicuity, discrete and reproducible osseous attachments are present in the glenohumeral joint and hip, facilitating the localization of musculotendinous pathologic changes. In the hip, four distinct facets, three of which have corresponding tendon attachment sites, have been described (Fig. 1) [14–19].

The first of these, the anterior facet, is located on the anterolateral surface of the trochanter. It is oval in shape and shares a medial border with the intertrochanteric line. The second, the lateral facet, has an inverted triangular shape, with the most caudal portion comprising the palpable part of the trochanter at physical examination. The posterior superior border of the lateral facet is in contact with the superoposterior facet. This facet forms the most cranial part of the greater trochanter and has an oblique transverse orientation. The posterior facet is composed of the most

* Corresponding author.
*E-mail address:* cbchung@ucsd.edu (C.B. Chung).

1064-9689/05/$ - see front matter 
doi:10.1016/j.mric.2005.08.004

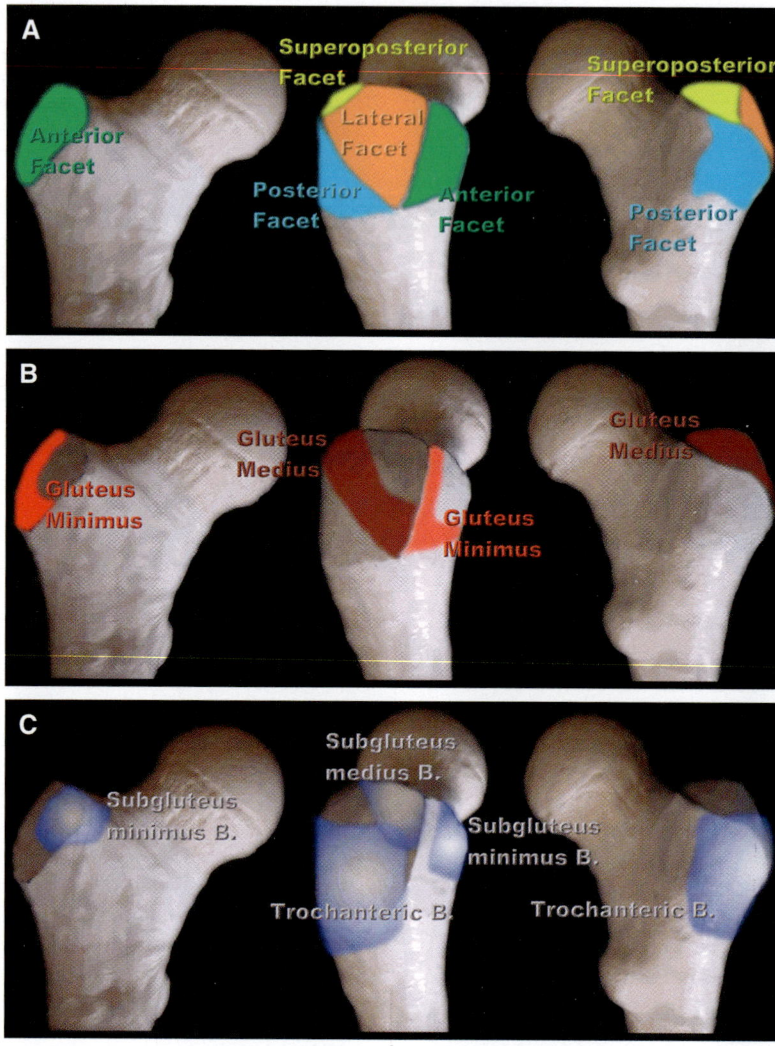


Fig. 1. Schematics of the proximal part of the femur in the frontal view (*left image*), lateral view (*middle image*), and posterior view (*right image*) display the four facets: anterior facet, lateral facet, posterior facet, and superoposterior facet (*A*); osseous attachment sites of the gluteus medius and gluteus minimus tendons (*B*); and locations of the bursae (*C*). (*Adapted from* Pfirrmann CW, Chung CB, Theumann NH, et al. Greater trochanter of the hip: attachment of the abductor mechanism and a complex of three bursae—MR imaging and MR bursography in cadavers and MR imaging in asymptomatic volunteers. Radiology 2001;221(2):470; with permission.)

posterior aspect of the trochanter. It borders the lateral and superoposterior facets and has a curved shape in a mediolateral direction. These facets, with their corresponding tendon attachments, march around the greater trochanter from its anterior to posterior extent, facilitating the wide range of motion elicited at this articulation.

The detectability of the facets of the greater trochanter as well as their MR imaging appearance has been described in cadaveric specimens as well as in asymptomatic volunteers [19]. The transverse imaging plane has been described as the optimal plane for visualization of the anterior facet. Its anterior border is formed by the intertrochanteric line just posterior to the capsular insertion of the hip. On transverse images, a distinct tubercle can be identified (Fig. 2). This facet corresponds to the insertion site of the gluteus minimus tendon.

The lateral facet has been localized to the posterior half of the greater trochanter on coronal oblique images through the hip (Fig. 3). It has

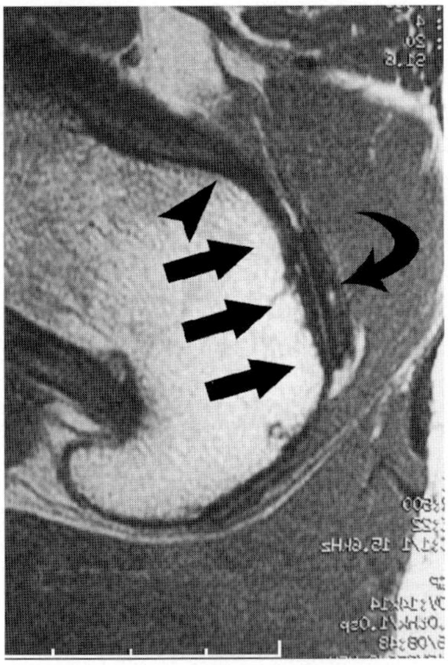

Fig. 2. T1-weighted axial MR image through the greater trochanter shows the attachment of the gluteus minimus tendon (*curved arrow*) onto the anterior facet (*arrows*) of the greater trochanter. This facet is optimally visualized in the axial plane and can be identified by localizing the lateral margin of the joint capsule (*arrowhead*).

been emphasized that care must be taken to distinguish this facet from the anterior facet. Both have a similar configuration in the coronal imaging plane but are distinguished on sequential images by an anterior versus posterior position. On transverse images, the lateral facet appears broader at its superior extent in keeping with its inverted triangular morphology. The superior border of the lateral facet contacts the superoposterior facet, the latter of which serves as the most cephalad portion of the trochanter. The lateral facet is reported to be best visualized in the sagittal imaging plane. It serves as the muscular attachment site for the gluteus medius, whereas the superoposterior facet serves as the primary tendon attachment for the gluteus medius (Fig. 4).

The posterior facet demonstrates a straight contour in the sagittal imaging plane and a curved contour in the transverse imaging plane. In some cases, it is difficult to distinguish the exact line of demarcation between the lateral and posterior facets. The sagittal imaging plane is noted to be the best plane of visualization for this facet. There is no tendon insertion present on this facet; rather, it is covered by the trochanteric bursa.

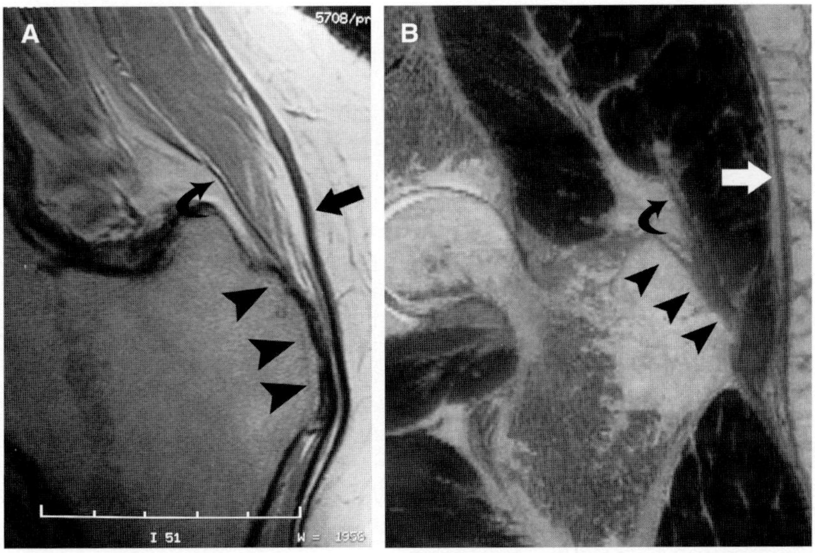


Fig. 3. T1-weighted coronal MR image (*A*) and corresponding specimen photograph (*B*) through the posterior part of the greater trochanter in a cadaveric specimen show the lateral facet (*arrowheads*), the lateral part of the gluteus medius tendon (*curved arrow*), and the iliotibial band (*straight arrow*). (*A*, *Adapted from* Pfirrmann CW, Chung CB, Theumann NH, et al. Greater trochanter of the hip: attachment of the abductor mechanism and a complex of three bursae—MR imaging and MR bursography in cadavers and MR imaging in asymptomatic volunteers. Radiology 2001;221(2):473; with permission.)

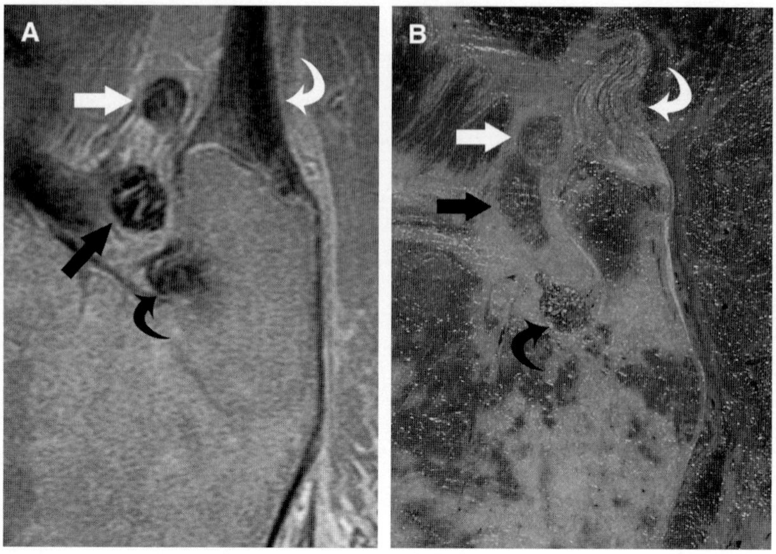


Fig. 4. Coronal MR image (*A*) and corresponding specimen photograph (*B*) show the superoposterior facet, with the main tendon (*curved white arrow*) of the gluteus medius tendon attached to it. The piriformis tendons (*straight white arrow*), obturator internus tendon (*straight black arrow*), and obturator externus tendon (*curved black arrow*) are also seen. (*A, Adapted from* Pfirrmann CW, Chung CB, Theumann NH, et al. Greater trochanter of the hip: attachment of the abductor mechanism and a complex of three bursae—MR imaging and MR bursography in cadavers and MR imaging in asymptomatic volunteers. Radiology 2001;221(2):473; with permission.)

## Abductor attachment anatomy

The designation of tendon and muscular attachments of the gluteus medius and minimus may be somewhat confusing (see Fig. 1). It is generally believed that muscular attachments to bone demonstrate four consistent zones composed of tendon, unmineralized fibrocartilage, mineralized fibrocartilage, and Sharpey fibers [20]. Although little variability is noted in the presence of these four zones, wide variability can be noted in the extent of the zones in different tendons. This variability can make macroscopic identification of distinct tendinous fibers difficult in some cases. In the following discussion, the term *tendon attachment* implies a macroscopically identifiable tendon that attaches to bone, whereas the term *muscle attachment* implies that the tendinous zone of the attachment to bone is not macroscopically identifiable.

The gluteus minimus attachment can be divided into two distinct components. The main tendon arises from the superficial part of the muscle fascia and demonstrates a consistent insertion to the anterior facet of the trochanter. The morphology of the tendon in the transverse plane is flat and biconcave. The second component of its distal insertion is a muscular and tendinous attachment to the ventral and superior capsule of the hip joint [16,21]. The latter attachment functions to stabilize the head of the femur in the acetabulum by tightening the capsule and applying pressure on the head.

The gluteus medius attachment can be divided into three parts. The main tendon arises from the central posterior portion of the muscle and has a strong insertion covering the superoposterior facet. In the transverse plane, the main tendon morphology is flat or slightly oval. The lateral part of the gluteus medius tendon arises from the undersurface of the muscle, is usually thin, and is purely muscular in nature. It attaches to the lateral facet, crossing it obliquely from a posterior-to-anterior direction. It continues anteriorly to comprise the third attachment of the gluteus medius, that covering the gluteus minimus tendon insertion to the anterior facet. This anterior portion of the gluteus medius tendon is not visible macroscopically.

## Trochanteric bursal anatomy

Three bursae are noted about the greater trochanter. The trochanteric bursa, also referred to as the subgluteus maximus bursa, is the largest of the three and covers the posterior facet as well as portions of the lateral facet. It does not extend over the anterior border of the lateral facet (Fig. 5). This bursa is located beneath the gluteus maximus muscle and iliotibial tract. The bursa is surrounded by fat on both sides and can be identified on nonenhanced transverse T1-weighted images as a fine linear structure paralleling the posterior facet. Variability in the number of subgluteus maximus bursae has been described in the literature [22]. The most common variation in multiplicity of the trochanteric bursa includes the description of a superficial component and a deep component. The superficial bursa lies deep to the fascia lata, intimately related to the gluteus maximus fibers. The deep bursa lies medial to the superficial bursa, separated from it by a well-defined intervening connective tissue plane. In a small number of cases, as many as four trochanteric bursal components have been identified occupying the same tissue planes as the superficial or deep bursae. Of note, anatomic dissections have identified branches of the inferior gluteal nerve entering the subgluteus maximus bursa and surrounding tissues. This provides a possible anatomic explanation for the sensation of pain distal to the knee, which has been reported in patients presenting with distention and inflammation of this bursa [22].

The second bursa noted about the trochanter is found deep to the lateral part of the gluteus medius tendon and is called the subgluteus medius bursa (Fig. 6). It covers the superior part of the lateral facet. Its superior border is the tip of the trochanter, its anterior border is the lateral facet, and its posterior and inferior border is the tendinous insertion of the gluteus medius. When collapsed, it is not readily visualized on MR images.

The third and final bursa about the trochanter is the subgluteus minimus bursa (Fig. 7). This bursa lies beneath the gluteus minimus tendon, medial and superior to its insertion. The bursa extends medially, covering the distal anterior portion of the joint capsule. In some cases, this bursa can be detected as a fine linear structure adjacent to the gluteus medius tendon on nonenhanced

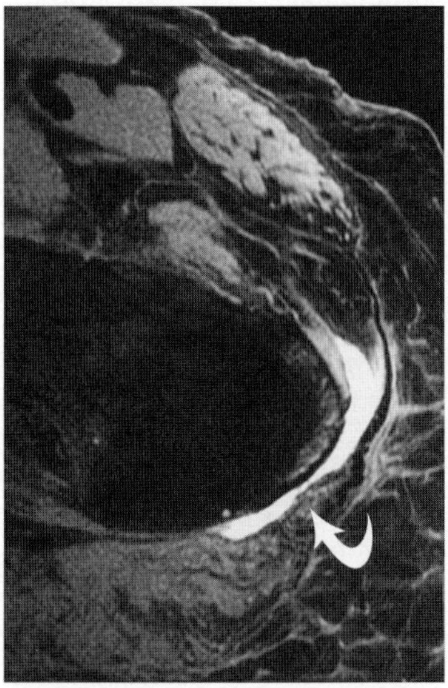

Fig. 5. Axial T1-weighted fat-suppressed MR image obtained in a cadaveric specimen after MR bursography shows the location of the trochanteric bursa (*curved arrow*) just superficial to the posterior facet. (*Adapted from* Pfirrmann CW, Chung CB, Theumann NH, et al. Greater trochanter of the hip: attachment of the abductor mechanism and a complex of three bursae—MR imaging and MR bursography in cadavers and MR imaging in asymptomatic volunteers. Radiology 2001;221(2):475; with permission.)

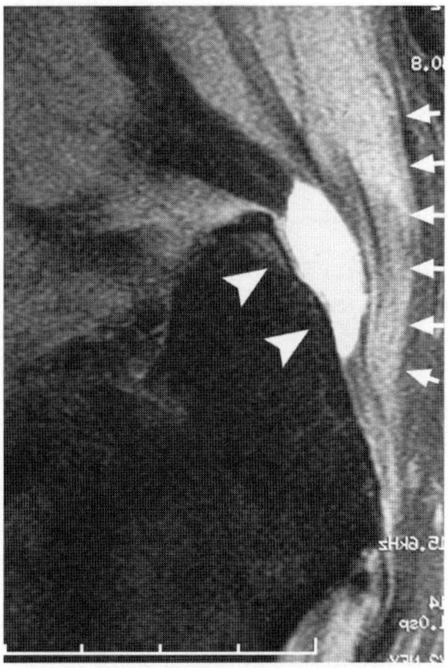


Fig. 6. Coronal T1-weighted fat-suppressed MR image obtained in a cadaveric specimen after MR bursography shows the location of the subgluteus medius bursa (*arrowheads*) deep to the lateral part of the gluteus medius tendon and muscle (*arrows*). (*Adapted from* Pfirrmann CW, Chung CB, Theumann NH, et al. Greater trochanter of the hip: attachment of the abductor mechanism and a complex of three bursae—MR imaging and MR bursography in cadavers and MR imaging in asymptomatic volunteers. Radiology 2001;221(2):476; with permission.)

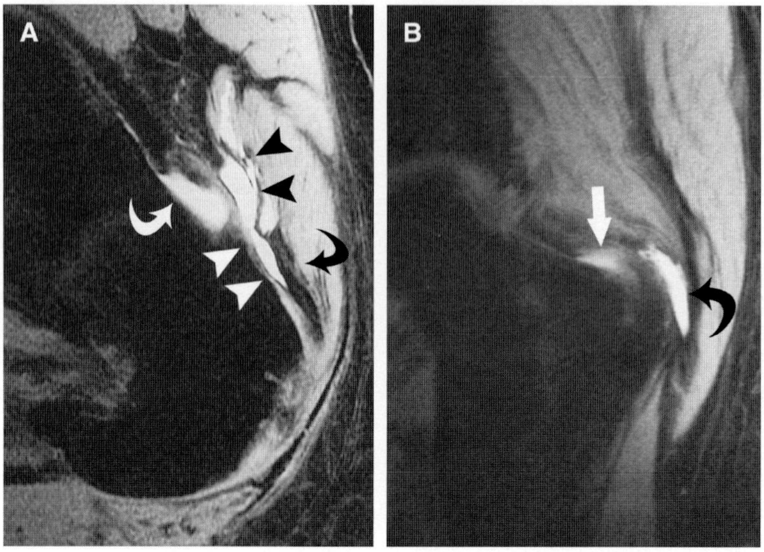


Fig. 7. (*A*) Axial T1-weighted fat-suppressed MR image obtained after bursography shows the subgluteus minimus bursa (*black and white arrowheads*) deep to the main tendon of the gluteus minimus (*curved black arrow*) and extending medially to merge with the hip capsule. Contrast material is present within the hip joint space (*curved white arrow*). (*B*) Corresponding coronal T1-weighted fat-suppressed MR image through the anterior part of the trochanter after subgluteus minimus bursography shows the relation between the contrast in the bursal space (*curved arrow*) and the contrast material in the joint space (*straight arrow*). (*Adapted from* Pfirrmann CW, Chung CB, Theumann NH, et al. Greater trochanter of the hip: attachment of the abductor mechanism and a complex of three bursae—MR imaging and MR bursography in cadavers and MR imaging in asymptomatic volunteers. Radiology 2001;221(2):474; with permission.)

transverse MR images. In most cases, however, it cannot be identified.

## Pathologic findings

Recently, pain about the greater trochanter has been characterized by the descriptive term *greater trochanter pain syndrome*. This entity is a common regional pain syndrome that is characterized by pain and point tenderness adjacent to the greater trochanter, and it is relieved by injection of an anesthetic or corticosteroids [7]. In the past, this clinical presentation was often attributed to trochanteric bursal inflammation, without further interrogation. In reality, however, the differential diagnosis for this clinical presentation is quite broad and requires consideration of articular, periarticular, and distant processes as sources of pain. This discussion focuses on the pathologic findings of the periarticular soft tissues about the greater trochanter.

### *Tendon*

#### *Rotator cuff tears of the hip*

It is becoming increasingly accepted that tears of the abductor tendons may be a common cause of the greater trochanteric pain syndrome [1–3, 7,23]. As noted previously, structural and functional similarities between the hip and shoulder do exist. The common anatomic features of the shoulder and hip include the presence of a powerful internal rotator that inserts into the lesser trochanter (iliopsoas) of the hip and the lesser tuberosity (subscapularis) of the shoulder. The hip and shoulder have two abductors that insert into the greater trochanter (gluteus minimus and medius) and into the greater tuberosity (supraspinatus and infraspinatus), respectively. In both cases, as noted in the anatomic section, the abductor attachments can be localized by the identification of discrete facets at the trochanter and tuberosity. Finally, the hip and shoulder have a tendon that crosses the head, as reflected in the head of the rectus femoris in the hip and in the biceps in the shoulder. It is for this reason that pathologic findings in the gluteus minimus and medius attachments to the greater trochanter have been likened to those encountered in the shoulder and referred to as "rotator cuff tears of the hip."

Specifically, the initial description of this pathologic finding discussed partial- or full-thickness tears of the gluteus minimus and medius tendons at their attachment to the greater trochanter. The lesions of the gluteal tendons predominated in an elderly (mean age = 83.4 years) female patient population undergoing surgical treatment of femoral neck fractures [1]. In this series, the incidence of lesions of the gluteus minimus and medius proved to be 22%. Tears of the tendons were described as interstitial, small (0.5–1 cm), and, most commonly, large (2–3 cm) in greater than 50% of cases. The appearance of the lesions was described as a circular or oval defect in the inserting tendon. The lesions were often associated with the presence of fluid in the trochanteric bursa. On surgical exploration, the osseous surface of the trochanter was visible through the defect in the tendon attachment. This has been referred to as the "bald trochanter" seen in the setting of chronic tears as well as acute spontaneous ruptures of the abductor tendons [24].

In subsequent studies, the MR imaging findings of rotator cuff tears of the hip were described [2,7]. In these studies, a spectrum of pathologic changes was identified in the gluteus minimus and medius tendons, including tendinosis, partial-thickness tears, and full-thickness tears (Figs. 8 and 9). One study further characterized tears of the tendons as avulsive in nature through the identification of bone fragments adjacent to the osseous attachment site of the tendon [2]. Furthermore, bursitis has been reported in up to 40% of patients with lesions of the gluteus minimus or medius tendons.

Tendon pathologic findings are diagnosed based on the analysis of morphology, signal intensity, and integrity of the tendon and adjacent bone. Tendinosis is characterized by abnormal tendon morphology in the form of thickening or attenuation and/or abnormal signal intensity. With regard to signal intensity changes, any increased signal intensity on fluid-sensitive sequences should not parallel the signal of simple fluid. Partial tears are diagnosed by abnormal high signal intensity on fluid-sensitive sequences (paralleling that of simple fluid) within tendon that may be normal in morphology, attenuated, or thickened. Full-thickness tendon tears are characterized by discontinuity of tendon fibers. In the setting of a full-thickness tear, further observations regarding the location of the tear, degree of retraction, and presence or absence of atrophy are generally made and help to determine the acuity of the lesion and its potential response to therapy.

Cvitanic and colleagues [3] evaluated the abductor tendons of the hip using five major criteria: tendon discontinuity, elongation of the tendon of the gluteus medius, atrophy of gluteus medius and gluteus minimus muscles, presence of an area of

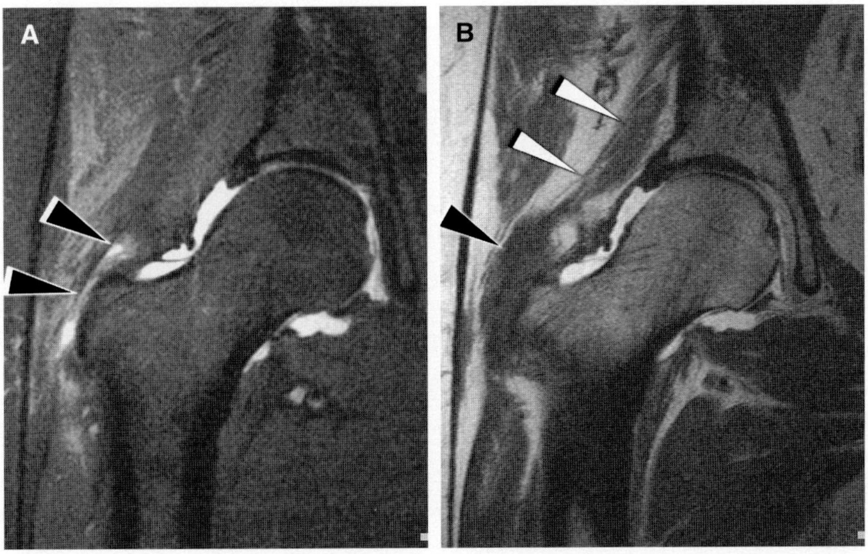


Fig. 8. (*A*) Coronal proton density–weighted fat-suppressed MR arthrography image in a 58-year-old woman with lateral hip pain demonstrates a high-grade partial tear of the gluteus minimus tendon. The defect is filled with fluid (*black arrowheads*). (*B*) Corresponding coronal T1-weighted MR arthrography image shows atrophy and retraction of the gluteus minimus muscle (*white arrowheads*). The fluid and the defect are represented by an area of intermediate signal (*black arrowhead*).

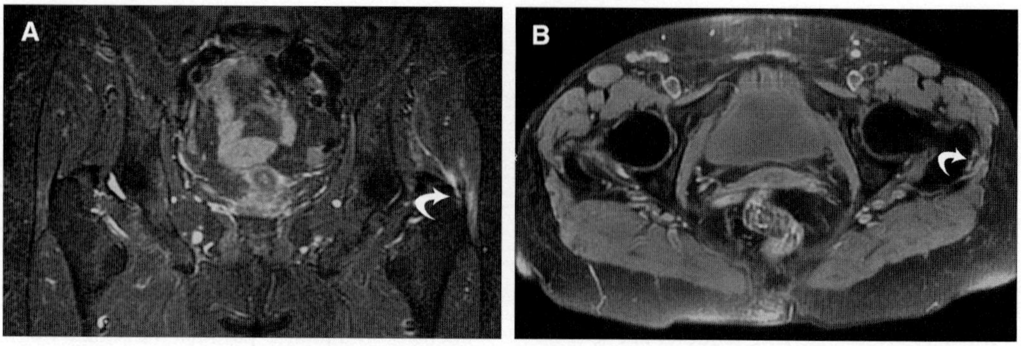


Fig. 9. Coronal T2-weighted fat-suppressed (*A*) and corresponding axial proton density–weighted fat-suppressed (*B*) MR images in a 62-year-old woman with sudden onset of hip pain show a partial tear of the muscular attachment of the gluteus medius tendon to the lateral facet. There is a small associated amount of fluid present (*curved arrow*) in the subgluteus medius bursa.

high signal intensity superior to the greater trochanter on T2-weighted images, and presence of an area of high signal lateral to the greater trochanter on T2-weighted images. Tendon discontinuity was considered to be present if the distal tendon of the gluteus medius or minimus was replaced by intermediate or high signal or was absent. The former finding suggested that the tendon was replaced by granulation tissue, fluid, or synovitis. Tendon elongation in the gluteus medius was diagnosed if the apparent length of the tendon, the distance between the greater trochanter and the musculotendinous junction, was greater than 2 cm on any single coronal slice and was longer than the tendon of the gluteus medius in the contralateral hip. The muscles were considered to be atrophic if there was a 25% or greater decrease in volume as compared with the opposite side. Areas of high signal intensity on T2-weighted images were placed into one of two categories based on location. Any high signal localized lateral to a vertical line drawn from the lateral margin of the greater trochanter on a coronal image was considered to be lateral in location and within the trochanteric bursa. Any high signal intensity localized superior to a horizontal line drawn from the lateral margin of the greater trochanter and between vertical lines drawn from the medial and lateral margins of the greater trochanter was considered to be superior in location. This region was considered to be within a tendon or between tendons in the subgluteus medius or subgluteus minimus bursa [3]. The authors concluded that focal areas of T2 hyperintensity superior to the greater trochanter were 46% more common than tendon discontinuity in hips with tears of the abductor tendons. Furthermore, patterns in which a focal area larger than 1 cm in diameter or in which a thin sheet enveloped the lateral and superior aspects of the greater trochanter were associated with tendon tears. If the region of signal hyperintensity was less than 1 cm in diameter, no association with tendon tear occurred. Tendon elongation in the gluteus medius was present in more than half of all tendon tears. No statistically significant relation was identified between abductor muscle atrophy and tendon tears. Areas of T2 hyperintensity lateral to the greater trochanter were commonly found in surgically confirmed tears of the abductor tendons but were noted in 20% of hips in the control group [3].

Although rotator cuff pathologic findings of the hip were initially believed to be asymptomatic, they are now recognized as an important cause of the trochanteric pain syndrome. Several studies have demonstrated that the pain associated with this entity responds poorly to conservative therapy [1–3,5–7]. In many cases, surgical repair of tendon ruptures has been reported, with subsequent resolution of patient symptoms.

The cause of tendinosis and tears of the gluteus medius and minimus is uncertain. It has been postulated that tension within the iliotibial band may result in frictional trauma to the gluteus medius and minimus tendons and their associated bursae, similar to the clinical entity of extrinsic impingement in the shoulder. Rheumatologic disorders like crystal deposition arthropathy have been implicated in gluteal tendon pathologic findings, as has simple tendon degeneration attributable to aging or altered biomechanics. More recently, chronic repetitive microtrauma resulting in tendon degeneration and macrotrauma attributable to direct and hyperadductive stresses have been reported as causes of rotator cuff pathologic changes of the hip [7]. In the acute setting, this injury has been described in recreational runners and those who perform step aerobics [12]. Whatever the cause, MR imaging has proven to be a useful tool for the accurate diagnosis, localization, and characterization of rotator cuff pathologic changes of the hip.

*Hydroxyapatite deposition*

Calcification within tendons and periarticular soft tissues associated with pain is a commonly encountered entity that has been well described. Specifically, hydroxyapatite deposition about the hip has been sporadically reported [10,25–33]. Although involvement of the tendons about the hip is most frequently reported in the gluteus maximus attachment, the gluteus minimus and medius can also be affected (Fig. 10) [30,33–36]. This entity has been described by a variety of names, perhaps most commonly, "calcific tendonitis," although a more appropriate name may be calcific tendinosis.

Tendon and periarticular soft tissue calcification can be classified by cause (idiopathic, hereditary, and disease-associated) as well as by imaging appearance. It is the latter that gives important information with regard to the consistency of the calcification, which, in turn, helps to guide therapy options. DePalma and Kruper [37] distinguished two morphologic types of calcification about the shoulder based on radiographic observation. These included type I (fluffy and amorphous) and type II (defined and homogeneous). Type I deposits are indicative of the acute stages of the disease, in which the calcific material may be liquid (consistency of milk) to semiliquid (consistency of toothpaste). In the acute stage of disease, reduction of pain and aspiration of the calcification have been advocated. Type II deposits are associated with subacute or chronic disease, with the calcific material forming a dry dense powder. In this stage of the disease, pain management as well as local injection with or without steroids has been considered standard therapy [37–39].

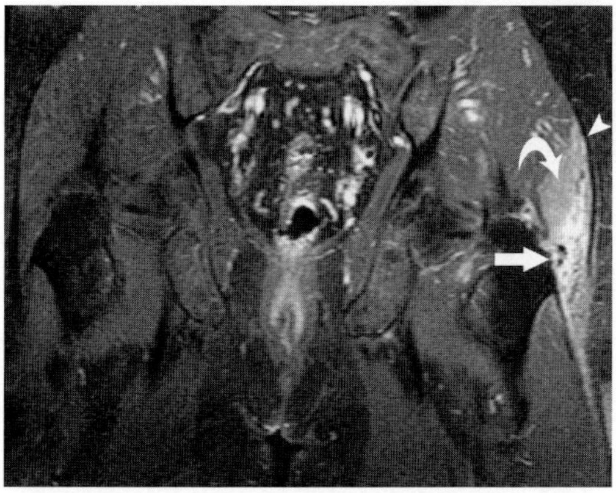

Fig. 10. Coronal T2-weighted fat-suppressed MR image in a 45-year-old man with acute-onset hip pain shows a focus of low signal intensity (*arrow*) adjacent to the posterior facet of the greater trochanter consistent with hydroxyapatite deposition. There is extensive edema in the gluteus maximus muscle (*curved arrow*), demarcated by the tensor fascia lata (*arrowhead*).

Bone destruction is not considered to be a common feature of tendon or periarticular calcification, although it can occur. Hayes and coworkers [30] described a series of five cases of calcific tendinosis, three of which were located about the hip and pelvis, with radiographic evidence of adjacent cortical bone erosion. It was postulated that the erosive changes resulted from inflammation at the tendon insertion or simply from adjacent mass effect. In this series, biopsy was performed in four of five cases to exclude tumor [30].

Similarly, although bone marrow edema is not considered to be a common association with tendon or periarticular calcification, we have anecdotally encountered this finding on more than one occasion in our practice. Moreover, it has been reported in the gluteus medius as an imaging pitfall for osseous metastasis in a patient with a history of primary malignancy [27,33].

The entity of calcification in tendons and periarticular soft tissues is commonly encountered with classic imaging findings. Familiarity with this entity in locations such as the hip as well as with the MR imaging appearance of such calcifications and their associated findings is crucial for accurate diagnosis and to avoid imaging pitfalls in differential considerations. Moreover, a precise description of the morphology and location of the calcification as well its effect on surrounding structures may be helpful in guiding therapy.

*Postoperative evaluation*

Primary total hip arthroplasty (THA) is the second most common joint replacement performed in the United States after primary total knee replacement. Surgical hip replacement involves hip exploration and exposure through a transtrochanteric posterior or anterolateral

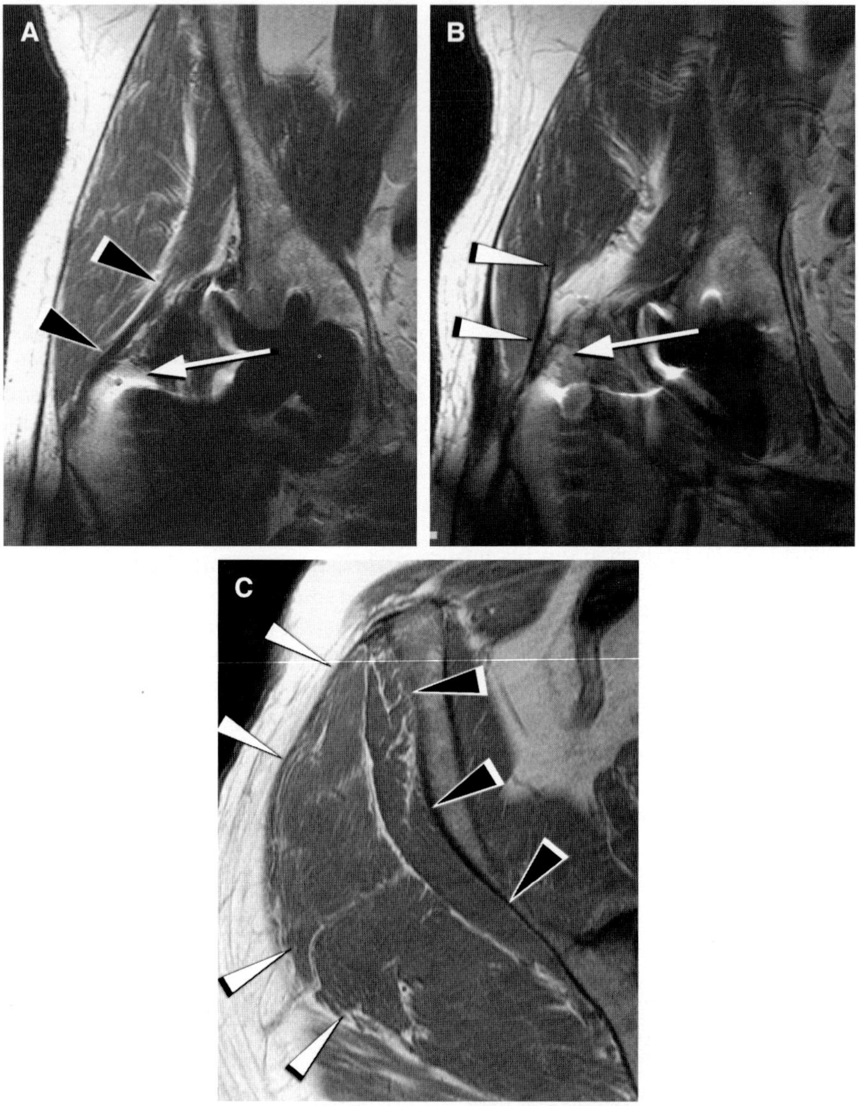


Fig. 11. (*A*) Coronal T2-weighted MR image at the anterior portion of the greater trochanter demonstrates a normal gluteus minimus tendon (*arrowheads*) attaching to the greater trochanter (*arrow*). (*B*) More posterior T2-weighted MR image at the central portion of the greater trochanter demonstrates a normal gluteus medius tendon (*arrowheads*) attaching to the greater trochanter (*arrow*). (*C*) Corresponding transverse T1-weighted MR image shows normal muscle tissue of the gluteus medius (*white arrowheads*) and gluteus minimus (*black arrowheads*). The patient is a 60-year-old asymptomatic person 1 year after THA.

approach. The transtrochanteric approach involves trochanteric osteotomy with reattachment via Kirchner cerclage wire. This approach restores hip abductor function but may be complicated by wire fracture. The posterior approach involves incision of the glutei, which leads to posterior joint laxity and postoperative hip subluxation and dislocation despite repair. To avoid these complications, many physicians advocate an anterolateral approach to expose the hip joint at the time of surgery [40–42]. With the anterolateral approach, the glutei are reattached at their insertion sites to the greater trochanter.

Residual pain after THA is a common clinical problem and can be attributable to soft tissue abnormalities, including tendon tears and muscle atrophy. Abductor dysfunction in this setting can be attributable to tendon detachment or superior

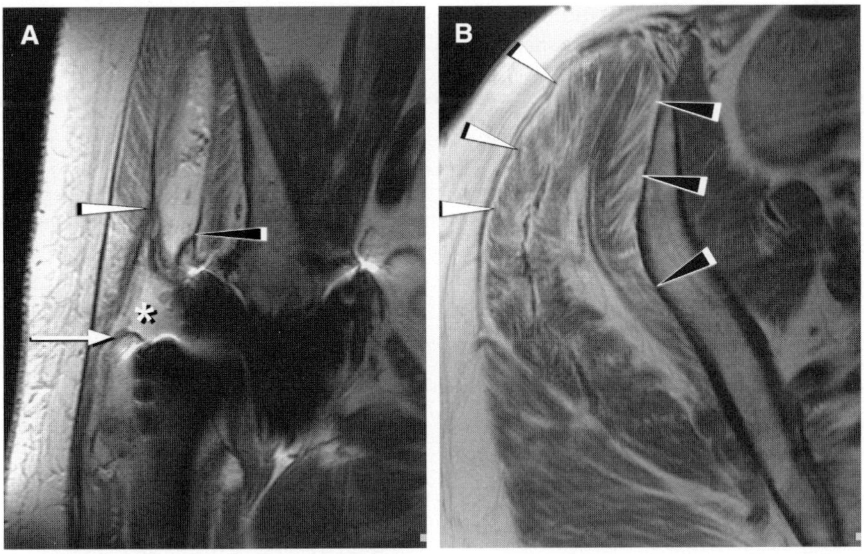


Fig. 12. (*A*) Coronal T2-weighted MR image demonstrates detachment of the gluteus minimus tendon (*black arrowhead*) and gluteus medius tendon (*white arrowhead*). Atrophic change is noted along the expected course of the gluteus medius tendon (*). Both tendons are retracted from the greater trochanter (*arrow*). (*B*) Corresponding transverse T1-weighted MR image shows marked fatty atrophy of the muscle tissue of the gluteus medius (*white arrowheads*) and gluteus minimus (*black arrowheads*). The patient is a 60-year-old woman with pain and weakness 1 year after THA.

gluteal nerve damage at the time of surgery [43]. In tendon failure and nerve damage, patients present with Trendelenburg gait and secondary muscle atrophy. Electrophysiologic studies may prove equivocal, and radiologic evaluation is limited for soft tissue pathologic findings. Because of its excellent soft tissue contrast, MR imaging has emerged as the imaging study of choice when this differential set of considerations is encountered, despite the potential problem of metal artifact in the postsurgical patient.

In the past, MR imaging has played a limited role in the evaluation of patients after THA primarily because of susceptibility artifacts related to metallic implants. Modifications of traditional MR imaging sequences can be used to manipulate such artifacts to optimize visualization of the structures of interest as well as image quality. The spin-echo technique with high bandwidth (at least 130 Hz per pixel), a high-resolution matrix (512×512), sequences with multiple refocusing pulses, and a frequency-encoding axis parallel to the long axis of the prosthesis can help to do so. Other techniques used to reduce susceptibility artifact include manipulation of slice-select orientation and frequency-encoded gradient orientation in conjunction with tissue excitation using rapid acquisition with relaxation enhancement–based sequences [42,44,45]. Artifact reduction is particularly effective when prostheses are cobalt chrome– or titanium-based rather than steel-based. With such technique optimization, MR imaging has proven effective in accurately diagnosing abductor avulsions in patients with THA (Figs. 11 and 12) [42,45].

It is important to recognize that although they are more frequent in symptomatic patients, many

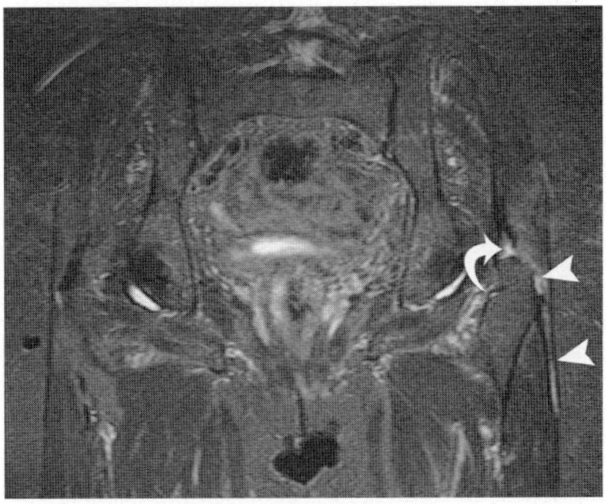

Fig. 13. Coronal T2-weighted MR image shows a partial intrasubstance tear (*curved arrow*) of the main tendon attachment to the superoposterior facet of the greater trochanter, with associated fluid in the trochanteric bursa (*arrowheads*).

MR findings, such as altered signal and diameter of the abductor tendons, bursal fluid collections and fatty atrophy of the anterior gluteus minimus muscle, are frequently found in asymptomatic patients after THA through a transgluteal approach. Defects of the abductor tendons and fatty atrophy of the gluteus medius and the posterior part of the gluteus minimus muscle are uncommon in asymptomatic patients after THA, however, and are therefore clinically relevant [45].

*Bursa*

*Trochanteric bursitis*

Trochanteric bursitis is a clinical condition that can simulate hip disease as well as low back pain. This entity is a common regional pain syndrome seen predominantly in middle age and in women [22]. It is believed to result from inflammation of the subgluteus maximus bursa. The major clinical findings are somewhat nonspecific, with tenderness localized to the lateral part of the hip, pain in the hip, and pain in the lateral thigh. This condition has been referred to as the greater trochanteric bursitis pain syndrome, referring to pain attributed to pathologic changes of the trochanteric or subgluteus maximus bursa. Because of the difficulty in distinguishing isolated bursal pathologic changes from tendon abnormalities and other soft tissue lesions, the clinical entity of lateral hip pain is appropriately referred to in more general terms as the greater trochanter pain syndrome.

The MR imaging diagnosis of trochanteric bursitis is made by the presence of high signal intensity within the bursa on fluid-sensitive sequences. In some cases, septations have been identified within a distended bursa [46]. After the administration of gadolinium, MR images show enhancement of the wall of the bursa with central low signal intensity. Because the bursa is lined by synovium, thickening, irregularity, and nodularity can be identified in the setting of chronic inflammation.

There have been many suggested causes of trochanteric bursitis. The concept that the primary lesion in trochanteric bursitis is damage to the gluteal tendons at their insertion onto the greater trochanter with secondary involvement of the bursa was described decades ago, although, as previously noted, it has gained increasing popularity in the orthopedic and imaging literature (Fig. 13) [47]. This concept involves the theory that tears in the tendons attaching to the greater trochanter induce inflammation in the contiguous bursae, much as subacromial-subdeltoid bursitis is encountered in the presence of rotator cuff tears in the glenohumeral joint [22]. Clearly, knowledge of the facet and bursal anatomy of the hip is helpful in localization of pathologic changes in the tendon attachments and adjacent soft tissues.

Other less common causes of trochanteric bursitis can include indolent infection, such as tuberculosis. In one study describing the imaging findings of tuberculous tenosynovitis and bursitis, the most commonly involved bursa in the body proved to be that of the trochanteric bursa. The presence of small abscess formation in a subset of the patient population helped to identify the process as infectious in nature. In some cases, however, nonspecific bursal distention was the only imaging finding [4].

Trochanteric bursitis has also been reported in the setting of rheumatoid arthritis. Not only can erosive changes in the adjacent bone be encountered in rheumatoid arthritis, but cyst formation emanating from the bursa extending into the subcutaneous soft tissues can occur. The presence of rice bodies within the bursa can be seen with rheumatoid arthritis and tuberculous bursal inflammation [48].

## References


[1] Bunker TD, Esler CN, Leach WJ. Rotator-cuff tear of the hip. J Bone Joint Surg Br 1997;79(4):618–20.

[2] Chung CB, Robertson JE, Cho GJ, et al. Gluteus medius tendon tears and avulsive injuries in elderly women: imaging findings in six patients. AJR Am J Roentgenol 1999;173(2):351–3.

[3] Cvitanic O, Henzie G, Skezas N, et al. MRI diagnosis of tears of the hip abductor tendons (gluteus medius and gluteus minimus). AJR Am J Roentgenol 2004;182(1):137–43.

[4] Jaovisidha S, Chen C, Ryu KN, et al. Tuberculous tenosynovitis and bursitis: imaging findings in 21 cases. Radiology 1996;201(2):507–13.

[5] Kagan A II. Rotator-cuff tear of the hip. J Bone Joint Surg Br 1998;80(1):182–3.

[6] Kagan A II. Rotator cuff tears of the hip. Clin Orthop 1999;368:135–40.

[7] Kingzett-Taylor A, Tirman PF, Feller J, et al. Tendinosis and tears of gluteus medius and minimus muscles as a cause of hip pain: MR imaging findings. AJR Am J Roentgenol 1999;173(4):1123–6.

[8] Little H. Trochanteric bursitis: a common cause of pelvic girdle pain. Can Med Assoc J 1979;120(4):456–8.

[9] Lonner JH, Van Kleunen JP. Spontaneous rupture of the gluteus medius and minimus tendons. Am J Orthop 2002;31(10):579–81.

[10] Sakai T, Shimaoka Y, Sugimoto M, et al. Acute calcific tendinitis of the gluteus medius: a case report

with serial magnetic resonance imaging findings. J Orthop Sci 2004;9(4):404–7.
[11] Steinbach LS, Schneider R, Goldman AB, et al. Bursae and abscess cavities communicating with the hip. Diagnosis using arthrography and CT. Radiology 1985;156(2):303–7.
[12] Walsh G, Archibald CG. MRI in greater trochanter pain syndrome. Australas Radiol 2003;47(1):85–7.
[13] Zacher J, Gursche A. Regional musculoskeletal conditions: 'hip' pain. Best Pract Res Clin Rheumatol 2003;17(1):71–85.
[14] Nazarian S, Tisserand P, Brunet C, et al. Anatomic basis of the transgluteal approach to the hip. Surg Radiol Anat 1987;9(1):27–35.
[15] Armbuster TG, Guerra J Jr, Resnick D, et al. The adult hip: an anatomic study. Part I: the bony landmarks. Radiology 1978;128(1):1–10.
[16] Beck M, Sledge JB, Gautier E, et al. The anatomy and function of the gluteus minimus muscle. J Bone Joint Surg Br 2000;82(3):358–63.
[17] Duparc F, Thomine JM, Dujardin C, et al. Anatomic basis of the transgluteal approach to the hip-joint by anterior hemimyotomy of the gluteus medius. Surg Radiol Anat 1997;19(2):61–7.
[18] Gottschalk F, Kourosh S, Leveau B. The functional anatomy of tensor fasciae latae and gluteus medius and minimus. J Anat 1989;166:179–89.
[19] Pfirrmann CW, Chung CB, Theumann NH, et al. Greater trochanter of the hip: attachment of the abductor mechanism and a complex of three bursae—MR imaging and MR bursography in cadavers and MR imaging in asymptomatic volunteers. Radiology 2001;221(2):469–77.
[20] Resnick D, Niwayama G. Entheses and enthesopathy. Anatomical, pathological, and radiological correlation. Radiology 1983;146(1):1–9.
[21] Walters J, Solomons M, Davies J. Gluteus minimus: observations on its insertion. J Anat 2001;198(Pt 2): 239–42.
[22] Dunn T, Heller CA, McCarthy SW, et al. Anatomical study of the "trochanteric bursa." Clin Anat 2003;16(3):233–40.
[23] Bird PA, Oakley SP, Shnier R, et al. Prospective evaluation of magnetic resonance imaging and physical examination findings in patients with greater trochanteric pain syndrome. Arthritis Rheum 2001; 44(9):2138–45.
[24] LaBan MM, Weir SK, Taylor RS. 'Bald trochanter' spontaneous rupture of the conjoined tendons of the gluteus medius and minimus presenting as a trochanteric bursitis. Am J Phys Med Rehabil 2004;83(10): 806–9.
[25] Berney JW. Calcifying peritendinitis of the gluteus maximus tendon. Radiology 1972;102(3):517–8.
[26] Chow HY, Recht MP, Schils J, et al. Acute calcific tendinitis of the hip: case report with magnetic resonance imaging findings. Arthritis Rheum 1997;40(5): 974–7.
[27] Chung CB, Gentili A, Chew FS. Calcific tendinosis and periarthritis: classic magnetic resonance imaging appearance and associated findings. J Comput Assist Tomogr 2004;28(3):390–6.
[28] Fam AG, Pritzker KP, Stein JL, et al. Apatite-associated arthropathy: a clinical study of 14 cases and of 2 patients with calcific bursitis. J Rheumatol 1979;6(4):461–71.
[29] Hayes CW, Conway WF. Calcium hydroxyapatite deposition disease. Radiographics 1990;10(6):1031–48.
[30] Hayes CW, Rosenthal DI, Plata MJ, et al. Calcific tendinitis in unusual sites associated with cortical bone erosion. AJR Am J Roentgenol 1987;149(5): 967–70.
[31] Holt PD, Keats TE. Calcific tendinitis: a review of the usual and unusual. Skeletal Radiol 1993;22(1):1–9.
[32] Wepfer JF, Reed JG, Cullen GM, et al. Calcific tendinitis of the gluteus maximus tendon (gluteus maximus tendinitis). Skeletal Radiol 1983;9(3):198–200.
[33] Yang I, Hayes CW, Biermann JS. Calcific tendinitis of the gluteus medius tendon with bone marrow edema mimicking metastatic disease. Skeletal Radiol 2002;31(6):359–61.
[34] Flemming DJ, Murphey MD, Shekitka KM, et al. Osseous involvement in calcific tendinitis: a retrospective review of 50 cases. AJR Am J Roentgenol 2003;181(4):965–72.
[35] Kandemir U, Bharam S, Philippon MJ, et al. Endoscopic treatment of calcific tendinitis of gluteus medius and minimus. Arthroscopy 2003;19(1):E4.
[36] Kraemer EJ, El-Khoury GY. Atypical calcific tendinitis with cortical erosions. Skeletal Radiol 2000; 29(12):690–6.
[37] DePalma AF, Kruper JS. Long-term study of shoulder joints afflicted with and treated for calcific tendinitis. Clin Orthop 1961;20:61–72.
[38] Maier M, Maier-Bosse T, Schultz CU, et al. Inter and intraobserver variability in DePalma's classification of shoulder calcific tendinitis. J Rheumatol 2003;30(5):1029–31.
[39] Moseley HF. The natural history and clinical syndromes produced by calcified deposits in the rotator cuff. Surg Clin North Am 1963;43:1489–93.
[40] Frankel A, Booth RE Jr, Balderston RA, et al. Complications of trochanteric osteotomy. Long-term implications. Clin Orthop 1993;288:209–13.
[41] Frndak PA, Mallory TH, Lombardi AV Jr. Translateral surgical approach to the hip. The abductor muscle "split." Clin Orthop 1993;295:135–41.
[42] Twair A, Ryan M, O'Connell M, et al. MRI of failed total hip replacement caused by abductor muscle avulsion. AJR Am J Roentgenol 2003;181(6): 1547–50.
[43] van der Linde MJ, Tonino AJ. Nerve injury after hip arthroplasty. 5/600 cases after uncemented hip replacement, anterolateral approach versus direct lateral approach. Acta Orthop Scand 1997;68(6): 521–3.

[44] Eustace S, et al. A comparison of conventional spin-echo and turbo spin-echo imaging of soft tissues adjacent to orthopedic hardware. AJR Am J Roentgenol 1998;170(2):455–8.
[45] White LM, et al. Complications of total hip arthroplasty: MR imaging-initial experience. Radiology 2000;215(1):254–62.
[46] Varma DG, Parihar A, Richli WR. CT appearance of the distended trochanteric bursa. J Comput Assist Tomogr 1993;17(1):141–3.
[47] Gordon EJ. Trochanteric bursitis and tendinitis. Clin Orthop 1961;20:193–202.
[48] Tanaka H, et al. Trochanteric bursitis in rheumatoid arthritis. J Rheumatol 2002;29(6):1340–1.

ELSEVIER
SAUNDERS

Magn Reson Imaging Clin N Am
13 (2005) 705–716

MAGNETIC
RESONANCE
IMAGING CLINICS
of North America

# MR Imaging of Iliopsoas Musculotendinous Injuries

Nogah Shabshin, MD[a,*], Zehava Sadka Rosenberg, MD[b], Conrado F.A. Cavalcanti, MD[b]

[a]*Department of Diagnostic Imaging, Chaim Sheba Medical Center, Tel-Hashomer, Israel 52561*
[b]*Department of Radiology, Hospital for Joint Diseases, Bernard Aronson Plaza, 301 East 17th Street, 6th Floor, New York, NY 10003, USA*

Ailments of the iliopsoas musculotendinous unit, although relatively uncommon, are becoming more frequently recognized because of the escalating athletic activity in the general population as well as the ever increasing demands placed on professional athletes. Iliopsoas tendon injuries are also encountered in the elderly population and are a well-known complication of total hip arthroplasties. Most iliopsoas diseases, including tendinosis, avulsion injuries, snapping tendon, and bursitis, can present as groin pain, a symptom that carries an extensive differential diagnosis, and thus are often clinically overlooked. Additionally, abnormalities of the iliopsoas tendon and bursa are usually present simultaneously, making the diagnosis even more challenging. The greater use of cross-sectional imaging modalities, such as MR imaging and ultrasound (US), has allowed increased accuracy in the diagnosis of iliopsoas disease. This article focuses on the normal MR imaging anatomy and on the MR imaging characteristics of diseases of the iliopsoas musculotendinous unit.

## Normal anatomy of the iliopsoas compartment

The iliopsoas muscle compartment consists of three muscles: the psoas major, the psoas minor, and the iliacus [1–8]. The compartment functions as a thigh flexor and as a lateral flexor of the lumbar spine, with the psoas muscle flexing the thigh on the pelvis, aided by the iliacus. Based on electromyographic studies, the iliopsoas muscle compartment also participates in lateral rotation of the hip and provides balance to the trunk while sitting down. The psoas and iliacus muscles, when acting bilaterally, flex the trunk and pelvis against resistance and raise the trunk from a recumbent to sitting position [1].

The psoas major, the longest muscle in the compartment, extends from the posterior mediastinum to the thigh. Its main origin is from the lumbar vertebral column. The muscle passes deep to the arcuate ligament of the diaphragm proximally and is in contact more distally with the posterior pararenal fascia and psoas fascia. This allows the spread of disease, such as infection, between the mediastinum, retroperitoneum, and thigh. The main origin of the iliacus muscle is from the inner iliac fossa. The muscle is fan shaped at its origin and tapers as it descends lateral to the psoas muscle.

The psoas major and iliacus muscles merge at the level of the L5 to S2 vertebrae, underneath the inguinal ligament, to form the iliopsoas muscle (Fig. 1) [9]. The muscles are covered by the iliopsoas fascia, which acts to separate them from the extraperitoneal tissues and peritoneum [1].

The psoas major tendon migrates from within the muscle belly into a posterior position located immediately anterior to the hip joint. A more slender iliacus tendon is located lateral to the psoas tendon. The two tendons usually converge into a single tendon a few centimeters above the lesser trochanter attachment. The conjoined tendon attaches to and slightly inferior to the lesser trochanter. The iliacus muscle also has direct muscular attachment into the anterior femur at and slightly below the lesser trochanter [9].

* Corresponding author.
*E-mail address:* nogah.shabshin@sheba.health.gov.il (N. Shabshin).

1064-9689/05/$ - see front matter 
doi:10.1016/j.mric.2005.08.010

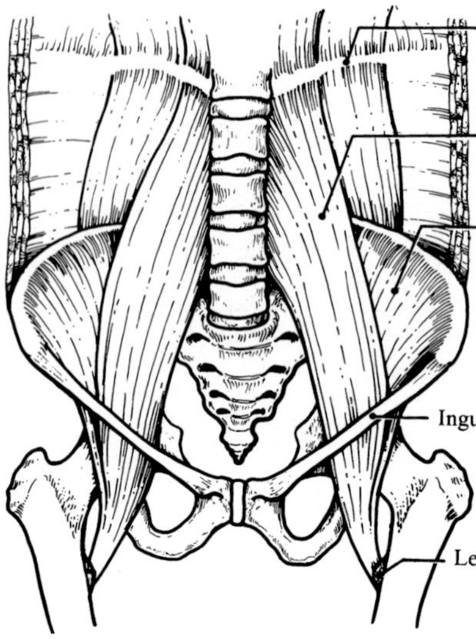


Fig. 1. Drawing of the normal anatomy of the iliopsoas musculotendinous complex. (*From* Muttarak M, Peh WC. CT of unusual iliopsoas compartment lesions. Radiographics 2000;20:S54; with permission.)

The iliopsoas bursa, the largest synovial bursa in human beings [1,2,8], separates the iliopsoas tendon from the hip joint capsule and the pubis [1]. The bursa often communicates with the hip joint. It may extend proximally into the pelvis and distally to the region of the lesser trochanter of the femur.

The psoas minor muscle, a long slender muscle present in 60% of individuals, originates from T12 and L1 [2]. It descends anterior to the psoas major toward its main insertion into the iliopectineal eminence of the iliac bone lateral to the iliac fascia. The psoas minor muscle acts as a weak flexor of the thigh [1].

## MR imaging anatomy of the iliopsoas musculotendinous unit

In general, the iliopsoas musculotendinous unit is best seen on axial images (Fig. 2). The muscle and tendon can also be followed a little less consistently on sagittal images. Because of partial volume averaging, the proximal aspect of the iliopsoas tendon is not always visualized on coronal images. The coronal images as well as the axial images, however, are quite useful for visualizing the tendon's attachment to the lesser trochanter. MR arthrography, although not necessary for visualizing the tendon, is nevertheless useful in highlighting the tendon as it descends, superficial to the anterior hip capsule.

In the pelvic area, axial and coronal images serve to depict the psoas major and iliacus muscles as they approximate each other to form the iliopsoas muscle. As the muscles join, the psoas major tendon becomes imbedded into the muscle belly to form the major iliopsoas tendon. An additional slender tendon slip, best seen on axial images, is noted more laterally within the iliacus muscle (Fig. 3). This second tendon usually converges with the main iliopsoas tendon just above the insertion to the lesser trochanter.

The iliopsoas muscle can be optimally followed on axial images as it proceeds downward obliquely from a medial and anterior location to a lateral and posterior location. Concomitantly, the main iliopsoas tendon migrates from within the muscle belly until it lays posterior and medial to the muscle. At the level of the hip joint, the tendon is first noted anterior and then lateral to the anterior labrum. A thin fat plane found between the tendon and the labrum is noted on axial images and should not be confused with a labral tear.

The iliopsoas tendon can be followed as it continues anterior to the femoral head and neck and curves toward its direct lesser trochanter attachment. The tendon is accompanied by the more laterally located residual iliacus muscle fibers. The attachment of the tendon inferior to the lesser trochanter results in a C-shaped linear low signal structure best seen on axial and coronal images. A direct muscular attachment of the remaining iliacus muscle into the anterior aspect of the lesser trochanter is best visualized on axial images.

## Iliopsoas compartment injuries

Groin pain in athletes is clinically challenging and can be difficult to evaluate even by experienced physicians, because the anatomy of the region is complex and two or more disorders often coexist. The cause of the pain remains unclear in approximately 30% of cases [10,11]. The differential diagnosis is extensive and includes numerous sports-related disorders, such as adductor strains, sports hernia, iliopsoas strains and bursitis, snapping hip, osteitis pubis, pubic stress fractures, avulsion fractures, and nerve entrapment syndromes. Nonathletic causes of groin pain, such as intra-abdominal pathology, genitourinary abnormalities, referred lumbosacral pain, and hip joint disorders (eg, arthritis, synovitis,

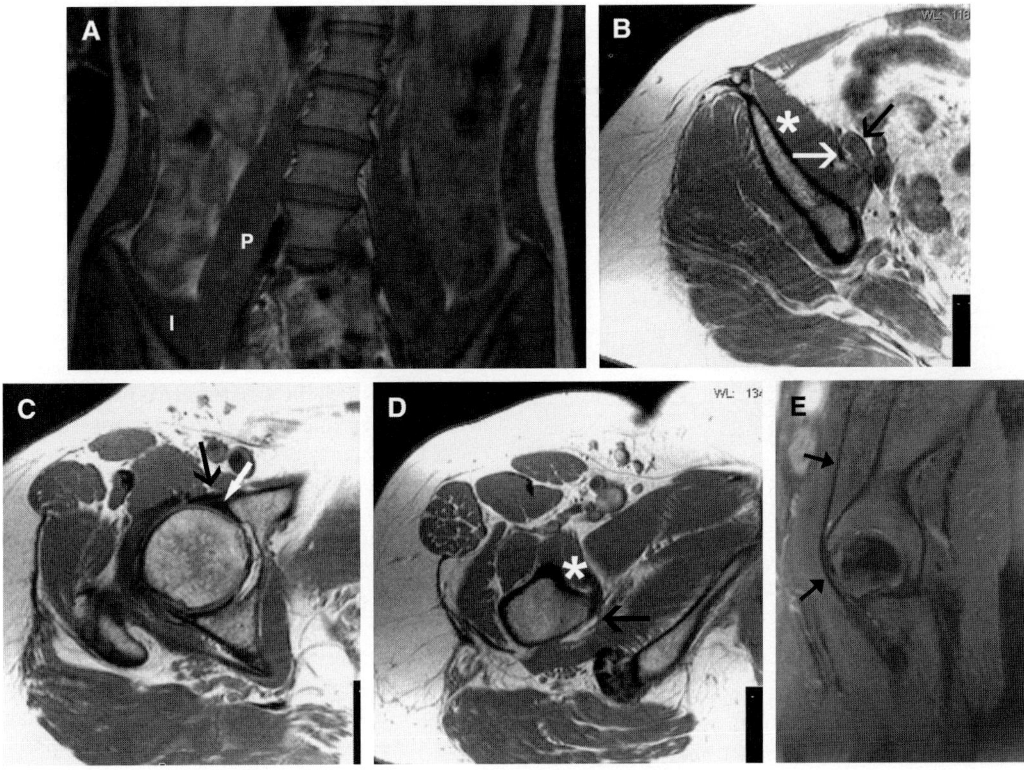


Fig. 2. Normal MR imaging anatomy of the iliopsoas musculotendinous unit on T1-weighted spin echo images. (*A*) Coronal image demonstrate the psoas muscle (P) and the iliacus muscle (I) as they join together in the lower pelvis. (*B*) Axial image at the level of the iliac fossa demonstrates the iliacus muscle (*) against the iliac bone. The psoas muscle (*black arrow*) and tendon (*white arrow*) are noted more medially. (*C*) At the level of the hip joint, the flat thin iliopsoas tendon (*black arrow*) is anterior to the anterior labrum (*white arrow*). Occasionally, the linear gap between the tendon and labrum can mimic a labral tear. (*D*) Axial image at the level of the lesser trochanter of the femur demonstrates the psoas tendon inserting on the lesser trochanter (*black arrow*). Direct insertion of the iliacus muscle to the bone without an apparent tendon is noted (*). (*E*) On a sagittal T-2 weighted fat-suppressed image, the tendon is seen anterior and parallel to the hip joint capsule (*black arrows*).

avascular necrosis), must also be considered [10,11].

Thus, it is not surprising that iliopsoas musculotendinous pathology, an uncommon cause of acute or chronic groin pain, is often clinically overlooked and requires extra vigilance on the part of the treating physician. Johnston and colleagues [12] suggested that iliopsoas musculotendinous injuries, such as tendinosis, tears, bursitis and snapping iliopsoas tendon, should be called "the iliopsoas syndrome," because abnormalities of the tendon and bursa are often present simultaneously. These entities reflect a spectrum of disease, especially when related to sports and other types of overuse activities. Most frequently affected are athletes who participate in sports like soccer, ice hockey, fencing, handball, cross-country skiing, hurdling, and high jumping [13]. Cross-sectional imaging, such as MR imaging and US, have provided us with a greater understanding of these disorders and have allowed means for presurgical planning and treatment guidance.

## Iliopsoas tendinosis

The prevalence of iliopsoas tendinosis is not fully agreed on in the orthopedic literature, but the entity may be a more common sport injury than is presently recognized. Despite this, there are only a few articles in the English literature describing this entity [14]. The injuries are seen more frequently in kicking-related sports, such as soccer and hockey, and in other high-energy sports [15]. Tight hip flexors and overuse predispose to the injury. Shin and coworkers [16] found

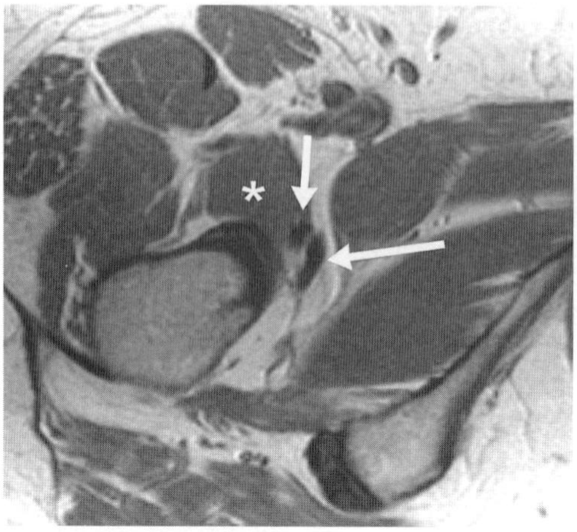

Fig. 3. Iliacus and psoas components of the iliopsoas tendon. Axial T1-weighted image at the level of the lesser trochanter demonstrates two distinct psoas (*long arrow*) and iliacus (*short arrow*) tendons. More laterally, iliacus muscle fibers (*) insert directly on the femur.

MR imaging to be useful in the evaluation of high-endurance–related hip pain and discovered one case of iliopsoas muscle tear and one case of bilateral iliopsoas tendinosis in 21 hips of soldiers with hip and groin pain.

Tendinopathy of the iliopsoas is also encountered after total hip arthroplasty and is related to impingement of the anterior rim of a malpositioned acetabular cup on the tendon [17]. An enlarged cup and pelvic cement may also produce impingement on the tendon. At surgery, enlargement, fraying, and inflammation of the tendon adjacent to the cup may be encountered.

Iliopsoas tendinopathy is manifested clinically as chronic groin or trochanteric pain that is exacerbated with active flexion and adduction of the hip and is associated with sports activities, such as kicking, or even simple daily activities, such as descending stairs, getting in and out of a car, or turning in bed. Tenderness along the course of the tendon as it travels through the lateral aspect of the inguinal canal is also encountered. A snapping sensation at the hip and radiation of the pain to the knee have been described. The treatment is usually conservative, with rest, anti-inflammatory medication, and stretching exercises. Local corticosteroid injection of the tendon may produce pain relief [17,18].

On MR imaging, iliopsoas tendinosis is depicted as thickening or attenuation of the tendon along its course or at its insertion to the lesser trochanter (Fig. 4). This is best seen on axial images. Peritendonal high signal intensity on T2-weighted or inversion recovery images and distention of the iliopsoas bursa can also be seen. US can play a complementary role to MR imaging in the diagnosis of iliopsoas tendinosis and is particularly useful for guiding local injection of long-acting corticosteroids [15].

### Iliopsoas tendon avulsion injuries

Because the lesser trochanter is protected by surrounding muscles and bone, fracture secondary to

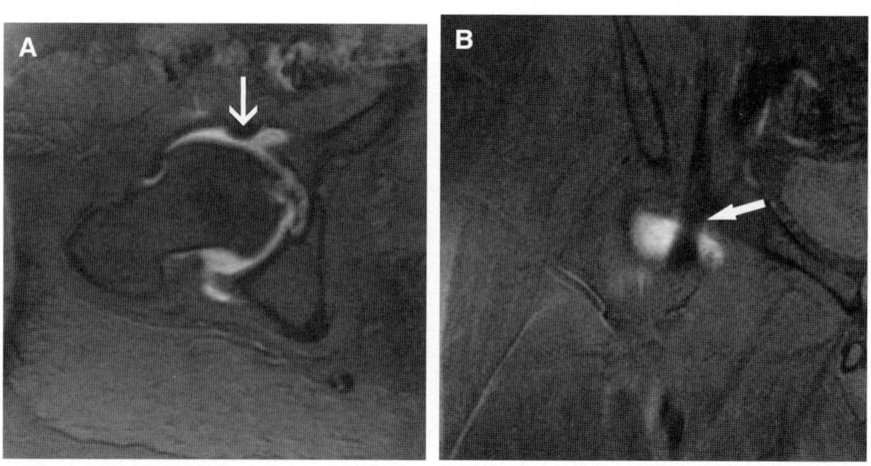



Fig. 4. Tendinosis of the iliopsoas tendon in a 37-year-old man with a history of Legg-Calvé-Perthes disease. Axial (*A*) and coronal (*B*) T1-weighted fat-suppressed MR arthrographic images demonstrate a thickened tendon (*arrow*) that indents the anterior capsule of the hip joint. On the coronal image, the thickened iliopsoas tendon (*arrow*) is outlined by the hyperintense intra-articular gadolinium.

direct trauma is uncommon. Sports-related isolated avulsion of the iliopsoas tendon with detachment of the lesser trochanter is a more common occurrence. The greatest incidence is observed in male adolescent patients before fusion of the lesser trochanteric apophysis because of an imbalance between iliopsoas muscular strength and the weaker apophyseal-bone interphase [19,20].

An avulsion injury is usually caused by sudden traction of the iliopsoas muscle on the tendinous insertion. This usually occurs during forceful adduction and flexion of the hip against the thigh, which is fixed or forced into extension (Fig. 5) [21].

Clinically, patients with iliopsoas tendon avulsion describe a snap at the time of injury, followed by acute pain in the inguinal region and limping. On physical examination, tenderness, with or without ecchymosis, in the groin area is common. Pain is reproduced by passive multidirectional movement of the hip. It is most severe in maximum external rotation of the hip with extension and is relieved when the patient is seated [19]. In children, avulsion of the lesser trochanter may clinically mimic transient synovitis of the hip or Legg-Calvé-Perthes disease [20]. Standard therapy is nonsurgical, with bed rest and immobilization of the leg even if the avulsed fragment is displaced away from the bone [22].

Avulsion of the lesser trochanter has been described to occur as an isolated fracture in the osteoporotic population [23]. When it is seen in an adult without significant trauma, however, it should be regarded as secondary to metastatic neoplasm until proven otherwise (Fig. 6) [22,24–26].

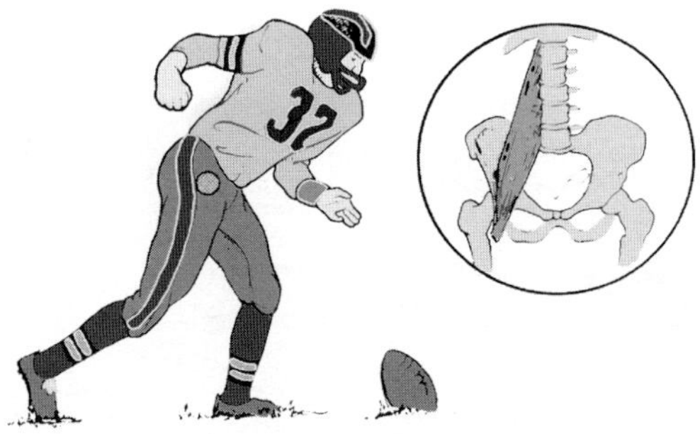


Fig. 5. Mechanism of iliopsoas tendon tear. The right iliopsoas muscle contracts while the hip is extended and the foot is fixed against the ground (right toes caught in turf). (*From* Sim FH, Rock MG, Scott SG. Pelvis and hip injuries in athletes: anatomy and function. In: Nicholas JA, Hershman EB, editors. The lower extremity and spine in sports medicine. 2nd edition. London: Mosby; 1995. p. 1048; with permission.)

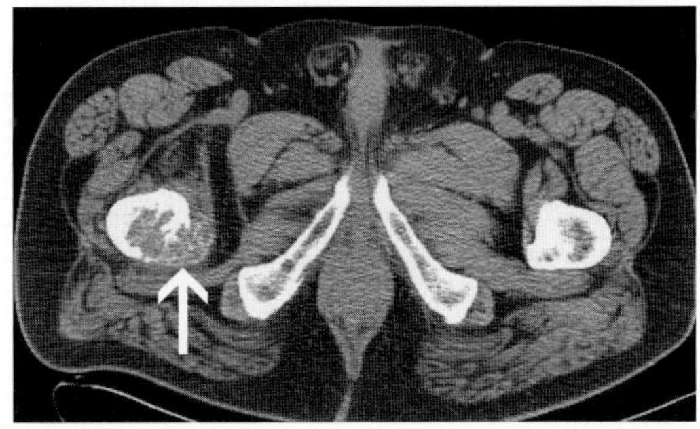

Fig. 6. Iliopsoas tendon avulsion secondary to metastatic carcinoma. CT image (soft tissue windows) demonstrates a lytic lesion (*arrow*) of the lesser trochanter with calcifications at the insertion of the iliopsoas tendon.

Bony avulsion of the iliopsoas tendon can be easily detected on plain radiographs and typically does not require advanced cross-sectional imaging. A fracture of the lesser trochanter with or without displacement of the apophyseal fragment is noted. Chronic or healed injuries can depict extensive ossification within the distal tendon close to its insertion to the lesser trochanter (Fig. 7).

In children, widening and increased signal at the lesser trochanteric apophysis, best seen on coronal or axial MR images, is typically encountered during the acute phase of the injury [27]. Fluid signal consistent with soft tissue edema in the region of the distal tendon and distention of the iliopsoas bursa are other frequent MR imaging findings.

In the adult athletic patient, an iliopsoas tendon tear typically occurs without an avulsion

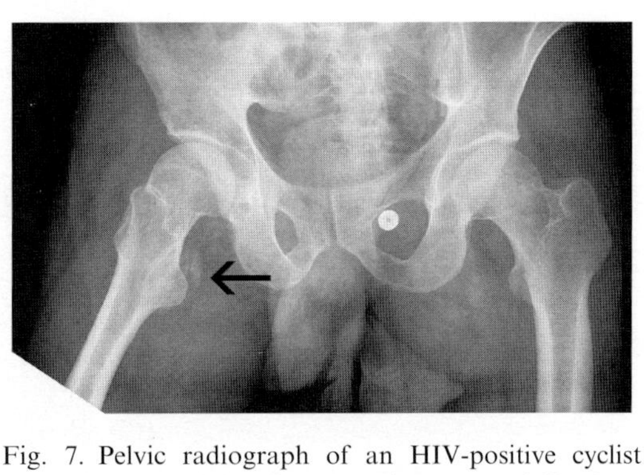

Fig. 7. Pelvic radiograph of an HIV-positive cyclist complaining of right hip pain. There are calcifications and ossifications in the iliopsoas tendon (*arrow*) adjacent to the lesser trochanter, likely related to repetitive trauma.

fracture of the lesser trochanter, and thus can be a more clinically difficult diagnosis. The clinical presentation is similar to that of patients with an avulsion fracture, where an acute snapping sensation is followed by persistent groin pain and tenderness. An anterior thigh mass, ecchymosis, and limitations in hip flexion and extension may also be encountered.

In the elderly population, an iliopsoas tendon tear may occur after a fall but can present with minimal or no history of trauma. Spontaneous rupture of the tendon in two elderly women without any history of trauma has recently been reported [28]. Rarely, tendon tears can be associated with an intra-articular hip infection, which can extend, via the iliopsoas bursa, into the iliopsoas tendon.

Iliopsoas tendon tears are best visualized on axial and coronal MR images, but sagittal images can be of use in demonstrating the extent of tendon retraction. Partial or complete discontinuity of the tendon, tendon retraction, hematoma, and edematous high T2 signal in the adjacent soft tissues as well as mass effect on the anterior hip joint capsule and iliopsoas bursitis are common findings. The tear usually involves the tendinous attachment of the iliopsoas close to or at the lesser trochanter attachment. The more lateral direct iliacus muscular attachment to the lesser trochanter, best appreciated on axial images, however, is usually preserved (Figs. 8–10) [28,29]. The latter finding may be related to the greater disposition of the tendinous attachment to degeneration or age-related attrition. Complete absence of the tendon and muscle fatty atrophy can be seen in old or chronic tears (Fig. 11) [28].

## Iliopsoas hematoma

Iliopsoas hematomas can cause femoral neuropathy or vascular compromise because of compression of the neurovascular bundle against the rigid walls of the inguinal canal [9,30–34]. The course can be benign but may necessitate prompt surgery.

Described causes of isolated iliopsoas hematomas include high-energy and contact sports injuries [30,35,36]. Bleeds after catheterization of femoral artery puncture [31] and secondary to bleeding disorders, such as disseminated intravascular coagulation and hemophilic conditions, have also been described [32–34]. The muscle is commonly involved in elderly people after a fall [29]. In a series of four reported posttraumatic hematomas with femoral nerve compression, the mechanism of injury was a fall on the back [33].

MR imaging is useful for detecting iliopsoas hematomas and for presurgical planning in cases with neurovascular compression. MR imaging can also exclude other entities that can cause neurologic symptoms, such as spinal disease, hip disorders, or muscular lesions [30]. Acute hematomas usually demonstrate low signal on all pulse sequence because of the presence of deoxyhemoglobin, whereas subacute hematomas depict high T1 and T2 signal because of the presence of methemoglobin. Fluid-fluid levels may occasionally be seen [29]. Chronic hematomas are usually of intermediate to low heterogeneous signal on all

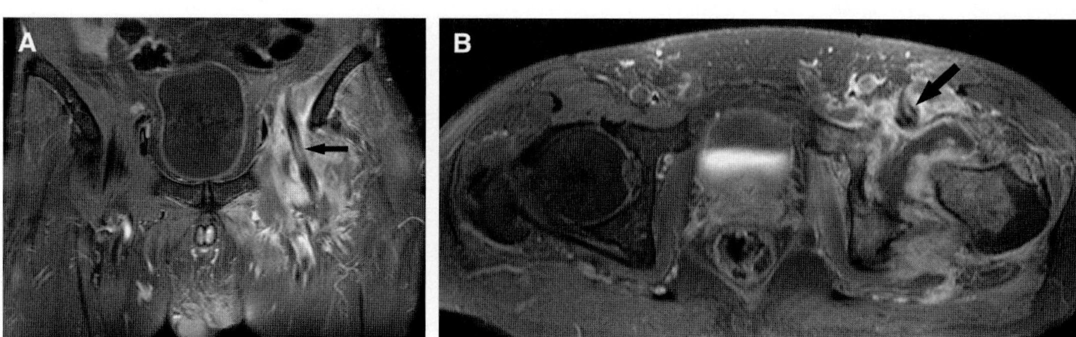


Fig. 8. Fraying of the iliopsoas tendon in a 62-year-old man with a left septic hip joint. Coronal (*A*) and axial (*B*) T1-weighted fat-suppressed images after intravenous administration of gadolinium demonstrate a thickened and heterogeneous tendon (*arrow*) embedded in infected soft tissues. Enhancement of the proximal femur, capsule, and adjacent soft tissues is seen.

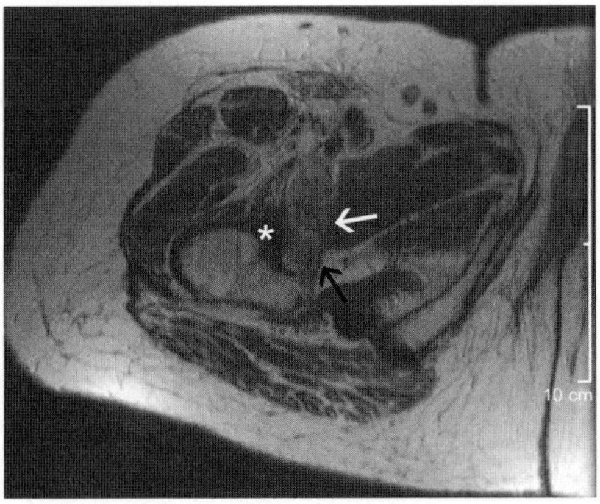


Fig. 9. Near-complete tear of the iliopsoas tendon at the insertion to the lesser trochanter. Axial T1-weighted image demonstrates only a few intact fibers (*black arrow*) inserting on the bone. There is a high signal intensity hematoma (*white arrow*) adjacent to the intact iliacus muscular attachment (*).

pulse sequences and may be difficult to distinguish from hemorrhagic soft tissue tumors.

## Myositis ossificans

Posttraumatic myositis ossificans is a condition of heterotopic nonneoplastic bone formation. Myositis ossificans of the iliopsoas muscles has been reported to be a rare cause of chronic groin pain in soccer players and ballet dancers [37,38]. In two reported cases of myositis ossificans of the iliopsoas muscle, the condition developed after trauma [39,40]. Recently, a case of myositis ossificans in the psoas muscle without a history of trauma was reported [41].

Myositis ossificans should be differentiated from malignant bone and soft tissue tumors. In its early stages, the lesion can mimic a soft tissue sarcoma, such as synovial sarcoma, rhabdomyosarcoma, or malignant fibrous histiocytoma. In its more mature stage, myositis ossificans should be distinguished from extraskeletal bone-forming tumors, such as osteosarcoma [42]. Myositis ossificans is usually self-limiting and resolves spontaneously. Treatment tends to be conservative; however, involvement of a tendon or muscle insertion, a painful mass, or function impairment may necessitate surgery [42].

Posttraumatic myositis ossificans follows a typical radiographic course. Initially, a nonspecific soft tissue mass is present. Within 7 to 14 days, thin periosteal new bone formation may be seen. Fluffy calcifications, denser at the periphery, are formed within the mass after 3 to 4 weeks. As the lesion matures, within 6 to 8 weeks, the calcifications coalesce into a lacy bone formation with a sharp peripheral cortex. Trabecular bone formation may be present [42]. Gradually, the center enlarges until the mass shows the typical appearance of an "eggshell." The final "zonal phenomena" is pathognomonic for the diagnosis.

MR imaging is the most sensitive imaging modality for diagnosing myositis ossificans but is nonspecific early on before the formation of peripheral calcifications. The MR images evolve throughout the course of the condition. Initially, the T1 signal can be normal or isointense to muscle. An inhomogeneous mass with a hyperintense center relative to fat is noted on T2-weighted images. A thin rim of low signal, when present, reflects early peripheral calcifications. Extensive muscle edema around the lesion, with low T1 and

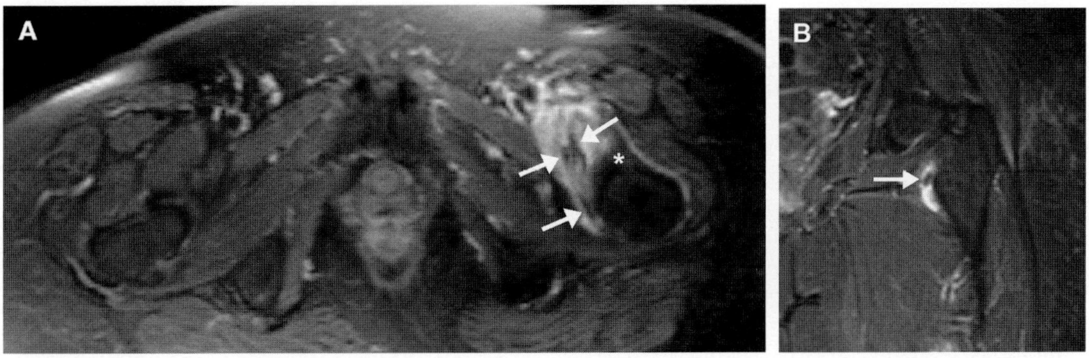


Fig. 10. Near-complete left iliopsoas tendon tear off the lesser trochanter on fluid-weighted axial (*A*) and coronal (*B*) fat-suppressed images. The iliopsoas tendon (*arrows*) is thickened and heterogeneous close to its insertion. The more lateral iliacus muscle fibers (*) are intact.

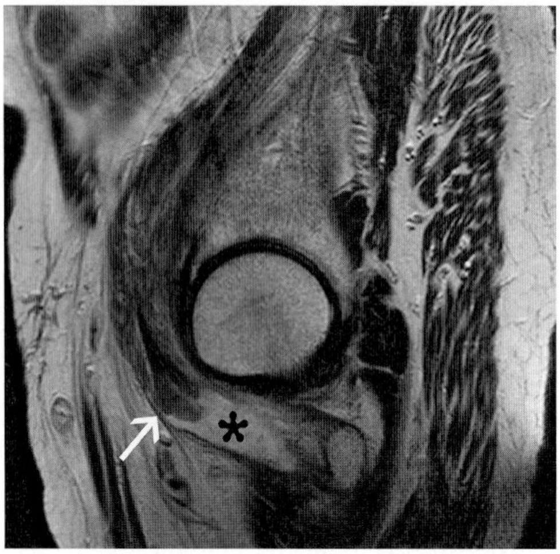

Fig. 11. Complete tear of the iliopsoas tendon. On a sagittal proton density–weighted image, there is complete interruption and retraction of the tendon (*arrow*), with a hyperintense hematoma (*) filling the gap. (Courtesy of W. Palmer, MD, and E. Nelson, MD, Boston, MA.)

high T2 signal, supports the diagnosis. With further ossification, the zonal pattern of the mass becomes evident, making the MR imaging diagnosis easier. Peripheral bone signal is noted on all pulse sequences, without surrounding edema. Rim enhancement after intravenous administration of gadolinium is nonspecific and may also be seen in tumors with central necrosis and abscesses. Not infrequently, CT is more specific than MR imaging for the diagnosis of myositis ossificans and is quite useful in demonstrating the zonal pattern of peripheral calcifications.

## Snapping hip

Snapping hip is a condition in which an audible snapping sound of variable intensity is produced during motion of the hip or during walking [43]. The causes may be intra- or extra-articular. The extra-articular snapping hip can be subdivided into two types: snapping of the iliotibial band or gluteus maximus muscle over the greater trochanter of the femur (external or lateral snap) and snapping of the iliopsoas tendon (internal or medial snap) against a bony ridge [44–47].

Iliopsoas snapping (also called internal coxa saltans) can be painful or asymptomatic [43,48–52]. When painful, it is commonly associated with iliopsoas tendinosis or bursitis [12,43,44]. Suggested mechanisms are snapping of the iliopsoas tendon over a prominent iliopectineal eminence, over the anteroinferior iliac spine, or over a bony ridge at its insertion at the lesser trochanter (Fig. 12) [53]. Accessory iliopsoas tendinous slips and iliopsoas stenosing tenosynovitis can also produce snapping of the tendon [44,54].

The diagnosis of an iliopsoas snap is based on dynamic studies in which a snapping sensation or jerk is felt during hip motion. Dynamic US during provocative motion consisting of hip flexion, abduction, and external rotation may reveal abrupt mediolateral motion of the iliopsoas tendon relative to the iliopectineal eminence [43]. Fluoroscopy after bursography or tenography is an alternative, albeit invasive, diagnostic study.

The role of MR imaging in diagnosing a snapping iliopsoas tendon is limited because of its inadequate dynamic capabilities. MR imaging is useful for excluding other extra- or intra-articular hip abnormalities [54]. MR imaging may also show concomitant iliopsoas tendinosis or bursitis.

Conservative treatment, such as rest, stretching exercises, anti-inflammatory drugs, and local steroid injection, is usually sufficient for a snapping iliopsoas tendon. In refractory cases, surgical partial release and lengthening of the tendon can be performed [43,44,55,56].

## Iliopsoas bursitis

The iliopsoas bursa, also known as the iliopectineal bursa, is present in 98% of hips [3,8,

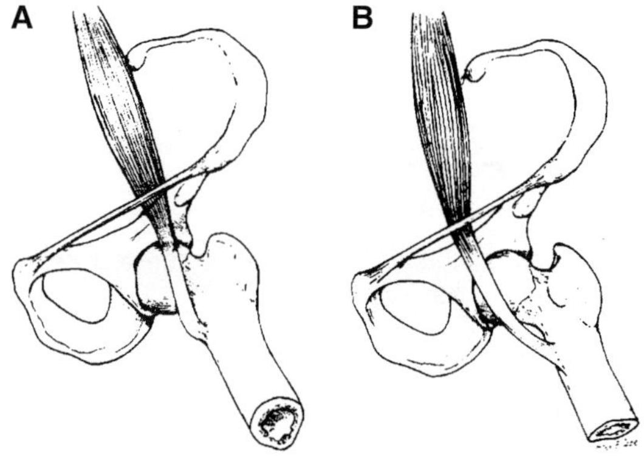

Fig. 12. Illustration of a snapping iliopsoas tendon. The tendon snaps from lateral (*A*) to medial (*B*) over the iliopectineal eminence during hip motion. (*From* Wahl CJ, Warren FR, Adler RS, et al. Internal coxa saltans [snapping hip] as a result of overuse. Am J Sports Med 2004;32(5):1304; with permission.)

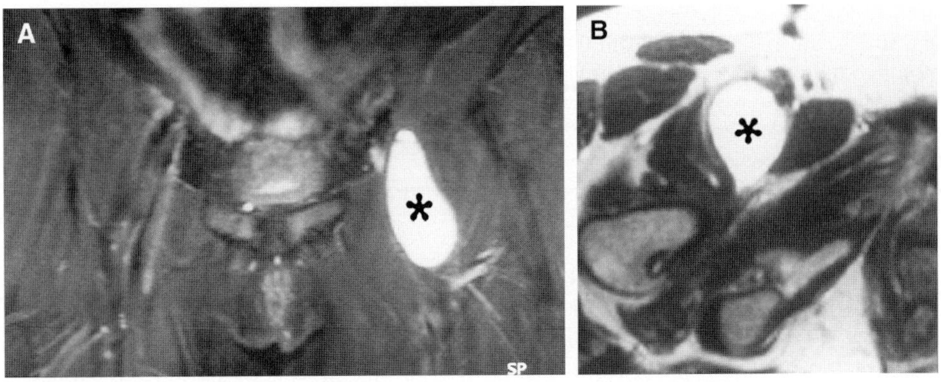


Fig. 13. Iliopsoas bursitis. Coronal T2-weighted fat-saturated (*A*) and axial T2-weighted non-fat saturated (*B*) images demonstrate an enlarged iliopsoas bursa (*).

57–59]. In 15% of the population, it communicates with the hip joint [8,57–60] via a congenital defect in the anterior capsule between the iliofemoral and pubofemoral ligaments. The gap is usually collapsed and can open when excessive intra-articular pressure is present [57–59].

Major causes of iliopsoas bursitis include acute trauma and overuse injuries as well as intra-articular diseases like rheumatoid arthritis and osteoarthritis. Less common causes include pigmented villonodular synovitis, infection, synovial chondromatosis, and gout. The cause of iliopsoas bursitis can also be idiopathic [57–61].

Overuse bursitis is caused by repetitive friction of the tendon over the iliopectineal eminence of the pubis. The condition is associated with extensive use of the hip flexors, such as in soccer, ballet, uphill running, hurdling, and jumping [62].

Detection of bursitis is often difficult on physical examination. Patients experience deep groin pain that may be hard to localize and may radiate to the anterior hip or thigh. An occasional limp may be encountered [58]. Pain is passively reproduced on deep palpation over the femoral triangle (adjacent to the femoral artery) at the musculotendinous junction of the iliopsoas [57, 62]. Pain is aggravated by active extension of the hip or, with the patient supine, by raising the heels approximately 15° off the table.

Alternatively, patients can present with a growing inguinal mass [59,63,64]. Compressive symptoms, such as leg edema, femoral neuropathy, and urinary symptoms, have been reported [59, 60,65–71]. With extreme distention, the bursa can present as a pelvic retroperitoneal, inguinal, or thigh mass [72]. Because the pain is often insidious

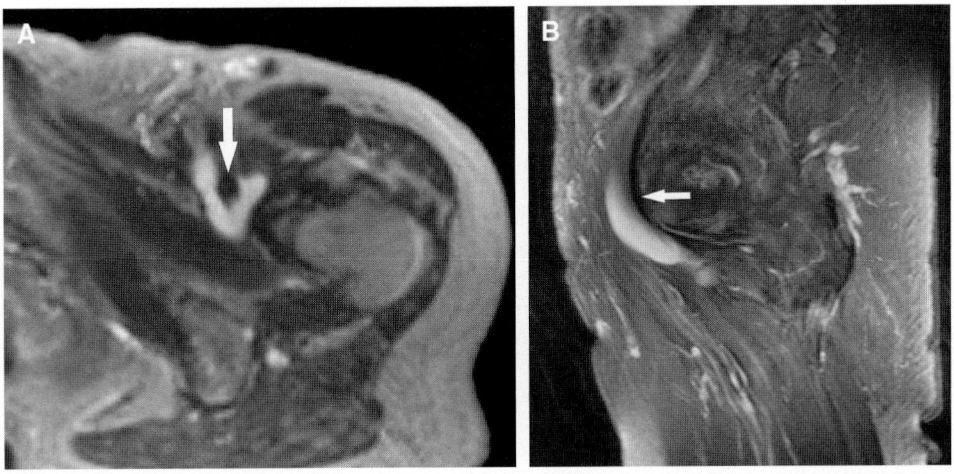


Fig. 14. Iliopsoas bursitis. Axial (*A*) and sagittal (*B*) fluid-weighted images demonstrate a hyperintense distended iliopsoas bursa surrounding the iliopsoas tendon (*arrow*).

in onset and athletes are usually highly motivated to continue training, the average time from the onset of symptoms to diagnosis has been reported to be 31 to 42 months [12,62].

Treatment of iliopsoas bursitis is conservative and consists of rest, followed by stretching of the hip flexors and rotators and US-guided corticosteroid injections. Rarely, surgical management is indicated [12].

MR imaging is an accurate modality for assessment of iliopsoas bursitis [73]. The iliopsoas bursa is seen as an elongated fluid collection located medial and posterior to the iliopsoas muscle, anterior to the hip joint, and lateral to the femoral vessels [60]. The muscle itself may be displaced laterally. Typically, the bursa shows fluid characteristics of low signal on T1-weighted images and high signal on fluid-sensitive images (Fig. 13). Postcontrast sequences reveal a thin regular rim enhancement of the bursal wall. When large, the bursa may extend into the pelvis and downward along the course of the iliopsoas tendon (Fig. 14). Complex fluid may be seen in association with pigmented villonodular synovitis, chondromatosis, infection, and hematoma [57]. Communication between the bursa of the iliopsoas muscle and the hip cavity may be demonstrated by MR imaging or US [58,60,72]. Doppler analysis is useful in differentiating iliopsoas bursitis from a pseudoaneurysm of the femoral vessels when a patient presents with a pulsatile mass [57].

## Summary

The literature describing iliopsoas compartment injuries is based on case reports and small patient series, mostly in the orthopedic literature. Nevertheless, in recent years, there has been a growing recognition of these injuries. Because many intra-articular and extra-articular bony and soft tissue injuries in the groin may clinically mimic each other, because two or more pathologic entities may coexist, and because athletes are highly motivated to continue with their physical activity, diagnosis of iliopsoas injury is often delayed. Thus, cross-sectional imaging is highly important. MR imaging is most accurate for diagnosing nondynamic diseases of the iliopsoas compartment as well as for ruling out other abnormalities of the hip joint and surrounding structures. When a snapping hip is being investigated or corticosteroid injection is warranted, US can be of help in providing a dynamic study and by guiding the injection.

## References


[1] Williams PL, Warwick R. Fascia of the muscles and lower limbs. In: Gray's anatomy. 36th edition. Edinburgh (Scotland): Churchill Livingstone; 1980. p. 593–4.

[2] Gray H. Muscles and fascia. In: Clemente CD, editor. Gray's anatomy. Philadelphia: Lea & Febiger; 1985. p. 556–8.

[3] Torres GM, Cernigliaro JG, Abbitt PL, et al. Iliopsoas compartment: normal anatomy and pathologic processes. Radiographics 1995;15(6):1285–97.

[4] Muttarak M, Peh WC. CT of unusual iliopsoas compartment lesions. Radiographics 2000;20: 53–66.

[5] Lenchik L, Dovgan DJ, Kier R. CT of the iliopsoas compartment: value in differentiating tumor, abscess, and hematoma. AJR Am J Roentgenol 1994; 162(1):83–6.

[6] Feldberg MA, Koehler PR, van Waes PF. Psoas compartment disease studied by computed tomography. Analysis of 50 cases and subject review. Radiology 1983;148(2):505–12.

[7] Van Dyke JA, Holley HC, Anderson SD. Review of iliopsoas anatomy and pathology. Radiographics 1987;7(1):53–84.

[8] Harper MC, Schaberg JE, Allen WC. Primary iliopsoas bursography in the diagnosis of disorders of the hip. Clin Orthop 1987;221:238–41.

[9] Tatu L, Parratte B, Vuillier F, et al. Descriptive anatomy of the femoral portion of the iliopsoas muscle. Anatomical basis of anterior snapping of the hip. Surg Radiol Anat 2001;23(6):371–4.

[10] Roos HP. Hip pain in sport. Sports Med Arthroscopy Rev 1997;5:292–300.

[11] Ekberg O, Persson NH, Abrahamsson PA, et al. Longstanding groin pain in athletes. A multidisciplinary approach. Sports Med 1988;6:56–61.

[12] Johnston CAM, Wiley JP, Lindsay DM, et al. Iliopsoas bursitis and tendinitis. Sports Med 1998;25: 271–83.

[13] Westlin N. Groin pain in athletes from Southern Sweden. Sports Med Arthroscopy Rev 1997;5: 280–4.

[14] Fredberg U, Hansen LB, Kissmeyer-Nielsen P, et al. Iliopsoas tendinitis in athletes. Diagnosis and treatment. Ugeskr Laeger 1995;157(28):4031–3.

[15] Fredberg U, Hansen LB. Ultrasound in the diagnosis and treatment of iliopsoas tendinitis: a case report. Scand J Med Sci Sports 1995;5(6):369–70.

[16] Shin AY, Morin WD, Gorman JD, et al. The superiority of magnetic resonance imaging in differentiating the cause of hip pain in endurance athletes. Am J Sports Med 1996;24(2):168–76.

[17] Della Valle CJ, Rafii M, Jaffe WL. Iliopsoas tendinitis after total hip arthroplasty. J Arthroplasty 2001; 16(7):923–6.
[18] Wank R, Miller TT, Shapiro JF. Sonographically guided injection of anesthetic for iliopsoas tendinopathy after total hip arthroplasty. J Clin Ultrasound 2004;32(7):354–7.
[19] Giacomini S, Di Gennaro GL, Donzelli O. Fracture of the lesser trochanter. Chir Organi Mov 2002; 87(4):255–8.
[20] Theologis TN, Epps H, Latz K, et al. Isolated fractures of the lesser trochanter in children. Injury 1997;28(5–6):363–4.
[21] Sim FH, Rock MG, Scott SG. Pelvis and hip injuries in athletes: anatomy and function. In: Nicholas JA, Hershman EB, editors. The lower extremity and spine in sports medicine. 2nd edition. London: Mosby; 1995. p. 1025.
[22] Phillips CD, Pope TL Jr, Jones JE, et al. Nontraumatic avulsion of the lesser trochanter: a pathognomonic sign of metastatic disease? Skeletal Radiol 1988;17(2):106–10.
[23] Bonshahi AY, Knowles D, Hodgson SP. Isolated lesser trochanter fractures in elderly—a case for prophylactic DHS fixation. A case series. Injury 2004; 35(2):196–8.
[24] James SL, Davies AM. Atraumatic avulsion of the lesser trochanter as an indicator of tumour infiltration. Eur Radiol 2005 Feb 9; [Epub ahead of print].
[25] Edmonds LD, Ly JQ, Carter MC, et al. Quiz case. Nontraumatic avulsion of the lesser trochanter secondary to metastatic adenocarcinoma of the colon. Eur J Radiol 2003;47(1):57–9.
[26] Afra R, Boardman DL, Kabo JM, et al. Avulsion fracture of the lesser trochanter as a result of a preliminary malignant tumor of bone. A report of four cases. J Bone Joint Surg Am 1999;81(9): 1299–304.
[27] Pisacano RM, Miller TT. Comparing sonography with MR imaging of apophyseal injuries of the pelvis in four boys. AJR Am J Roentgenol 2003;181(1): 223–30.
[28] Lecouvet FE, Demondion X, Leemrijse T, et al. Spontaneous rupture of the distal iliopsoas tendon: clinical and imaging findings. Eur Radiol 2005 Jun 16; [Epub ahead of print].
[29] May DA, Purins JL, Smith DK. MR imaging of acute traumatic fractures and muscular injuries of the hip and pelvis in elderly population. AJR Am J Roentgenol 1996;166:1075–8.
[30] Maffulli N, So WS, Ahuja A, et al. Iliopsoas haematoma in an adolescent Taekwondo player. Knee Surg Sports Traumatol Arthrosc 1996;3(4):230–3.
[31] Ozcakar L, Isik M, Erol O, et al. Iliopsoas muscle injury during a femoral artery puncture: benign but disabling. J Crit Care 2003;18(4):259–60.
[32] Turk EE, Tsokos M. Iliopsoas muscle bleeding as a complication of septic disseminated intravascular coagulation. Virchows Arch 2003;443(1):106–7.
[33] Gertzbein SD, Evans DC. Femoral nerve neuropathy complicating iliopsoas haemorrhage in patients without haemophilia. J Bone Joint Surg Br 1972; 54(1):149–51.
[34] Ashrani AA, Osip J, Christie B, et al. Iliopsoas haemorrhage in patients with bleeding disorders: experience from one center. Haemophilia 2003; 9(6):721–6.
[35] Lorei MP, Hershman EB. Peripheral nerve injuries in athletes. Treatment and prevention. Sports Med 1993;16(2):130–47.
[36] Berlusconi M, Capitani D. Post-traumatic hematoma of the iliopsoas muscle with femoral nerve entrapment: description of a rare occurrence in a professional cyclist. Ital J Orthop Traumatol 1991; 17(4):563–6.
[37] Cetin C, Sekir U, Yildiz Y, et al. Chronic groin pain in an amateur soccer player. Br J Sports Med 2004; 38(2):223–4.
[38] Petropoulos AS, Sferopoulos NK. Post traumatic myositis ossificans of the iliopsoas muscle. Apropos of a case with review of the literature. Rev Chir Orthop Reparatrice Appar Mot 1997;83(8):747–51.
[39] Ceccarelli F, Morici F, Berti L, et al. Circumscribed myositis ossificans of the iliopsoas muscle. Description of a case followed-up after 1 and 14 years. Chir Organi Mov 2004;89(2):151–9.
[40] Thorseth K. A case of traumatic myositis ossificans in the iliopsoas muscle. Acta Orthop Scand 1968; 39(1):73–5.
[41] Sirvanci M, Ganiyusufoglu AK, Karaman K, et al. Myositis ossificans of psoas muscle: magnetic resonance imaging findings. Acta Radiol 2004;45(5): 523–5.
[42] Parikh J, Hyare H, Saifuddin A. The imaging of post-traumatic myositis ossificans with emphasis on MRI. Clin Radiol 2002;57(12):1058–66.
[43] Pelsser V, Cardinal É Hobden R, et al. Extraarticular snapping hip: sonographic findings. AJR Am J Roentgenol 2001;176:67–73.
[44] Schaberg JE, Harper MC, Allen WC. The snapping hip syndrome. Am J Sports Med 1984;12:361–5.
[45] Nunziata A, Blumenfeld I. Cadera a resorte: a proposito de una variedad. Prensa Med Argent 1951; 32:1997–2001.
[46] Jones FW. The anatomy of snapping hip. J Orthop Surg (Hong Kong) 1920;2:1–3.
[47] Mayer L. Snapping hip. Surg Gynecol Obstet 1919; 29:425–9.
[48] Lyons JC, Peterson LFA. The snapping iliopsoas tendon. Mayo Clin Proc 1984;59:327–9.
[49] Dickinson AM. Case reports by Dr. Arthur M. Dickinson: bilateral snapping hip. Am J Surg 1929; 6:97–101.
[50] Howse AJG. Orthopaedists aid ballet. Clin Orthop 1972;89:52–63.
[51] Silver SF, Connell DG, Duncan CP. Case report 550: snapping right iliopsoas tendon. Skeletal Radiol 1989;18(4):327–8.

[52] Allen WC, Cope R. Coxa saltans: the snapping hip revisited. J Am Acad Orthop Surg 1995;3(5):303–8.
[53] Wahl CJ, Warren FR, Adler RS, et al. Internal coxa saltans (snapping hip) as a result of overuse. Am J Sports Med 2004;32(5):1302–9.
[54] Janzen DL, Partridge E, Logan PM, et al. The snapping hip: clinical and imaging findings in transient subluxation of the iliopsoas tendon. Can Assoc Radiol J 1996;47(3):202–8.
[55] Jacobson T, Allen WC. Surgical correction of the snapping iliopsoas tendon. Am J Sports Med 1990; 18:470–4.
[56] Brignall CG, Stainsby GD. The snapping hip: treatment by Z-plasty. J Bone Joint Surg Br 1991;73:253–4.
[57] Pritchard RS, Shah HR, Nelson CL, et al. MR and CT appearance of iliopsoas bursal distention secondary to diseased hips. J Comput Assist Tomogr 1990;14(5):797–800.
[58] Aliabadi P, Baker ND, Jaramillo D. Hip arthrography, aspiration, block, and bursography. Radiol Clin North Am 1998;36(4):673–90.
[59] Guerra J Jr, Armbuster TG, Resnick D, et al. The adult hip: an anatomic study. Part II: the soft-tissue landmarks. Radiology 1978;128(1):11–20.
[60] Lupetin AR, Daffner RH. Rheumatoid iliopsoas bursitis: MR findings. J Comput Assist Tomogr 1990;14(6):1035–6.
[61] Salmeron I, Cardenas JL, Ramirez-Escobas MA, et al. Idiopathic iliopsoas bursitis. Eur Radiol 1999;9(1):175.
[62] Morelli V, Smith V. Groin injuries in athletes. Am Fam Physician 2001;64(8):1405–14.
[63] Cheung YM, Gupte CM, Beverly MJ. Iliopsoas bursitis following total hip replacement. Arch Orthop Trauma Surg 2004;124:720–3.
[64] Byrne PA, Rees JI, Williams BD. Iliopsoas bursitis—an unusual presentation of metastatic disease. Br J Rheumatol 1996;35(3):285–8.
[65] Pellman E, Kumari S, Greenwald R. Rheumatoid iliopsoas bursitis presenting as unilateral leg edema. J Rheumatol 1986;13(1):197–200.
[66] Letourneau L, Dessureault M, Carette S. Rheumatoid iliopsoas bursitis presenting as unilateral femoral nerve palsy. J Rheumatol 1991;18(3):462–3.
[67] Rodriguez-Gomez M, Willisch A, Fernandez L, et al. Bilateral giant iliopsoas bursitis presenting as refractory edema of lower limbs. J Rheumatol 2004;31(7):1452–4.
[68] Yoon TR, Song EK, Chung JY, et al. Femoral neuropathy caused by enlarged iliopsoas bursa associated with osteonecrosis of femoral head—a case report. Acta Orthop Scand 2000;71(3):322–4.
[69] Bystrom S, Adalberth G, Milbrink J. Giant synovial cyst of the hip: an unusual presentation with compression of the femoral vessels. Can J Surg 1995; 38(4):368–70.
[70] Lavyne MH, Voorhies RM, Coll RH. Femoral neuropathy caused by an iliopsoas bursal cyst. Case report. J Neurosurg 1982;56(4):584–6.
[71] Ford MJ, Martynoga AG, Nuki G. Iliopsoas bursitis in rheumatoid arthritis: an unusual cause of leg oedema. BMJ (Clin Res Ed) 1981;282(6268): 947–8.
[72] Bianchi S, Martinoli C, Keller A, et al. Giant iliopsoas bursitis: sonographic findings with magnetic resonance correlations. J Clin Ultrasound 2002; 30(7):437–41.
[73] Wunderbaldinger P, Bremer C, Schellenberger E, et al. Imaging features of iliopsoas bursitis. Eur Radiol 2002;12(2):409–15.

ELSEVIER
SAUNDERS

Magn Reson Imaging Clin N Am
13 (2005) 717–725

MAGNETIC
RESONANCE
IMAGING CLINICS
of North America

# MR Imaging of the Proximal Rectus Femoris Musculotendinous Unit

Marcelo Bordalo-Rodrigues, MD[a], Zehava Sadka Rosenberg, MD[b,*]

[a]*Department of Radiology, Instituto de Ortopedia e Traumatologia, Hospital das Clinicas, University of Sao Paulo Medical School, Rua Dr Ovídio Pires de Campos 333, Cerqueira César, Sao Paulo 05403-010, Brazil*
[b]*Hospital for Joint Diseases, New York University School of Medicine, Bernard Aronson Plaza, 301 East 17th Street, 6th Floor, New York, NY 10003, USA*

The rectus femoris is the most commonly injured muscle of the quadriceps muscle group [1–3]. The injuries occur during forceful hip extension and knee flexion, which are common in sprinting or kicking sports, such as running, soccer, and martial arts [4]. Four main types of rectus femoris injuries are seen at the hip region: tendinous avulsions, musculotendinous strains, muscle contusions, and lacerations. The injuries, particularly deep musculotendinous junction tears, can be difficult to diagnose clinically because of their deep location and because of the infrequency of muscle retraction. This article first focuses on the normal MR anatomy of the proximal rectus femoris. This will be followed by a discussion of MR imaging's role in the detection and assessment of common sports-related injuries of the proximal rectus femoris musculotendinous unit.

## Normal anatomy

The rectus femoris is the most superficial and anterior of all the quadriceps muscles. It functions to extend the knee, generate hip flexion torque, and stabilize the pelvis upon the weight-bearing femur. The muscle has two heads of origin: the direct or straight head, which arises from the anterior inferior iliac spine (AIIS), and the indirect or reflected head, which arises from the superior acetabular ridge (Fig. 1). The two heads form the conjoined tendon slightly below their origin. The direct head is involved in the beginning of hip flexion, whereas the reflected head plays a greater role while flexion is underway.

Hasselman and colleagues [5] were the first to describe in detail the normal anatomy of the proximal rectus femoris musculotendinous unit. Based on cadaveric dissections, they noted that the direct head contributes mostly to the superficial component of the conjoined tendon and blends anteriorly with the muscle's fascia. Conversely, the indirect head contributes to the fibers of the deep, intramuscular component of the conjoined tendon and forms a deep musculotendinous junction that extends downward approximately two thirds of the muscle belly of the rectus (Fig. 2). The deep intramuscular tendon is initially located medially and is "comma-shaped." As it travels more distally within the muscle, it flattens out and migrates more laterally.

## MR anatomy

The tendinous origins of the rectus femoris muscle are easily identified on axial, sagittal, and coronal MR images as low signal intensity structures that originate from the iliac bone (Figs. 3–5). The axial images are optimal for following the course of the deep and superficial components of the tendon (see Fig. 3). The most superior axial images at the AIIS level demonstrate the origin of the direct head. Slightly more distally, the more posterior origin of the indirect head from the acetabular ridge is visualized. The indirect head appears to blend with the hip capsule at its superior origin on posterior coronal images.

* Corresponding author.
*E-mail address:* Zehava@RAMtoGO.com (Z.S. Rosenberg).

1064-9689/05/$ - see front matter 
doi:10.1016/j.mric.2005.08.005

*mri.theclinics.com*

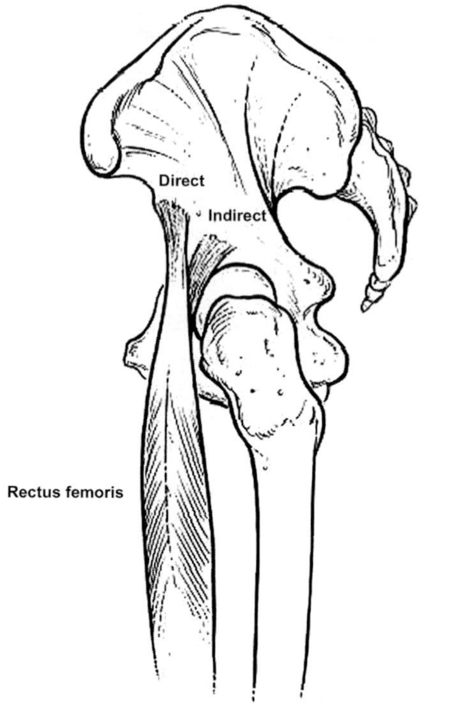


Fig. 1. Schematic drawing of the rectus femoris origin. The direct or straight head arises from the AIIS. The indirect or reflected head arises from the superior acetabular ridge. (*Adapted from* Hasselman CT, Best TM, Hughes CT, et al. An explanation for various rectus femoris strain injuries using previously undescribed muscle architecture. Am J Sports Med 1995;23:495; with permission.)

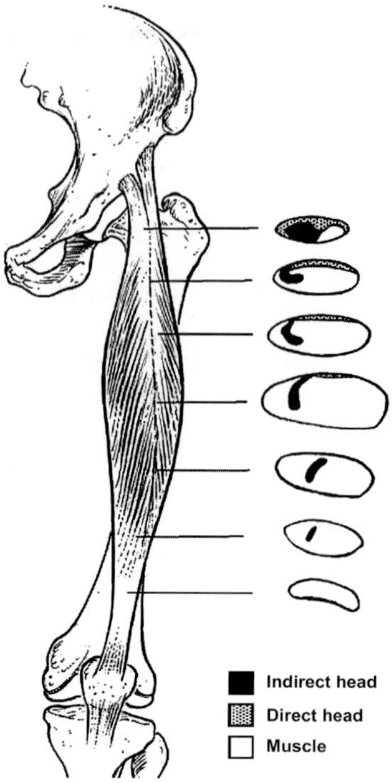


Fig. 2. Schematic drawing of the musculotendinous junction of the proximal rectus femoris. The direct head (*shaded*) and indirect head (*black*) form a conjoint tendon in the upper thigh. As the direct head migrates distally, it remains anterior to the muscle and blends with the anterior fascia in mid-thigh. The indirect head rotates from a horizontal to a more vertical orientation as it migrates into the muscle belly of the rectus. (*Adapted from* Hasselman CT, Best TM, Hughes CT, et al. An explanation for various rectus femoris strain injuries using previously undescribed muscle architecture. Am J Sports Med 1995;23:495; with permission.)

The two tendons can be followed as they move anteriorly to form the conjoined tendon on coronal and axial images (see Figs. 3 and 4). More distally, the direct head blends with the anterior fascia of the rectus femoris muscle. The indirect head rotates as it dives into the muscle belly of the muscle (see Fig. 3) and can be followed as it courses downward within the intrasubstance of the muscle into the thigh.

### Apophyseal avulsion injuries

Avulsion injury of the proximal rectus femoris is secondary to an uncoordinated powerful eccentric muscular contraction and is the third most common type of avulsion injury at the pelvis, surpassed only by hamstring and sartorius muscle injuries. In adults, the avulsion usually occurs at the tendon's attachment to the AIIS, whereas in adolescents, the avulsion is more likely to occur at the junction of the AIIS apophysis with the bone. Avulsion of the direct head at the AIIS is more frequent than avulsion of the indirect head at the superior acetabular rim because the direct head is taut in the beginning of hip flexion when tears are more likely to occur. In greater ranges of flexion, the indirect head is taut and the direct head becomes slack [6,7].

At the time of injury, patients may complain of a popping or tearing sensation in the groin and anterior thigh followed by severe pain, ecchymosis, and swelling. The pain tends to be more anterior in isolated tears of the direct head and more lateral when the indirect head is avulsed. On physical examination, tenderness at the origin of the tendons and painful decreased function of the extensor tendon mechanism are noted. A defect

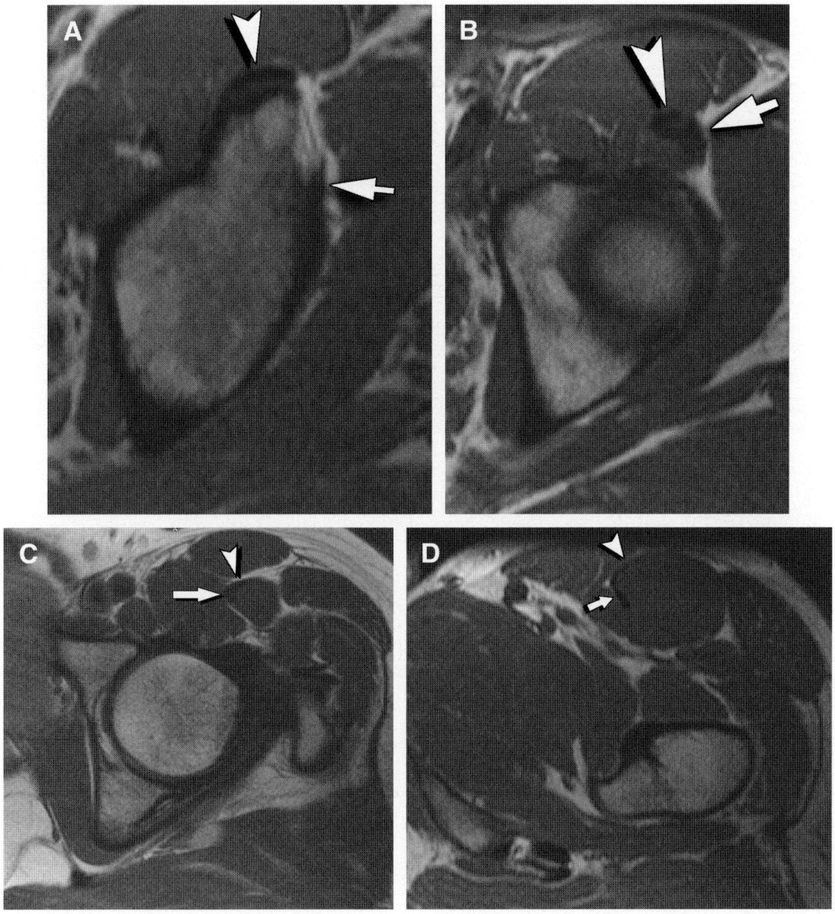


Fig. 3. Normal axial MR anatomy of the proximal rectus femoris. (*A*) Axial T1-weighted images demonstrate the origins of the direct (*arrowhead*) and indirect (*arrow*) heads. (*B*) In a slightly more distal image, the two heads form the conjoined tendon. (*C, D*) Further distally, the musculotendinous junction is depicted. The direct head (*arrowhead*) blends with the anterior fascia and the indirect head (*arrow*) rotates laterally and migrates into the muscle belly.

along the rectus femoris contour may be palpated if there is significant muscle retraction. The retracted muscle also may be present as an anterior thigh mass, more prominent during quadriceps contraction. Treatment varies depending on the extent of retraction. In adolescents, apophyseal avulsions are usually treated by rest with the hip and knee in semiflexed position [6,7].

On radiography, acute avulsions may demonstrate a displaced bone fragment, either from the AIIS or the superior acetabular ridge [8] (Fig. 6). Healing lesions may have an aggressive appearance with sclerosis and osteolysis, which can mimic infectious or tumoral processes [9,10]. Chronic avulsions that result from repetitive microtrauma also can lead to ominous looking prominent bone formation (Fig. 7).

Depiction of a displaced bone fragment at the insertion of the rectus femoris can be difficult on MR imaging (Fig. 8) and is best appreciated on plain films. MR imaging is useful for confirming the diagnosis of rectus femoris tendon avulsion, grading the tear, and determining the extent of retraction in grade 3 tears. In chronic cases, MR imaging is also useful for assessing the extent of tendon fibrosis and for presurgical planning of scar, hematoma, or pseudocyst resection.

## Musculotendinous junction injuries

Musculotendinous injuries or strains are common in the hip and pelvis and are related to excessive stretching during contraction [3]. The

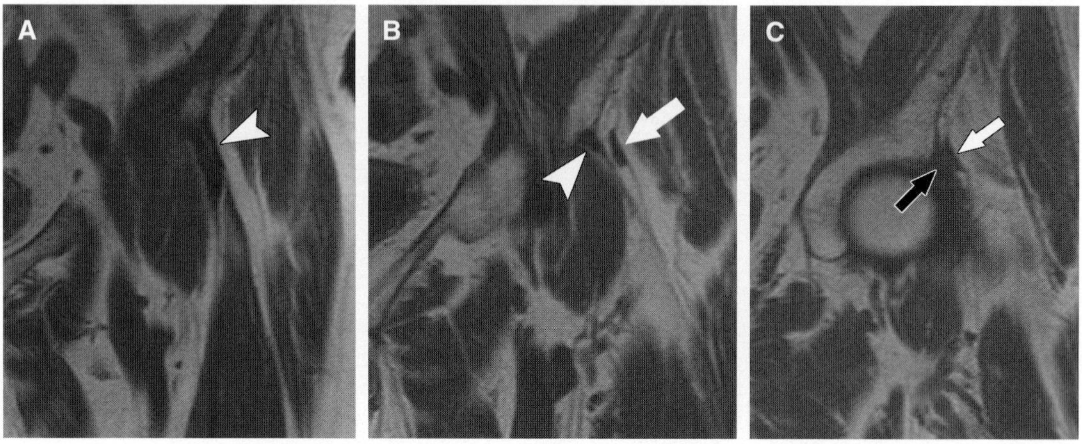


Fig. 4. Normal coronal MR anatomy of the rectus femoris origin. (*A*) Coronal T1-weighted images demonstrate the direct head origin at the AIIS (*arrowhead*). (*B, C*) The indirect head (*white arrow*) is depicted in more posterior coronal images. The acetabular labrum and the hip capsule (*black arrow*) are closely associated with the indirect head.

rectus femoris is the most commonly injured muscle of the quadriceps muscles because of its long fusiform shape, its tendency for eccentric muscle contraction, its high percentage of type II fibers, and its extension across two joints. Common predisposing factors for injury are a history of a previous tear, poor muscle conditioning, inadequate warm-up exercises, and muscle fatigue.

Classically the most common site of rectus femoris strain is at the distal musculotendinous junction at the knee level [1]. Proximal rectus femoris strains can occur at the junction of the conjoint tendon with the muscle belly. More commonly, however, proximal rectus femoris strains occur in the thigh at the deep musculotendinous junction. Rask and Lattig [11] described traumatic tears of the proximal rectus femoris at the thigh with secondary fibrotic mass. More recently, Hughes and colleagues [12] described a pattern of strain injury at the deep musculotendinous junction of the indirect head that consisted of an incomplete intrasubstance tear. This deep or central tear is probably the most commonly encountered tear of the rectus femoris tendon. A similar tear pattern also was described by De Smet and Best [13] in the hamstring muscles.

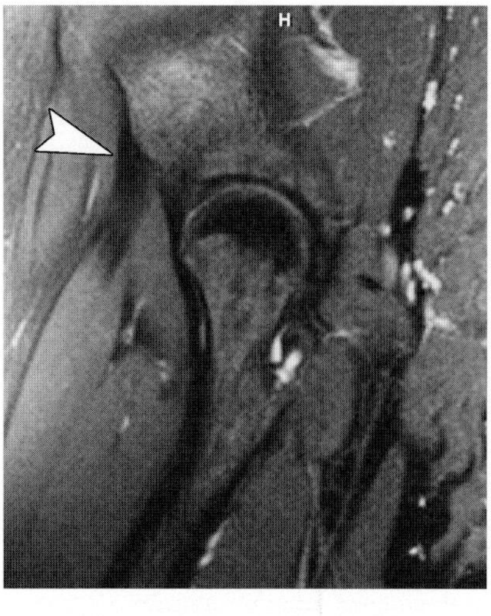


Fig. 5. Normal sagittal MR anatomy of the rectus femoris origin. Sagittal proton density-weighted image demonstrates the origin of the direct head from the AIIS (*arrowhead*).

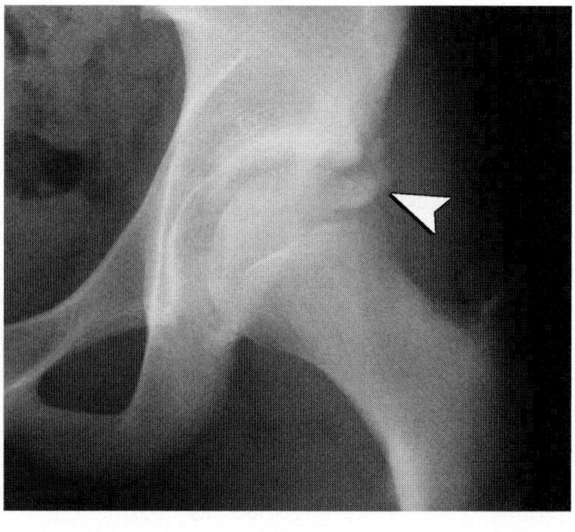

Fig. 6. Plain film of a rectus femoris avulsion. Anteroposterior radiograph of the left hip demonstrates a displaced AIIS apophysis (*arrowhead*).

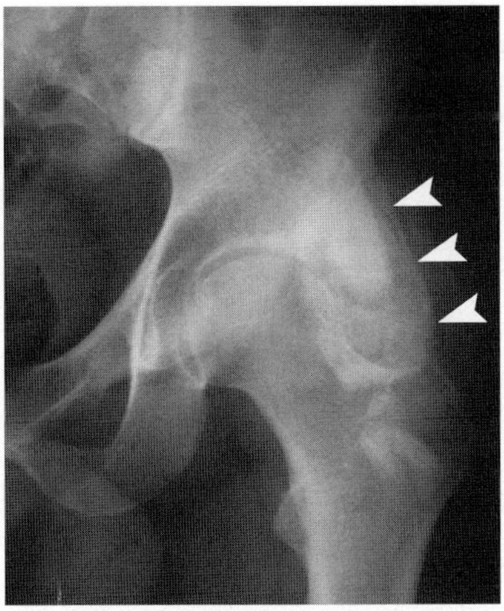

Fig. 7. Plain film of a chronic rectus femoris avulsion. Anteroposterior radiograph of the left hip shows extensive ossification at the AIIS (*arrowheads*).

The clinical presentation of proximal rectus femoris strain varies depending on the chronicity of the injury. Acutely, patients describe an acute onset of thigh pain associated with a tearing sensation. Ecchymosis, swelling, and tenderness are also noted. In the chronic or healing phase, the pain is usually aggravated by physical activity but the patient may be only mildly symptomatic during rest [12]. Atrophy with secondary girth discrepancy between the normal and injured thigh and an anterior thigh mass may be apparent. In complete tears, retraction of the mass toward the knee during muscle activation can be a distinguishing feature of proximal musculotendinous tears of the rectus femoris. In distal strains at the insertion site of the rectus to the quadriceps tendon, the mass retracts proximally during muscle activation [12].

The treatment of acute rectus femoris strains depends on the extent of injury. Most acute grade I and II strains are managed conservatively. Application of rest, ice, compression, elevation, and anti-inflammatory medication in the first 48 hours is strictly adhered to. A subsequent intensive, multistage physical therapy regimen is essential in professional athletes to prevent recurrence of the tear, because the greatest probable predisposing factor for reinjury is a history of a previous tear. Surgical intervention in grade I and II strains is uncommon except for resection of a chronic hematoma or a pseudocyst. Scar tissue can encase the tendon after deep strains and can be long, measuring up to 20 cm or more [11]. Secondary pain and tenderness, decreased extensor function, and limitation in knee flexion also may require surgical removal.

Cross categorized acute proximal rectus femoris strains into central tears, at the deep musculotendinous junction, and into the much less frequent peripheral tears, located at the periphery of the muscle [2]. Correlation of the location of the strain with recovery time indicates that deep musculotendinous injuries result in statistically longer rehabilitation time compared with peripheral ones. The mean rehabilitation interval is 26 days when the injury involves the deep tendon,

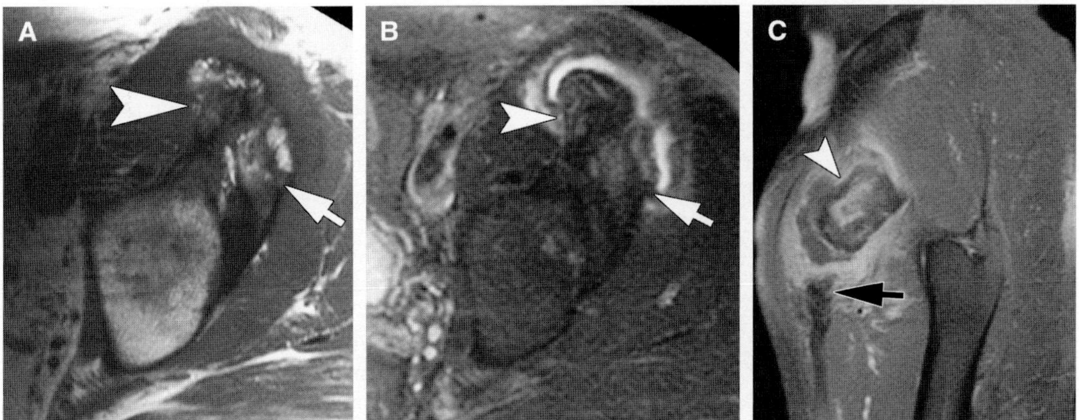


Fig. 8. MR images of heterotopic bone in chronic rectus femoris avulsion. Axial T1 (*A*) and T2-weighted (*B*) images demonstrate ossifications at the origins of the direct (*arrowhead*) and indirect (*arrow*) tendons. There is adjacent fluid collection. Sagittal T1-weighted image (*C*) obtained after intravenous administration of paramagnetic contrast media shows the ossification at the AIIS (*arrowhead*) and the retracted direct head tendon (*arrow*).

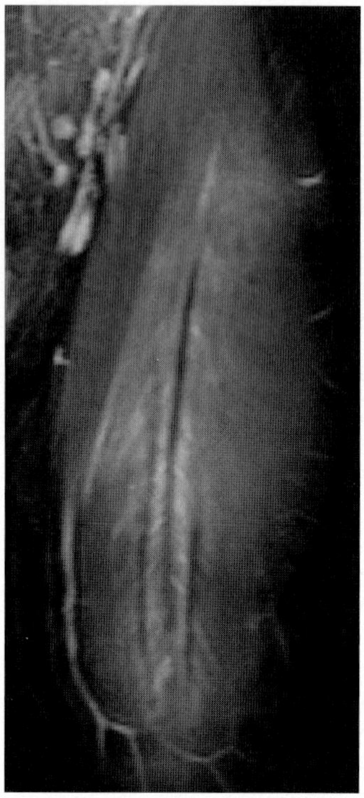

Fig. 9. Grade 1 strain at the deep musculotendinous junction of the rectus femoris. Coronal T2-weighted image shows the feathery appearance of edema around the deep tendon.

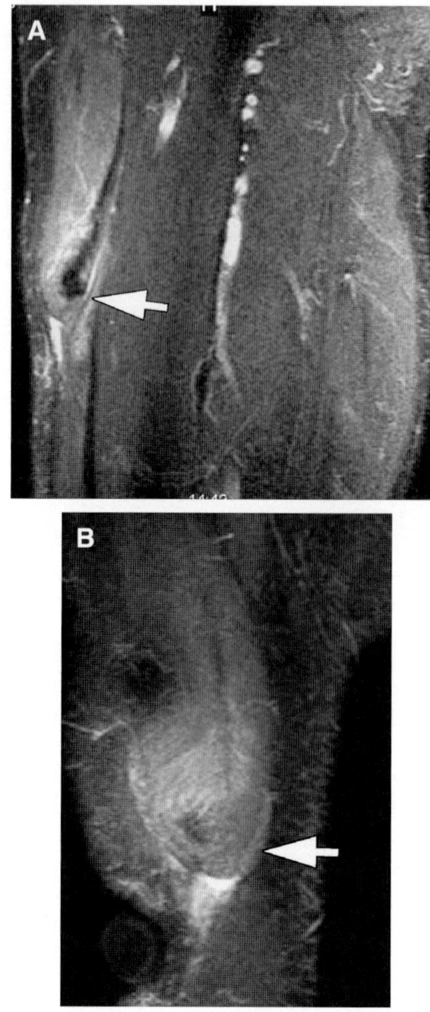


Fig. 11. Grade 3 strain of the rectus femoris. Sagittal (*A*) and coronal (*B*) T2-weighted images with fat-suppression demonstrate complete disruption at the musculotendinous junction with proximal retraction of the tendon and muscle belly (*arrow*).

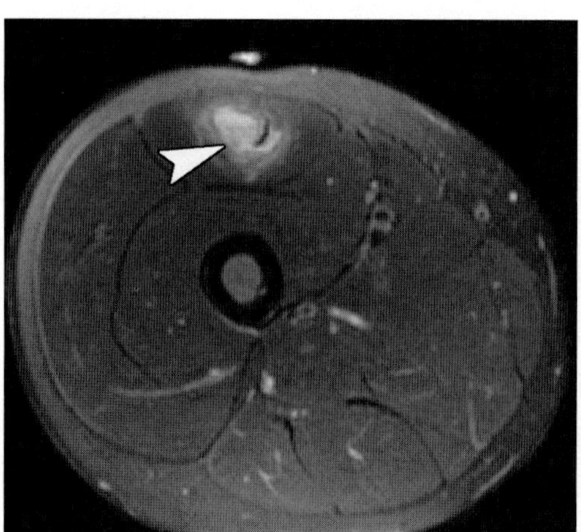

Fig. 10. Grade 2 rectus femoris strain. Axial T2-weighted image with fat suppression shows fluid collection around the deep musculotendinous junction of the rectus femoris (*arrowhead*).

whereas peripheral tears require a mean rehabilitation time of 9 days. Mid-thigh injuries have a worse prognosis than proximal injuries. Other predictive criteria for a worst prognosis are the cross-sectional area and length of muscle involvement as measured on axial MR images. Length of tendon injury more than 13 cm requires a mean of 20 days of rehabilitation, whereas shorter lengths require only 5 to 9 rehabilitation days. Similarly, cross-sectional area involvement of 15% and more indicates a mean rehabilitation time of 14 to 16 days compared with a smaller cross-sectional area, which requires 8 days of rehabilitation.

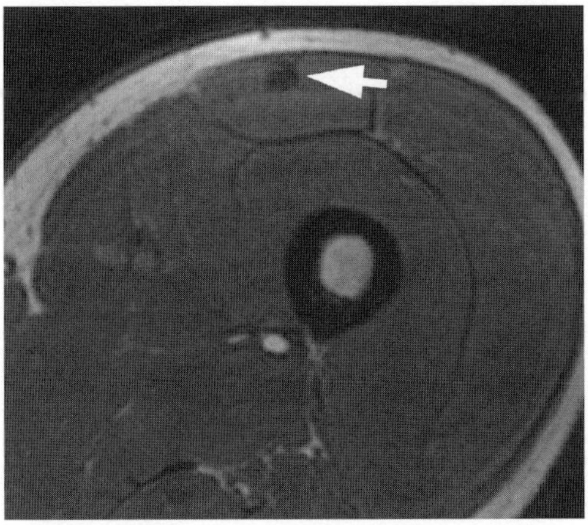

Fig. 12. Fibrous encasement of the deep tendon. Axial T1-weighted image demonstrates thickening of the deep tendon (*arrow*).

One hypothesis for the dysfunction and longer rehabilitation time associated with deep tendon injuries is that the deep and superficial tendons begin to act independently and create a shearing phenomenon [2,12].

Rectus femoris muscle strains can be graded by MR imaging [14]. A grade 1 strain is characterized by microscopic injury to the musculotendinous junction with no clinical loss of strength. MR imaging demonstrates focal or diffuse high signal intensity on fat-suppressed T2-weighted and short inversion time inversion-recovery sequences, which create a "feathery" appearance around the deep musculotendinous junction consistent with interstitial edema and hemorrhage (Fig. 9) [13,14].

Grade 2 strains are partial-thickness tears that can be associated with partial loss of muscle strength or decrease in range of motion. The MR imaging appearance varies depending on the extent of injury and chronicity of the injury. Hemorrhage and fluid around the deep musculotendinous junction greatly suggests an acute grade 2 strain (Fig. 10). A "bull's eye" appearance on fluid-sensitive sequences is often noted on multiple consecutive axial images, with the low signal deep tendon surrounded by bright signal fluid and hemorrhage [14]. A similar "bull's eye" appearance is also noted after intravenous gadolinium injection, secondary to increased vascularity and early scar tissue and healing around the centrally located, low signal tendon.

Grade 3 strains, fairly uncommon in the proximal rectus femoris [2], are complete tears with or without retraction and are associated with complete loss of strength and decreased range of motion. Diagnosis is usually made by clinical history and examination. MR imaging demonstrates a complete disruption of the deep musculotendinous junction with or without a hematoma (Fig. 11). Tendon retraction also may be seen.

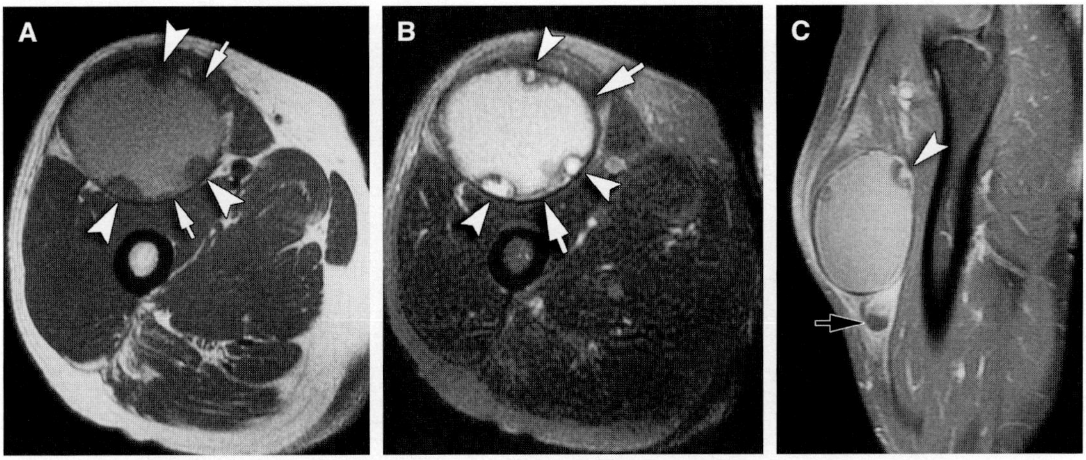


Fig. 13. Surgically proven rectus femoris hematoma that presented as a pseudotumor. Axial T1-weighted image (*A*) and T2-weighted image (*B*) show a cystic mass within rectus femoris, with a well-defined fibrous capsule (*arrows*) and some mural nodules (*arrowheads*). Contrast enhancement of the nodules (*arrowhead*) after intravenous administration of paramagnetic contrast media is noted on a sagittal T1-weighted fat suppressed image (*C*). Retraction of the distal tendon is also seen (*black arrow*).

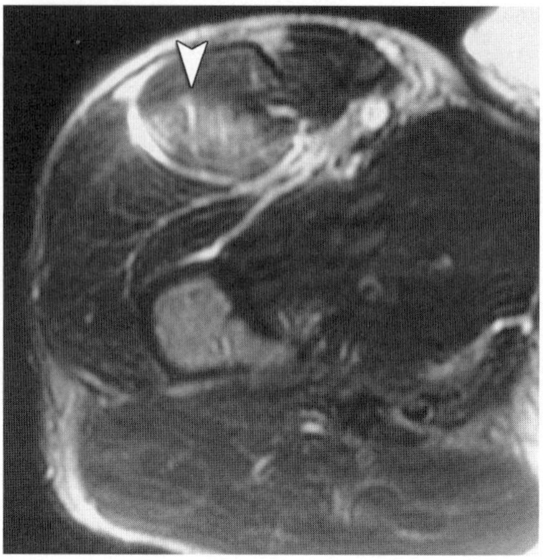

Fig. 14. Muscle contusion. Axial T2-weighted image of the mid-thigh shows increased signal within the posterior aspect of the muscle belly (*arrowhead*) with no lesion at the musculotendinous junction.

In chronic or healing rectus femoris strains, there may be a fibrous encasement of the deep tendon, characterized on MR imaging as T1 and T2 linear low signal around or adjacent to the deep tendon (Fig. 12). Muscle atrophy and fatty replacement also may be present. Occasionally, a pseudocyst, produced by serous fluid in the hematoma, is noted at the site of tear.

Not infrequently, rectus femoris tendon avulsions and strains present clinically as a soft tissue mass [11,15]. In such cases, clinical history and the association with a sport injury may elucidate the diagnosis. History of trauma may be absent, however, and MR imaging may be necessary to exclude a tumor. Chronic intramuscular hematoma, associated with rectus femoris strain, also can mimic a tumor. The hematoma can be large and can have heterogeneous signal within it because of the presence of blood products in different stages of degradation, mural nodules caused by neovascularity, and a low signal fibrous capsule (Fig. 13) [15,16]. Care should be taken to distinguish the hematoma from a soft tissue tumor. Not infrequently, however, follow-up MR imaging in a few months that depicts a decrease in the size of the hematoma may be the only way to distinguish it from a soft tissue malignancy.

## Muscle contusion and laceration

Because of its superficial location, the rectus femoris is susceptible to muscle contusions secondary to a nonpenetrating direct trauma [17,18]. Patients usually present with pain, swelling, and ecchymosis. At MR imaging, the muscle is swollen, and interstitial edema and hemorrhage without disruption are noted (Fig. 14). A common delayed complication of muscle contusion is myositis ossificans [19]. Muscle laceration is usually caused by penetrating trauma. MR imaging depicts a complete discontinuity of muscle fibers not related to the musculotendinous junction, hemorrhage, and interstitial edema (Fig. 15) [14].

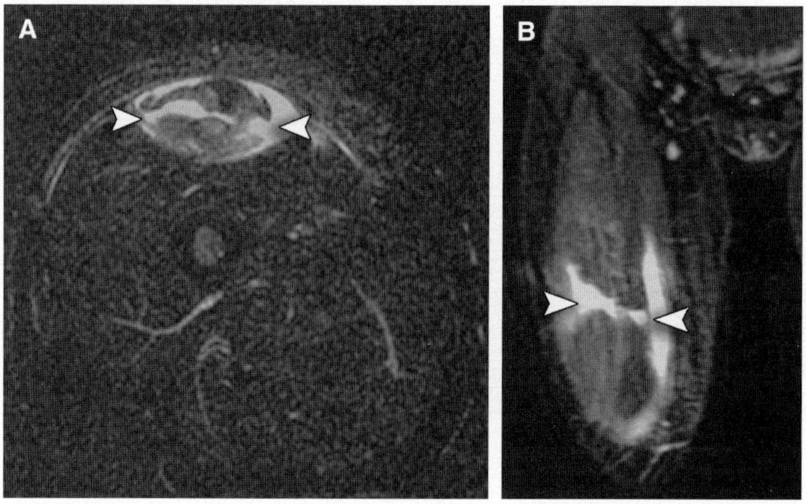


Fig. 15. Muscle laceration. Complete laceration of the midsubstance of the rectus femoris on axial (*A*) and coronal (*B*) T2-weighted images (*arrowheads*). (Courtesy of M. Schweitzer, MD, New York, NY.)

## Summary

MR imaging is a useful modality for diagnosing and grading proximal rectus femoris injuries. MR imaging is also valuable in predicting the length of recovery and rehabilitation time of musculotendinous strains and in presurgical planning when resection of a chronic hematoma, deep scar tissue, or a pseudocyst is contemplated.

## References

[1] Speer KP, Lohnes J, Garrett WE Jr. Radiographic imaging of muscle strain injury. Am J Sports Med 1993;21:89–95 [discussion: 96].
[2] Cross TM, Gibbs N, Houang MT, et al. Acute quadriceps muscle strains: magnetic resonance imaging features and prognosis. Am J Sports Med 2004;32: 710–9.
[3] Garrett WE Jr. Muscle strain injuries. Am J Sports Med 1996;24:S2–8.
[4] Renstrom PA. Tendon and muscle injuries in the groin area. Clin Sports Med 1992;11:815–31.
[5] Hasselman CT, Best TM, Hughes CT, et al. An explanation for various rectus femoris strain injuries using previously undescribed muscle architecture. Am J Sports Med 1995;23:493–9.
[6] Nanka O, Havranek P, Pesl T, et al. Avulsion fracture of the pelvis: separation of the secondary ossification center in the superior margin of the acetabulum. Clin Anat 2003;16:458–60.
[7] Deehan DJ, Beattie TF, Knight D, et al. Avulsion fracture of the straight and reflected heads of rectus femoris. Arch Emerg Med 1992;9:310–3.
[8] El-Khoury GY, Daniel WW, Kathol MH. Acute and chronic avulsive injuries. Radiol Clin North Am 1997;35:747–66.
[9] Brandser EA, el-Khoury GY, Kathol MH, et al. Hamstring injuries: radiographic, conventional tomographic, CT, and MR imaging characteristics. Radiology 1995;197:257–62.
[10] Metzmaker JN, Pappas AM. Avulsion fractures of the pelvis. Am J Sports Med 1985;13:349–58.
[11] Rask MR, Lattig GJ. Traumatic fibrosis of the rectus femoris muscle: report of five cases and treatment. JAMA 1972;221:268–9.
[12] Hughes CT, Hasselman CT, Best TM, et al. Incomplete, intrasubstance strain injuries of the rectus femoris muscle. Am J Sports Med 1995;23:500–6.
[13] De Smet AA, Best TM. MR imaging of the distribution and location of acute hamstring injuries in athletes. AJR Am J Roentgenol 2000;174:393–9.
[14] Boutin RD, Fritz RC, Steinbach LS. Imaging of sports-related muscle injuries. Radiol Clin North Am 2002;40:333–62.
[15] Temple HT, Kuklo TR, Sweet DE, et al. Rectus femoris muscle tear appearing as a pseudotumor. Am J Sports Med 1998;26:544–8.
[16] Jaovisidha S, Ryu KN, Hodler J, et al. Hemophilic pseudotumor: spectrum of MR findings. Skeletal Radiol 1997;26:468–74.
[17] Jackson DW, Feagin JA. Quadriceps contusions in young athletes: relation of severity of injury to treatment and prognosis. J Bone Joint Surg Am 1973;55: 95–105.
[18] Ryan JB, Wheeler JH, Hopkinson WJ, et al. Quadriceps contusions: West Point update. Am J Sports Med 1991;19:299–304.
[19] Huss CD, Puhl JJ. Myositis ossificans of the upper arm. Am J Sports Med 1980;8:419–24.

ELSEVIER
SAUNDERS

Magn Reson Imaging Clin N Am
13 (2005) 727–742

MAGNETIC RESONANCE IMAGING CLINICS of North America

# MR Imaging of Sports-Related Groin Pain

Erik N. Nelson, MD*, Ara Kassarjian, MD, FRCPC, William E. Palmer, MD

*Division of Musculoskeletal Radiology, Massachusetts General Hospital, 55 Fruit Street, YAW 6040, Boston, MA 02114, USA*

Sports-related groin pain is a common cause of disability and impaired activity among professional and recreational athletes. There is a particularly high incidence in sports that involve sprinting, kicking, and quick changes of direction, such as soccer, rugby, track, ice hockey, and football [1]. The extensive range of motion afforded by the hip and constant weight bearing result in repetitive stresses to the joint and to its supporting muscular and osseous structures in the pelvis, which make them particularly vulnerable to injury [2]. The complex musculoskeletal anatomy of the pelvis results in considerable overlap of clinical signs and symptoms, with many different entities causing pain referred to the hip or groin. Conditions may be acute or chronic and may involve muscle, tendon, bone, joint, nerve, or viscera.

The term "pubalgia" is applied when a patient presents with exertional pubic or groin pain in the absence of conclusive physical examination findings [1,3,4]. It is a clinical diagnosis that is invoked when no specific underlying cause for a patient's complaints can be determined by history and physical examination. This description may be replaced by a more specific diagnosis after further evaluation, including dedicated imaging evaluation of the hip and pelvis.

This article reviews these many varied causes of athletic-related groin pain and focuses on the musculoskeletal conditions most likely to be encountered during routine MR imaging.

## Techniques

### *Radiographs*

Conventional radiography remains the mainstay of initial imaging evaluation of musculoskeletal groin pain. A standard anteroposterior view of the pelvis and anteroposterior and frog-lateral views of the symptomatic hip are obtained. Particularly close attention should be paid in the assessment for subtle or nondisplaced fractures. The trabecular pattern of the acetabulum and proximal femur should be scrutinized for any discontinuity or focal areas of condensation. The anterior and posterior acetabular rims, medial walls of the acetabula, iliopubic line (anterior column), ilioischial line (posterior column), and obturator rings should be evaluated carefully. Joint space, alignment, and cortical integrity should be assessed on all views. The acetabular angle and degree of femoral head coverage can be measured [5].

The periarticular soft tissues are well demonstrated on a properly exposed conventional radiograph, and their conspicuity on digital radiography can be enhanced particularly by adjusting window and level settings. The periarticular fat pads may be displaced or effaced in the presence of a joint effusion. The gluteal, iliopsoas, obturator, and adductor muscles should be evaluated for asymmetry or other focal abnormality. Characteristic soft tissue calcifications may indicate myositis ossificans, synovial osteochondromatosis, or crystalline deposition.

### *MR imaging*

MR imaging evaluation of athletes with groin pain may begin with a survey of the pelvis and cover the sacrum, acetabula, and proximal femora

* Corresponding author.
*E-mail address:* ennelson@partners.org (E.N. Nelson).

1064-9689/05/$ - see front matter 
doi:10.1016/j.mric.2005.08.009

or may be tailored to address the symphysis pubis or a single hip. At our institution, routine MR imaging of the pelvis is performed with a torso array coil. Sequences include axial proton density (TR 3800, TE 18, slice thickness 3 mm), axial T2-weighted fat-suppressed (TR 4400, TE 78, slice thickness 3 mm), coronal inversion-recovery (TR 4000, TE 45, TI 150, slice thickness 4 mm), and coronal T1-weighted images (TR 400, TE 8, slice thickness 4 mm). In the absence of a joint effusion, evaluation of intra-articular structures of the hip is made much easier by the use of direct MR arthrography.

### *CT*

CT can be helpful for detecting or confirming nondisplaced or radiographically occult fractures or characterizing other osseous lesions. Multiplanar reconstructions assist in establishing the configuration of complex fractures and detecting intra-articular loose fragments. Soft tissue calcifications are also optimally detected and localized. CT and CT arthrography of the hip also can be useful in patients with contraindications to MR imaging.

### *Scintigraphy*

Although sensitive in the detection of fractures, bone scintigraphy lacks specificity, provides poor anatomic detail, and can be relatively time consuming in clinical practice [6,7]. A false-positive diagnosis of femoral neck stress fracture was reported one third of the time in one group of endurance athletes studied first with scintigraphy [8]. With increased availability and speed, precise anatomic detail, and the unique ability to evaluate nonosseous structures fully, MR imaging is preferred in most instances.

### *Ultrasound*

Sonographic evaluation is limited in the evaluation of adults with groin pain in the United States. Ultrasound can provide a quick and sensitive means of documenting the presence of a hip joint effusion or bursal fluid collection and may be helpful in guiding aspiration or therapeutic injections [6]. It allows the unique ability for dynamic evaluation of musculoskeletal conditions, such as in snapping hip syndromes. Real-time imaging also may be helpful in diagnosing inguinal hernias, with the ability to detect changes in the inguinal canal before and after patient straining [9]. Compared with MR imaging, ultrasound does not provide adequate evaluation of osseous structures and is considerably more operator dependent.

### *Herniography*

Before the advent of modern cross-sectional imaging, the only means by which a hernia sac could be demonstrated directly was herniography. In this procedure, positive contrast material is injected into the peritoneal cavity and fluoroscopic spot images and radiographs are obtained, which show the extension of contrast into the herniated sac. This procedure is relatively easy to perform and sensitive in hernia detection, but it is an invasive test and lacks the ability to characterize the relationship of the hernia with adjacent soft tissue structures [10]. In routine practice, herniography largely has been replaced by CT and MR imaging for the preoperative diagnosis of inguinal and femoral hernias.

## Anatomy

The ventral abdominal wall, inguinal canal, pubis, perineum, and femoral triangle come together at the groin to form an intricate intersection [11]. The hip joint and pubic symphysis are the primary articulations, and they allow complex movements and stabilize the junction of the lower extremities with the torso. The pubic symphysis is the articulation between the bodies of the two pubic bones. Hyaline cartilage lines the articular surfaces, which are separated by a thick fibrocartilaginous interpubic disc. The disc architecture is similar to that of the intervertebral discs, with a central cleft and a peripheral fibrous annulus. The annulus is well vascularized and contains numerous capillary loops, whereas the cleft is essentially avascular [12]. On average, the disc is thicker in women, which allows for increased mobility of the pelvic bones required during childbirth.

Superiorly, the symphysis is stabilized by the superior pubic ligament, which extends between the pubic tubercles of the superior pubic rami, and by the inguinal ligaments, which connect the pubic tubercle with the anterior superior iliac spine. Inferiorly, the arcuate pubic ligament spans the roof of the pubic arch and joins the lower margins of the pubic bones. Widening of the central portion of the pubic symphysis occurs among elderly persons as a result of progressive discal degeneration and increased ligamentous laxity [13].

The symphysis is stabilized anteriorly by the anterior pubic ligament and by the wide footprint that comprises the superficial fibers of the linea alba, the medial heads of the rectus abdominis muscle, and the pyramidalis muscle. This last muscle has a triangular shape, which arises from its tendinous attachment to the anterior pubic bones and anterior pubic ligament and tapers by varying degrees into the linea alba between the umbilicus and the pubis. The conjoined tendon represents the blended fibers of the inferior transversus abdominis aponeurosis and the internal oblique muscle. It passes anterior to the rectus abdominis muscle to insert on the anterior-superior aspect of the pubic bone [14].

The inguinal canal runs over a length of approximately 4 cm and extends obliquely parallel to the inguinal ligament. The anterior wall is formed by the external oblique aponeurosis and the internal oblique muscle. The posterior wall consists of the transversalis fascia and the conjoined tendon. The external (or superficial) inguinal ring is found anterior to the distal conjoined tendon [15].

At the junction of the pubis and the inferior pubic ramus there are attachments for the origins of the adductor longus, brevis, and magnus muscles, from medial to lateral. The pectineus attaches to the anterior aspect of the inferior pubic ramus. The obturator externus is a flat muscle that extends between the trochanteric fossa of the femur and the inferior pubic ramus and ischium at the medial aspect of the obturator foramen (Fig. 1) [14].

## Stress injury

Stress-related injury is a common cause of pain and limitation of activity among athletes, particularly as an individual suddenly increases the intensity or frequency of a repetitive exercise or changes the manner in which an activity is performed. It is estimated that stress-related injuries account for 10% of all presentations to sports medicine clinics and that stress fractures of the pelvis comprise up to 10% of all stress fractures [16]. Runners and jumpers are most prone to this type of injury, and women seem to be at higher risk than men [16,17]. Patients often complain of decreased range of motion and pain with weight bearing that improves with cessation of activity. In the pelvis, the proximal femur is the most common location in athletes, but one study of military conscripts showed that stress injuries of the sacrum and inferior pubic rami may be nearly as frequent [18]. A second study of military recruits also demonstrated a significant number of acetabular stress fractures that involved either the superior and lateral acetabular roof or the anterior column [16]. Lesions in any of these areas may cause pain centered primarily in the groin.

Regardless of location, the mechanism of stress injuries is the same. As normal bone is exposed to repeated loads, the accumulated forces stimulate regional remodeling, with an imbalance between osteoclastic resorption and osteoblastic new bone formation. The tensile strength of the bone is diminished, and there are multiple microtrabecular fractures. If this progresses to cortical disruption, the diagnosis of a stress fracture can be made. In addition to focal cortical discontinuity, radiographic findings of stress-related injuries include a condensation line of sclerosis typically oriented perpendicular to the long axis of the affected bone, periosteal new bone formation, and obscuration of the margins of the cortex. The MR imaging finding in an acute stress injury is a poorly marginated area of marrow edema in the affected bone—hypointense on T1-weighted images and hyperintense on short-tau inversion-recovery (STIR) or fat-suppressed T2-weighted sequences—without a discrete hypointense fracture line. With cessation of activity, these signal abnormalities typically resolve in 6 to 12 weeks [5].

If activity continues, the area of stress injury is at risk for progressing to a stress fracture, particularly in sites such as the superior and inferior pubic rami, the sacrum, and the medial femoral neck. On MR imaging, stress fractures appear as regions of marrow edema with linear hypointensities on T1- and T2-weighted sequences that often extend to a cortical surface (Fig. 2). This line is typically less distinct on the T1-weighted sequences and is more well defined on the T2-weighted images. Occasionally, the line is high in signal intensity on more heavily T2-weighted sequences. Rarely, parallel high and low intensity lines may be identified [19]. Focal periosteal new bone formation may be seen as segmental T2 hyperintensity adjacent to the cortex, and accompanying soft tissue edema or hemorrhage may be present.

## Musculotendinous injuries

Grouped together, injuries to the musculotendinous unit constitute the most common pelvic

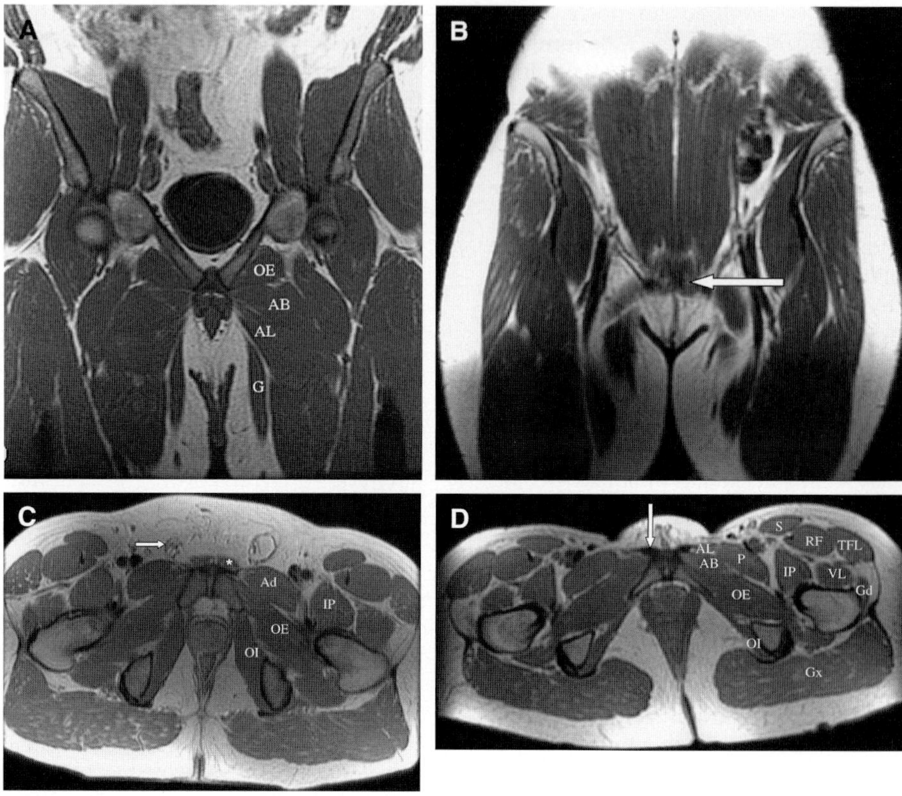


Fig. 1. Muscular anatomy of the groin. (*A, B*) Coronal T1-weighted images show the obturator externus (OE), adductor brevis (AB), adductor longus (AL), gracilis (G), and the rectus abdominis (*arrow*) muscles as they converge at the groin. (*C*) Axial proton density–weighted image at the level of the symphysis pubis shows the inguinal canal (*right, arrow*), rectus abdominis (*), adductor longus and brevis (Ad), obturator externus (OE), obturator internus (OI), and iliopsoas (IP) muscles. (*D*) A slightly more caudal image shows the adductor longus (AL), adductor brevis (AB) and their enthesis (*arrow*). The pectineus (P), sartorius (S), rectus femoris (RF), tensor fascia lata (TFL), vastus lateralis (VL), gluteus medius (Gd), and gluteus maximus (Gx) muscles are also well seen.

injuries encountered among competitive athletes, including avulsion injuries, muscle strain, tendon tear, muscle contusion, and musculofascial defects. MR imaging is ideally suited for evaluation of these injuries and it allows evaluation of the entire musculotendinous unit in multiple planes. Although radiographs and CT are still preferred for avulsion fractures and myositis ossificans, the unique inherent soft tissue resolution available on MR imaging provides a sensitive means of detecting subtle musculotendinous injuries and can evaluate for the presence of accompanying abnormalities, such as hemorrhage and muscle atrophy.

### *Avulsion*

Avulsion injuries occur at tendon attachment sites to bone after excessive muscle contraction or lengthening. The clinical presentation is focal tenderness to palpation and loss of muscle function. Radiographs of acute avulsion injuries show a discrete bone fragment adjacent to the tendon attachment site and some associated soft tissue thickening. MR imaging clearly demonstrates any marrow-containing fragments, but purely cortical avulsions may be difficult to appreciate. Stripping of the periosteum with associated edema is often visible at the tendon attachment, and a hematoma forms at the avulsion site. Laxity of the distal tendon and retraction also can be identified. Because multiple muscles often attach at a common point, the ability to demonstrate clearly the specific myotendinous unit involved is helpful. If there is compression of the sciatic nerve by an avulsed fragment or healing callous, the nerve may show enhancement on postcontrast images [19].

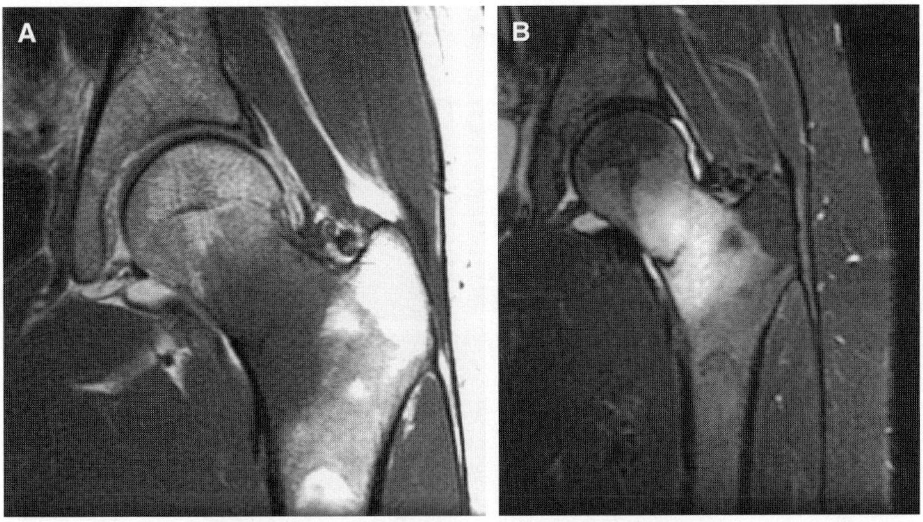


Fig. 2. Stress fracture in a 31-year-old woman training for a marathon. (*A*) Coronal T1-weighted image shows confluent hypointensity within the femoral neck, with a focal linear fracture line extending to the medial cortex. (*B*) Coronal STIR image confirms a hypointense nondisplaced fracture line within extensive marrow edema of the femoral neck.

Among athletes, pelvic avulsion injuries tend to involve characteristic locations related to their sports. Hamstring avulsion at the ischial tuberosity can occur after hyperflexion of the hip with the knee extended and is commonly seen among hurdlers, gymnasts, and dancers. The patient complains of pain referred to the buttocks and difficulty ambulating [20]. Management is usually conservative, with restricted activity for 6 to 12 weeks. Potential complications include sciatic nerve compression, either by the avulsed fragment or callous and fibrous union between the avulsed fragment and the parent bone [21].

Kicking athletes, such as soccer players, rugby players, and sprinters, may experience avulsion of the sartorius muscle from the anterior superior iliac spine or the rectus femoris muscle from the anterior inferior iliac spine. This injury typically causes focal tenderness, swelling, and skin ecchymosis, with reproduction of the pain on resisted muscle contraction [22]. Cheerleaders and other athletes who perform frequent "splits" may avulse the adductor magnus muscle from the anterior aspect of the inferior pubic ramus.

Chronic avulsion, or tenoperiosteal disease, at the symphysis pubis and inferior pubic rami occurs in runners and kicking athletes and can be a cause of groin pain. The adductor longus and gracilis are the most commonly implicated muscles, positioned in tandem at the symphysis [1,23]. With active enthesopathy, MR imaging shows marrow edema and enhancement at the anterior portions of the symphysis and often edema in the adjacent musculature that corresponds to the side of symptoms [1]. With repair, gross irregularity of the symphysis and inferior pubic rami becomes evident, with eventual development of sclerosis and subchondral cysts (Fig. 3).

The common adductor origin incorporates the adductors and gracilis muscles with the aponeurosis of the rectus abdominis muscle and provides anterior support for the symphysis pubis. An acute avulsion of this common origin can result in instability with anterior subluxation of the symphysis. Patients may present with a palpable mass at the external inguinal ring, which mimics a hernia [24]. Hockey players, skaters, and swimmers are particularly susceptible to this injury [2]. On MR imaging, the alignment abnormality of the symphysis is noted, and there may be asymmetry in size, convexity, and signal intensity of the ipsilateral rectus abdominis muscle [1]. Treatment consists of pelvic floor repair by a modified Bassini procedure and rectoplasty with or without adductor release [3,25].

A stress-related injury of the proximal femur, called the adductor insertion avulsion syndrome or "thigh splints," also may result in sports-related groin or inner thigh pain. Repetitive avulsive stress at the adductor insertion site results in a traction periostitis, which may progress to stress reaction or overt stress fractures. Patients present with tenderness to palpation over the adductor muscles and

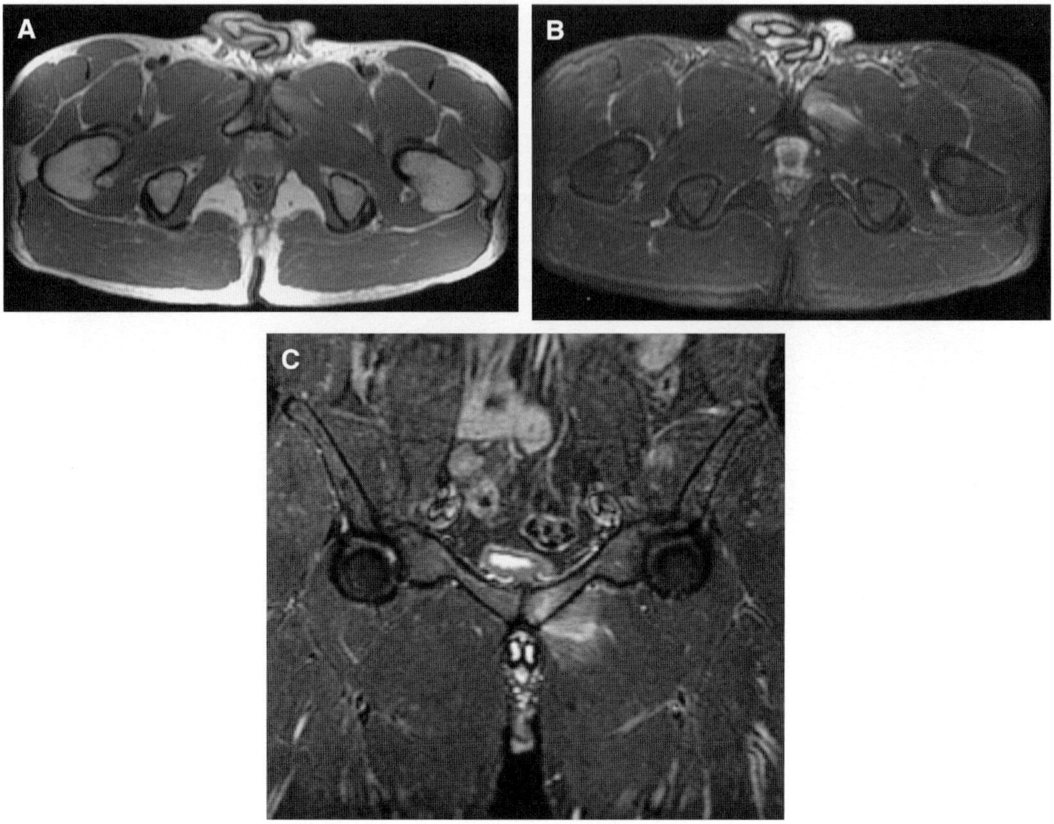


Fig. 3. Adductor avulsion in a 40-year-old man with sports-related left groin pain. Axial proton density–weighted (*A*), fat-suppressed axial T2-weighted (*B*), and coronal STIR images (*C*) demonstrate "feathery" edema within the medial adductor brevis and adductor longus muscles. T2 hyperintense edema is present within the marrow of the left pubis.

pain with resisted adduction. Radiographs may show segmental periosteal reaction along the medial aspect of the proximal femoral diaphysis, and MR imaging reveals a longitudinally oriented thin rim of T2 hyperintensity along the medial periosteum of the proximal femoral diaphysis (Fig. 4). There may be signal abnormality within the underlying marrow (stress reaction) or within the adjacent cortex (stress fracture). A pitfall in imaging is that the abnormality may be only partially included at the inferior limit of a conventional pelvic or thigh MR imaging field of view. In the absence of a fracture, thigh splints respond well to rest and limitation of activity, with return to sports in 4 to 8 weeks [22].

Avulsions of the greater (gluteus) and lesser (iliopsoas) trochanters may be seen in children and adolescents, whose apophyses are incompletely fused and weaker than the muscle or tendon. In adults, acute traumatic trochanteric avulsions are rare, and an underlying insufficiency of the bone should be suspected, such as in neoplasm or other infiltrative process [21].

### *Muscle strain*

Muscle strains occur at the myotendinous junction, which extends into the muscle belly well proximal to the apparent tendon termination. Strains at the myotendinous junction typically occur after a single traumatic event rather than as the result of a chronic overuse syndrome [26]. They are classified according to the degree of muscle function lost, ranging from none (first degree, a stretch injury), to mild (second degree, partial tear), to complete (third degree, rupture) [27]. On MR imaging, first-degree strains show hemorrhage at the myotendinous junction and a characteristic "feathery" pattern of edema that extends from the myotendinous junction along the muscle fascicles. Second-degree strains also present with a hematoma centered at the myotendinous junction,

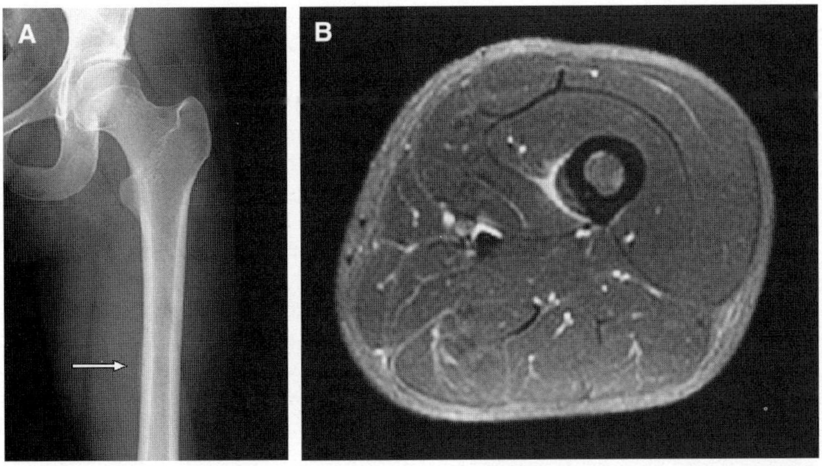


Fig. 4. Adductor insertion avulsion syndrome in a 19-year-old soccer player with left medial thigh pain. (*A*) Anteroposterior radiograph shows focal periosteal reaction along the medial aspect of the mid-left femoral diaphysis (*arrow*). (*B*) Axial T2-weighted image confirms periostits at the adductor insertion site, with associated thin rim of hyperintensity. There is no accompanying cortical signal abnormality.

and there is increased fluid adjacent to the fascicles, without tendon retraction. MR imaging of third-degree strains shows complete disruption of the myotendinous unit and is useful for assessing the extent of tendon retraction for preoperative planning (Fig. 5). It has been suggested that the presence of edema that involves more than 50% of the muscle's cross-sectional area, focal fluid collections, and deep fiber tears are associated with a prolonged recovery time [28,29].

The most commonly strained muscles at the pelvis and hip are the hamstrings (semimembranosus, semitendinosus, and biceps femoris) and the rectus femoris [28,30]. Both groups span two joints and are commonly injured during sprinting or kicking, with sudden forceful hip flexion or resisted extension [21]. Rectus femoris muscle strains can occur either distally at the quadriceps myotendinous junction or more proximally at the anterior superficial tendon of the direct head or deep intramuscular tendon of the indirect head. Distal strains present with swelling and tenderness of the posterior thigh and pain on hip flexion [28]. Hamstring strains typically occur at the proximal myotendinous junctions, near the ischial tuberosities; the biceps femoris is the muscle most commonly affected (Fig. 6) [26].

Adductor muscle dysfunction may result from tenoperiosteal disease or may be caused by myotendinous strain, especially involving the complex architecture of the adductor longus muscle [21]. Distinguishing the two is important, because aggressive rehabilitation of adductor strain injuries is often effective, whereas enthesopathic disease

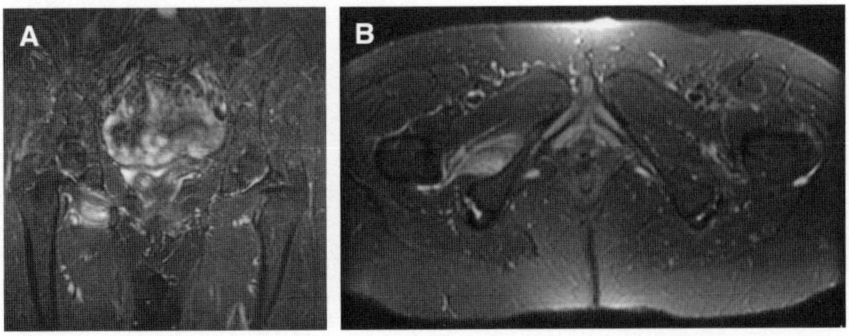


Fig. 5. Second-degree strain of the obturator externus muscle in a patient with right groin pain. Coronal STIR (*A*) and fat-suppressed axial T2-weighted (*B*) images show extensive edema within the right obturator externus muscle, with hemorrhage and perifascicular extension.

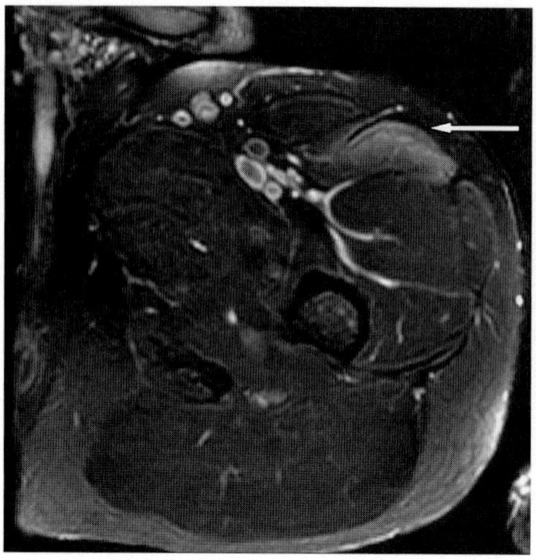

Fig. 6. A 32-year-old runner with first-degree strain of the rectus femoris. There is geographic edema surrounding the anterior superficial tendon of the direct head (*arrow*).

often progresses to prolonged, chronic groin pain [1,31]. Treatment of muscle strains consists of rest, ice, and compression, with the goal of limiting hemorrhage and soft tissue swelling. Progressive range-of-motion and strengthening exercises commence only when the patient is pain free [28].

### *Tendon tear*

Although muscle strains tend to occur after a single abrupt traumatic event, injuries of the tendons themselves more frequently result from chronic overactivity. There is progressive tendinosis, with degeneration and internal accumulation of myxoid material, which leads to weakening of the tendon with decreased tensile strength, which predisposes to partial- and full-thickness tears. On MR imaging, the normally homogeneously hypointense tendon shows focal or diffuse increased signal intensity, often with thickening. Tears appear as partial- or full-thickness tendon defects filled with T2-hyperintense fluid. Tendon retraction and muscular atrophy may be present (Fig. 7) [26,27].

Runners and dancers experience tendinosis and tears of the gluteus medius and minimus muscles and accompanying inflammation of the adjacent greater trochanteric bursa. This injury results in diffuse discomfort referred to the hip and buttocks, which is labeled the greater trochanteric pain syndrome (Fig. 8). This constellation of findings is also commonly discovered in elderly women with hip pain referred for MR imaging to exclude occult fracture. Impingement with friction from the overlying iliotibial tract is one postulated mechanism; treatment with injection of corticosteroids and local anesthesia into the bursa is often effective [32].

### *Muscle contusion*

Muscle contusions are caused by a direct blow, with injury to the deep layers of the muscle belly as the muscle is compressed against the underlying bone [33]. Among athletes, the gluteal muscles and the muscles of the anterior compartment are most frequently affected, such as in the well-known "charley horse" contusion of the quadriceps. American football players are also prone to contusions of the muscles of the iliac crest, the so-called "hip pointer" [28]. With enough force, a contusion may be accompanied by development of an intramuscular hematoma, with myonecrosis and myositis ossificans being potential complications. The femoral or lateral femoral

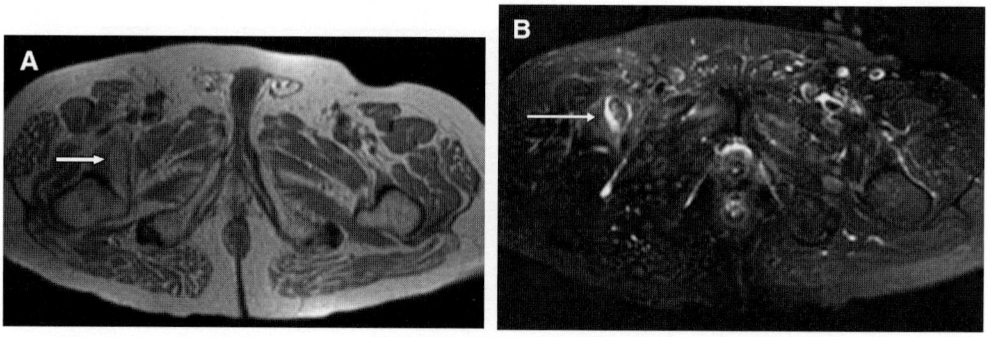


Fig. 7. Left iliopsoas tendon avulsion. (*A*) Axial proton density–weighted image shows retraction of the iliopsoas tendon with a hematoma (*arrow*) filling the gap. The retracted tendon is thickened and contains abnormal elevated T2-related signal. (*B*) Fat-suppressed T2-weighted axial image shows tendon retraction with surrounding hemorrhage (*arrow*).

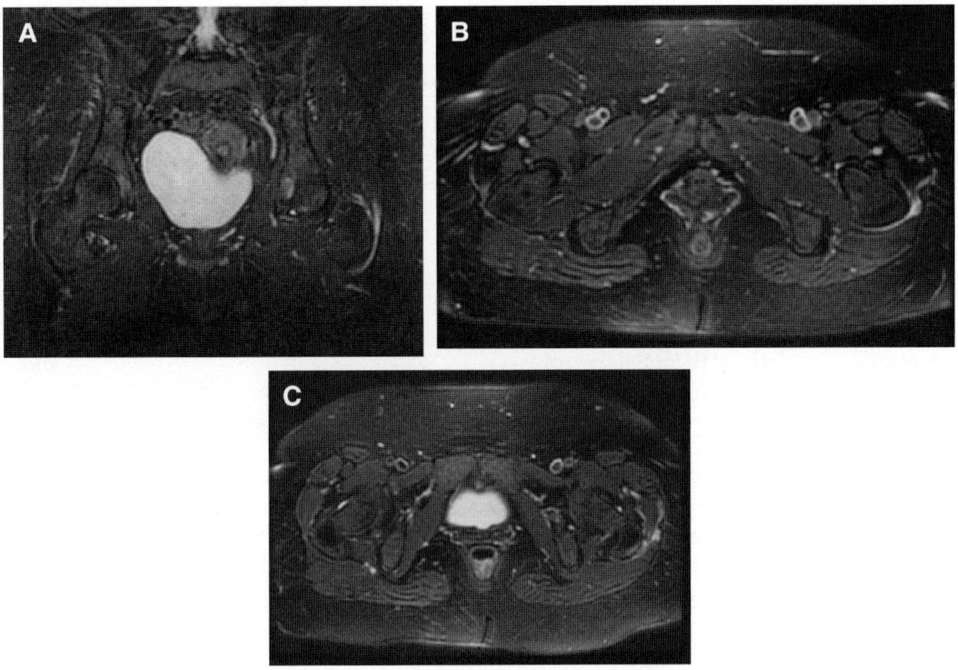


Fig. 8. Greater trochanteric pain syndrome. Coronal STIR (*A*) and fat-suppressed axial T2-weighted (*B, C*) images show a thin sheet of bursal fluid enveloping the superior and lateral aspects of the greater trochanter. There is thickening of the distal gluteus medius and minimus tendons, with intrinsic signal abnormality (*C*).

cutaneous nerve may be compressed, which results in progressive pain referred to the groin, or in meralgia paresthetica (severe burning sensation along the lateral aspect of the thigh) [28]. The sartorius and ilipsoas are the most common muscular sites of lateral femoral cutaneous nerve compression [34]. Contusions are managed conservatively with compression, ice, and non–weight bearing to limit hematoma formation followed by gradual rehabilitation; large areas of myositis ossificans may require surgical treatment.

On MR imaging, contusions appear as ill-defined areas of diffuse edema within the muscle belly, with asymmetric enlargement of the affected muscle [33]. The appearance of an intramuscular hematoma varies primarily with the age of the lesion, with acute hematoma typically isointense to adjacent muscle on T1-weighted images and hypointense on T2-weighted sequences. As the hematoma becomes subacute, the proportion of extracellular methemoglobin increases, which results in relative T1 hyperintensity and progressively increased T2 hyperintensity. With hemosiderin deposition in chronic hematoma, there is heterogeneous hypointensity on T1- and T2-weighted sequences (Fig. 9) [5]. The MR imaging appearance of myositis ossificans can be nonspecific and sometimes confusing. Some lesions have an aggressive appearance, and neoplasm may be suspected. Biopsy results also can be confounding, with areas of necrosis and hemorrhage surrounded

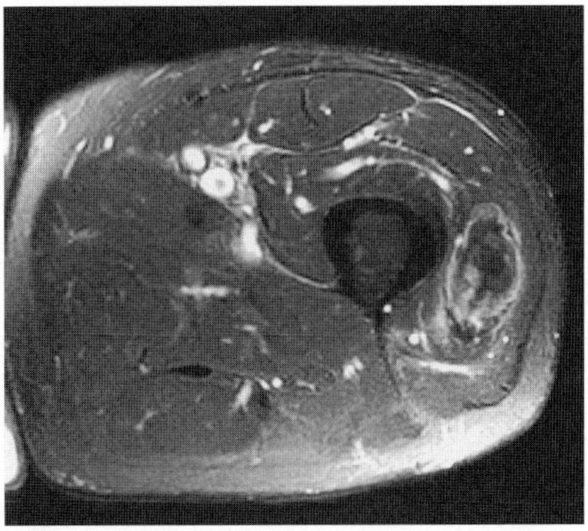

Fig. 9. Muscle contusion. Fat-suppressed axial T2-weighted image demonstrates a heterogeneous hematoma within the proximal vastus lateralis muscle. Central hypointensity represents early hemosiderin deposition.

by immature osteoblasts. Because a similar appearance can be seen in primary osteogenic sarcoma, distinguishing the two is problematic. Radiographs and CT in these instances can be helpful, because they better demonstrate the progressive peripheral calcification that is characteristic of myositis ossificans and not typical of osteosarcoma [33].

### *Musculofascial abnormalities and the "sportsman's hernia"*

In one group of athletes with pubalgia, investigators recently described abnormalities of the rectus abdominis muscle that seem to be the primary cause of the patients' groin pain. In these patients with "pubalgia caused by abdominal musculofascial abnormalities," MR imaging demonstrates attenuation or focal convexities of the abdominal wall musculature and thinning or macroscopic defects of the accompanying fascial layers. The rectus muscle may show diffuse bulge, focal tapering at the insertion, atrophy with fatty infiltration, or asymmetry in size, which correlates highly with the side and level of symptoms. These findings may occur alone or in combination with either common adductor tenoperiosteal disease or strains of the adductor and obturator muscles. Groin pain improves with pelvic floor repair; preoperative imaging is helpful in planning a unilateral versus bilateral procedure (Fig. 10) [3,4].

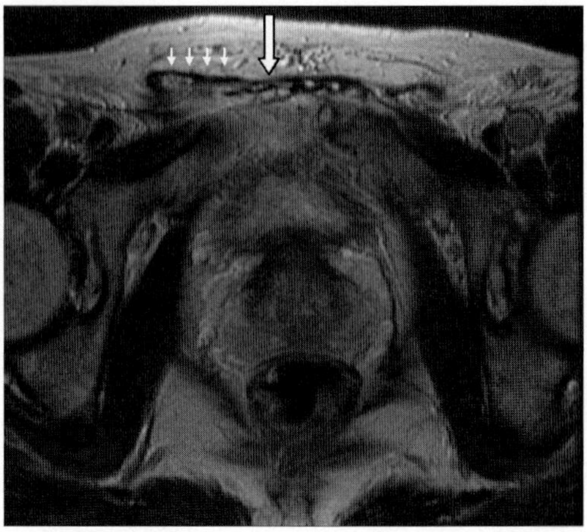

Fig. 10. Pubalgia caused by abdominal musculofascial abnormalities. Axial proton density–weighted image shows asymmetric tapering and fatty replacement of the right rectus abdominis muscle at its insertion on the pubic tubercle (*long arrow*). The patient has undergone inguinal hernia repair, with mesh in place (*short arrows*).

Pubalgia caused by abdominal musculofascial abnormalities likely represents one manifestation of a diverse entity commonly referred to as the "sportsman's hernia." Alternate names for this condition include "sports hernia," "conjoined tendon tear," "the pre-hernia complex," and "Gilmore's groin" [2,24]. The clinical presentation is chronic groin pain centered at the pubic tubercle that increases after a provoking activity or on Valsalva. Weakness on adduction can be demonstrated. Although the precise anatomic abnormality remains controversial, disruption of the inguinal canal is suspected, and a dilated external inguinal ring often can be palpated on physical examination. It is suggested that imbalance between the strong hip adductor and flexor muscles and the weaker abdominal muscles leads to chronic laxity of the transversalis fascia, disruption of the conjoined tendon, and enthesopathy of the rectus abdominis or internal oblique insertions [28]. Discrete tears in the external oblique aponeurosis can result in widening of the external ring [15]. Compression of the ilioinguinal or genitofemoral nerves near the external ring may contribute to a patient's symptoms [35,36].

As with acute avulsions at the pubic tubercle, a palpable bulge at the inguinal ring may or may not be present. Unlike an inguinal hernia, a true herniation sac is typically not present. Surgical approaches include isolated reinforcement of the transversalis fascia, reattachment of the conjoined tendon to the pubic tubercle or inguinal ligament, and standard inguinal herniorrhaphy, which is often performed laparoscopically. Resolution of symptoms after surgery has been reported in 63% to 97% of patients [4,37–40]. Proposed mechanisms by which surgery works are correction of the imbalance between the muscles of the lower abdominal wall and those of the hip, reduction in local compartmental pressures, and the implementation of an enforced period of inactivity and rehabilitation [11].

An additional overuse injury that may result in lower abdominal or groin pain is chronic tearing of the external oblique aponeurosis (which forms the anterior wall of the inguinal canal) and muscle. This injury has been described among a group of professional ice hockey players who complained of groin pain and paresthesia. Tears of the aponeurosis or muscle of varying severity were surgically confirmed, with accompanying entrapment of the ilioinguinal nerve. Return to activity was made possible by repair of the external oblique muscle and ablation of the ilioinguinal nerve [41].

Although a true inguinal hernia and its relationship with the inguinal rings and inferior epigastric vessels can be well characterized by modern MR imaging, the sportsman's hernia has fewer reliable imaging findings. The confluence of the numerous potentially involved structures at and near the pubic symphysis is complex in axial and coronal planes, and the soft tissue resolution often is inadequate in assessing for subtle abnormalities of the muscular insertions, fascia, and conjoined tendon. Dynamic images may suggest posterior inguinal canal insufficiency by demonstrating focal convexity or attenuation. Although further development of dedicated groin-imaging MR imaging techniques will occur, the diagnosis remains largely clinical [1].

## Osteitis pubis

The clinical diagnosis of osteitis pubis is based on a history of increasing groin, pubic, or lower abdominal pain and the presence of tenderness to palpation focally over the symphysis pubis, the superior pubic ramus, or the proximal adductor muscles. First described in fencers, it is also commonly encountered in runners, skaters, and soccer, rugby, and Australian rules football players, as related to kicking, twisting, and frequent lateral movements. There is increased mechanical stress across the symphysis pubis, which may compromise the ligamentous and capsular integrity of the joint and allow abnormal mobility. Over time, this laxity allows excessive impaction at the articular surfaces, and secondary degenerative changes with vertical instability may develop. Similar changes are seen with hormonally mediated ligamentous laxity in pregnant women [42]. Among athletes, the term "symphysis pubis stress injury" may be more accurate, distinguishing this entity from the osteitis pubis that is prevalent in elderly persons. This latter condition is frequently associated with infection, a finding notably absent among athletes with symphyseal stress injury [43,44]. Given the similarity in inciting mechanisms, it is not surprising that osteitis pubis often coexists with adductor tenoperiosteal disease and sportsman's hernia, and elements of these conditions may be seen concurrently. Chronic traction on the pubic ramus by the adductor muscle, gracilis muscle, or conjoined tendon may lead directly to disruption of the fibrocartilaginous symphyseal disc [45].

On radiographs, there is variable diastasis of the symphysis pubis, periarticular cortical irregularity and erosions, and sclerosis and cyst formation within the subchondral bone. Standard radiographs may be augmented by "flamingo views," performed anteroposteriorly with alternating unilateral lower extremity weight bearing. Instability is suggested when the symphysis is widened more than 7 mm or when the top surfaces of the superior pubic rami move more than 2 mm [21,42]. CT demonstrates the subchondral changes and may show "stamp erosions" or periarticular calcifications. MR imaging confirms subperiosteal resorption at the medial aspect of the pubic bones with articular surface irregularity and shows marrow edema on each side of the symphysis. Subchondral cysts may be present. Often there is deformity of the superior aspect of the symphysis with "beaking," which may extend far enough to impress on the lower surface of the urinary bladder (Fig. 11) [46]. One study showed a correlation between the extent of bone marrow edema and symphyseal beaking with the degree of clinical symptoms [44]. Sagittal images also may depict asymmetry of pubic anteversion at the symphysis [21]. There is often increased fluid intensity within the joint and edema throughout the periarticular soft tissues [19,44]. A secondary cleft sign may be identified, analogous to annular tears of the intervertebral disc, which is best seen on coronal STIR images, with the hyperintense secondary cleft contiguous with the fluid-filled primary (central) cleft and extending in an oblique linear fashion to one side. In the initial report of this finding, the side of the secondary cleft correlated in all patients with the side of symptoms, and signal abnormality was observed to continue into the ipsilateral adductor and gracilis entheses, which further supported the notion that chronic adductor enthesopathy and osteitis pubis are related conditions (Fig. 12) [45].

The osseous ring of the pelvis is interrupted at three points: the symphysis pubis and the left and right sacroiliac joints. Abnormal motion at one of these joints causes altered biomechanics with increased stress at the other two. In patients who have stress injury at the symphysis pubis, there may be simultaneous sacral stress fracture or degenerative change and instability at the sacroiliac joints. This possibility should be considered in athletes with osteitis pubis who also complain of low back or sciatic pain [43].

Treatment for osteitis pubis is usually conservative, with cessation of the inciting activity. Promising results have been reported with image-guided injection of corticosteroids and local anesthesia into the symphyseal cleft. Symphysography

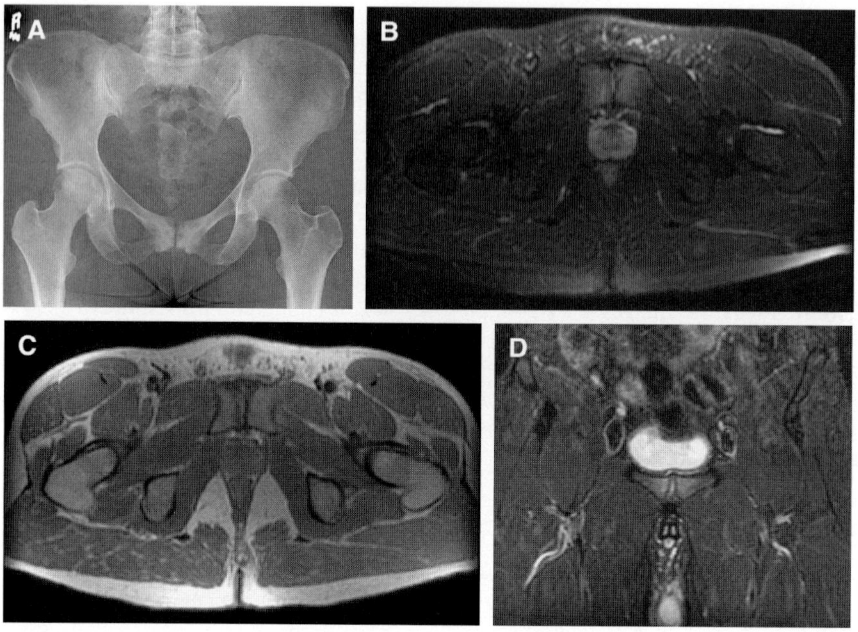


Fig. 11. Osteitis pubis. (*A*) A 26-year-old woman with pubalgia. Anteroposterior radiograph of the pelvis shows bilateral periarticular sclerosis at the pubic symphysis, subchondral lucency, articular surface irregularity, and slight superior offset of the right pubis. (*B–D*) A 35-year-old male basketball player with left groin pain. Fat-suppressed axial T2-weighted (*B*) and axial T1-weighted (*C*) images reveal sclerosis at the anterior symphysis, bilateral marrow edema, fluid in the disc, and posterior beaking. (*D*) Coronal STIR image confirms marrow edema on each side of the symphysis, fluid within the disc, and superior beaking with mild impression on the base of the bladder.

performed at the time of therapeutic injection also may be helpful in confirming the diagnosis by reproducing symptoms and demonstrating disruption of the fibrocartilaginous disc [42,45]. Surgical intervention with symphyseal arthrodesis is reserved for patients who fail conservative therapy with ongoing symptoms and imaging abnormalities [47].

## Bursa

Inflammation of the bursa can occur after direct blunt trauma or as the result of chronic irritation secondary to friction syndromes. The greater trochanteric pain syndrome is an example of the latter, with the iliotibial tract rubbing over the trochanter and causing bursitis of the subgluteus minimus, medius, and maximus bursae and tendinosis and partial-thickness tears of the distal gluteus medius and minimus tendons [32,48]. Athletes who have a wide pelvis or who adduct beyond midline are more commonly affected; running on a banked track also may predispose one to this condition [28]. Clinically, there may be a discernible "snap" as the iliotibial tract or anterior portion of the gluteus maximus muscle drags over the greater tuberosity (external snapping hip syndrome). A patient may or may not experience pain, which typically is located at the lateral aspect of the thigh or buttocks and rarely radiates to the groin [21]. MR imaging shows T2 hyperintensity superior to the greater trochanter as either a focal collection or a thin sheet covering the superior and lateral aspects of the greater trochanter [48]. Tendon thickening or apparent elongation, particularly of the gluteus medius, may be present, and there may be discernible atrophy of the gluteal muscles.

An audible snap also can occur commonly secondary to friction of the iliopsoas tendon on the iliopectineal eminence (internal snapping hip syndrome). There is usually accompanying iliopsoas bursitis, with pain referred to the hip or groin. Iliopsoas bursitis also may cause mechanical irritation of the femoral nerve, which results in pain in the anterior thigh and knee [6]. Distension of the iliopsoas bursa also can occur in the setting of degenerative joint disease of the hip, rheumatoid arthritis, or simply in the presence of a hip joint

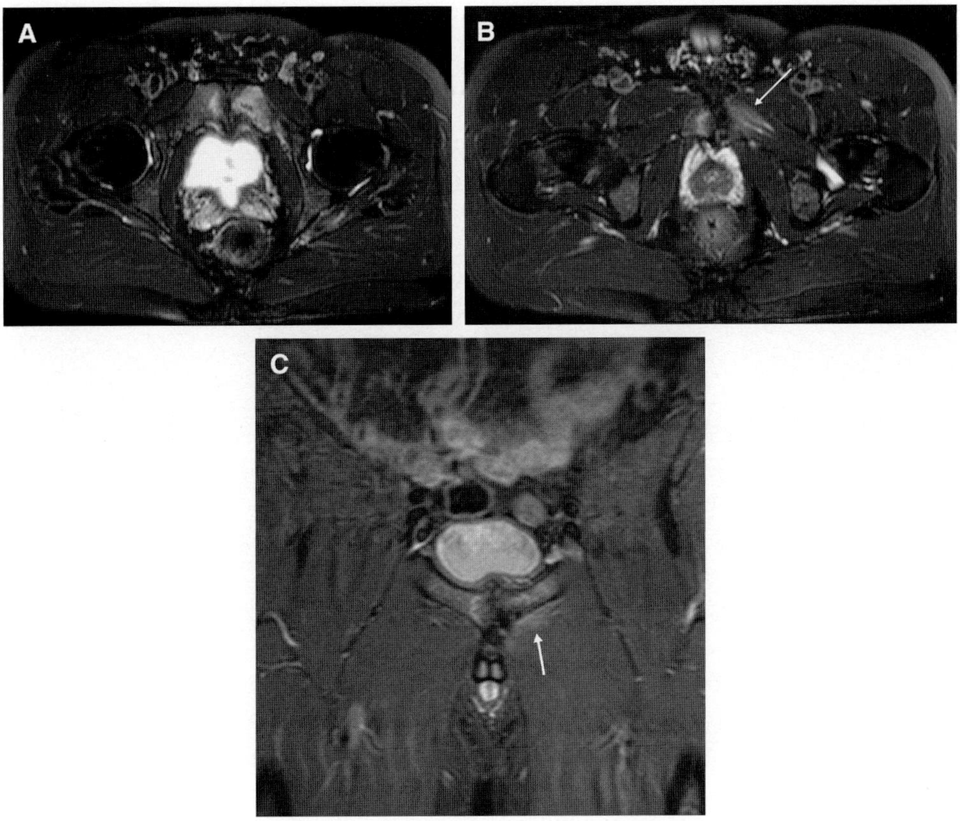


Fig. 12. Osteitis pubis. (*A*) Fat-suppressed axial T2-weighted image shows edema and articular surface irregularity within each pubic bone. Fat-suppressed axial T2-weighted (*B*) and coronal STIR (*C*) images show abnormal signal extending into the enthesis and proximal fibers of the obturator externus muscle (*arrow*).

effusion (Fig. 13). Ischiogluteal bursitis may result from friction of the long head of the biceps femoris tendon over the ischial tuberosity (posterior snapping hip syndrome) but is more frequently caused by direct trauma to the tuberosity.

## Other causes

Lumbar disc or facet joint abnormalities may result in radicular symptoms referred to the pelvis or groin. The genitofemoral nerve originates from the L1 and L2 roots, the ilioinguinal nerve from the T12 and L1 roots, and the pudendal nerve from S2, S3, and S4. Symptoms may be provoked with side- or femoral nerve stretch tests [21,28]. In cyclists, the pudendal nerve or genitofemoral nerve may be damaged by compression between the symphysis pubis and the bicycle seat, which results in neuropathy with groin pain and paresthesia. Athletes in contact sports may experience blunt trauma to the lateral femoral cutaneous nerve, with resulting anterolateral thigh pain and numbness. Skaters may experience paresthesia of the medial thigh secondary to compression of the obturator nerve by overdeveloped adductor muscles. An anomalous or hypertrophied piriformis muscle may entrap the sciatic nerve, reproducible with internal rotation of the hip.

The number of nonmusculoskeletal causes of groin pain is vast, and athletes may present with any of the potential causes of pelvic, lower abdominal, or inguinal discomfort masquerading as a sports-related injury. Inguinal, femoral, or inguinofemoral hernias occur frequently among athletes and nonathletes and may be difficult to palpate depending on size, location, or contents [3,4]. The position of the internal and external inguinal rings may be established by following the course of the spermatic cord or round ligament.

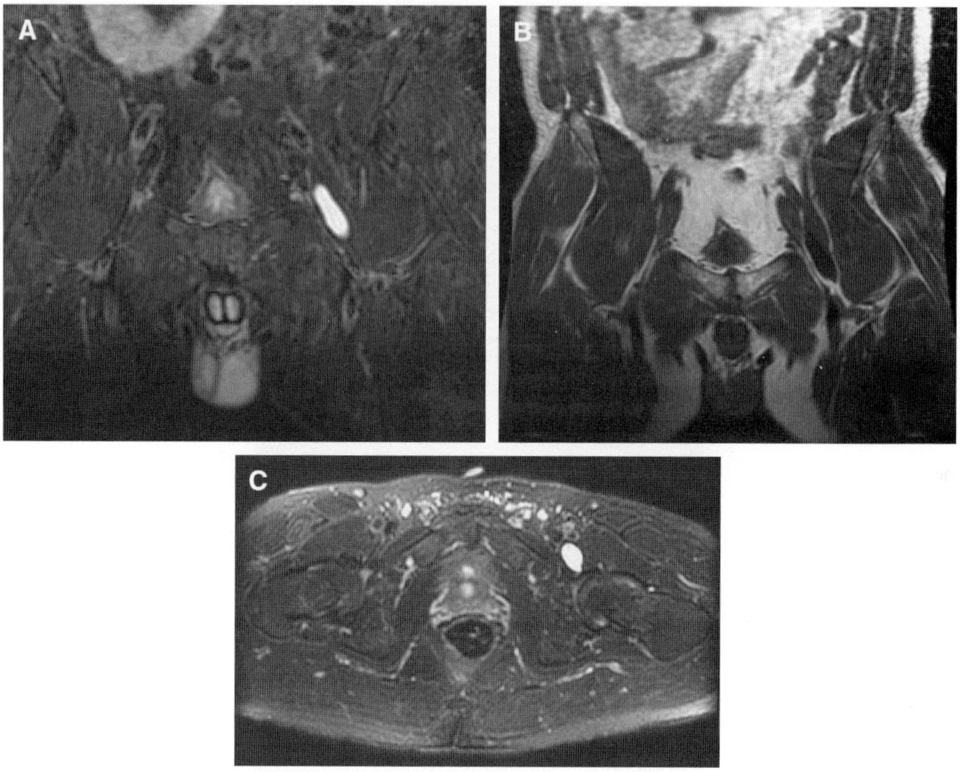



Fig. 13. Iliopsoas bursitis in a patient with left groin pain and audible snapping. Coronal STIR (*A*), coronal T1-weighted (*B*), and fat-suppressed axial T2-weighted (*C*) images show fluid distending the left iliopsoas bursa.

The inferior epigastric vessels are usually visible on axial T1- and proton density–weighted images; indirect hernias pass lateral to the inferior epigastric vessels, whereas direct hernias are medial to the vessels. Femoral hernias extend within the femoral canal medial to the femoral vein (Fig. 14) [10].

Infectious processes, such as septic arthritis and soft tissue abscess, may present initially with groin pain, with additional signs absent or subclinical in severity. Sacroiliitis, either infectious or inflammatory in nature, can produce pain referred to the groin or lower extremity. Genitourinary pathology is also notoriously difficult to localize accurately, with nephroureterolithiasis, endometriosis, ovarian cysts, epididymo-orchitis, and ovarian or testicular torsion all potentially causing groin symptoms that may initially be hard to distinguish from a musculoskeletal source. A thorough history and physical examination in combination with selected laboratory and imaging are usually sufficient in differentiating among these entities.

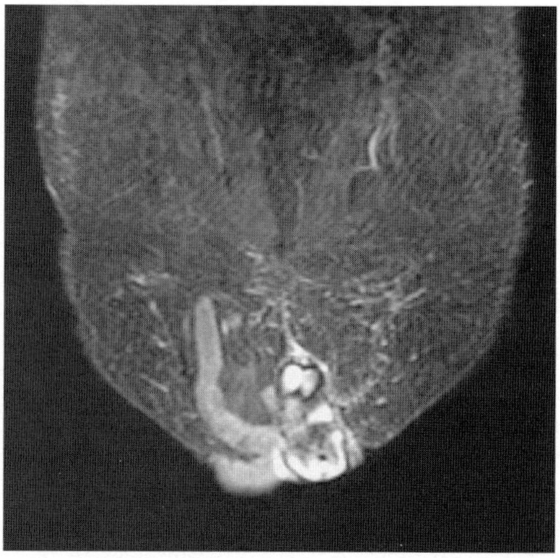

Fig. 14. Inguinal hernia in a patient with right groin pain. Coronal STIR image shows a large right inguinal hernia that contains bowel and extends into the right hemiscrotum.

## Summary

With increasing participation in professional and recreational athletics, activity-limiting pelvic and groin pain presents a growing challenge for patients and health care providers. The causes of musculoskeletal-related groin pain among athletes are diverse, with considerable overlap in history and physical examination findings. Pubalgia is a clinical diagnosis invoked when no more specific cause of a patient's symptoms can be determined on history and physical examination. In many cases, dedicated MR imaging of the hip and pelvis can provide a prompt and specific diagnosis, which allows for early treatment and return to participation.

## References

[1] Robinson P, Barron D, Parsons W, et al. Adductor-related groin pain in athletes: correlation of MR imaging with clinical findings. Skeletal Radiol 2004; 33:451–7.

[2] Rupp TJ, Purcell C. Groin injury. Available at: http://www.emedicine.com/sports/topic162.htm. Accessed June 20, 2005.

[3] Albers S, Spritzer C, Garrett W, et al. MR findings in athletes with pubalgia. Skeletal Radiol 2001;30: 270–7.

[4] Taylor D, Meyers W, Moylan J, et al. Abdominal musculature abnormalities as a cause of groin pain in athletes: inguinal hernias and pubalgia. Am J Sports Med 1991;19:239–43.

[5] Bencardino J, Kassarjian A, Palmer W. Magnetic resonance imaging of the hip: sports-related injuries. Top Magn Reson Imaging 2003;14(2):145–60.

[6] Fang C, Teh J. Imaging of the hip. Imaging 2003;15: 205–16.

[7] Holder L. Clinical radionuclide bone imaging. Radiol 1990;176(3):607–14.

[8] Shin A, Morin W, Gorman J, et al. The superiority of magnetic resonance imaging in differentiating the cause of hip pain in endurance athletes. Am J Sports Med 1996;24(2):168–76.

[9] Orchard J, Read J, Neophyton J, et al. Groin pain associated with ultrasound finding of inguinal canal posterior wall deficiency in Australian Rules footballers. Br J Sports Med 1998;32(2):134–9.

[10] Van den Berg J. Inguinal hernias: MRI and ultrasound. Semin Ultrasound CT MR 2002;23(2): 156–73.

[11] Orchard J, Read J, Verrall G, et al. Pathophysiology of chronic groin pain in the athlete. Int J Sports Med 2000;1:1.

[12] da Rocha RC, Chopard R. Nutrition pathways to the symphysis pubis. J Anat 2004;204(3):209–15.

[13] Sgambati E, Stecco A, Capaccioli L, et al. Morphometric evaluation of the symphysis pubis joint. Ital J Anat Embryol 1996;101(3):195–201.

[14] Gray H, Pick P, Howden R. Anatomy of the human body. Philadelphia: Lea & Febiger; 1985.

[15] Kemp S, Batt M. The sports hernia: a common cause of groin pain. Phys Sportsmed 1998;26(1):36–42.

[16] Williams T, Puckett M, Denison G, et al. Acetabular stress fractures in military endurance athletes and recruits: incidence and MRI and scintigraphic findings. Skeletal Radiol 2002;31:221–81.

[17] Bencardino J, Palmer W. Imaging of hip disorders in athletes. Radiol Clin North Am 2002;40:267–87.

[18] Kiuru M, Pihlajamaki H, Ahovuo J. Fatigue stress injuries of the pelvic bones and proximal femur: evaluation with MR imaging. Eur Radiol 2003;13: 605–11.

[19] Kneeland J. MR imaging of sports injuries of the hip. Magn Reson Imaging Clin N Am 1999;7(1):105–15.

[20] Stevens M, El-Khoury G, Kathol M, et al. Imaging features of avulsion injuries. Radiographics 1999;19: 655–72.

[21] De Paulis F, Cacchio A, Michelini O, et al. Sports injuries in the pelvis and hip: diagnostic imaging. Eur J Radiol 1998;27:S49–59.

[22] Anderson M, Kaplan P, Dussault R. Adductor insertion avulsion syndrome (thigh splints). AJR Am J Roentgenol 2001;177:673–5.

[23] Wiley J. Traumatic osteitis pubis: the gracilis syndrome. Am J Sports Med 1983;11(5):360–3.

[24] Holmich P, Uhrskou P, Ulnits L, et al. Effectiveness of active physical training as treatment for long-standing adductor-related groin pain in athletes: randomized trial. Lancet 1999;353:439–43.

[25] Meyers W, Foley D, Garrett W, et al. Management of severe lower abdominal or inguinal pain in high performance athletes: PAIN (Performing Athletes with Abdominal or Inguinal Neuromuscular Pain Study Group). Am J Sports Med 2000;28:2–8.

[26] Palmer W, Kuong S, Elmadbouh H. MR imaging of myotendinous strain. AJR Am J Roentgenol 1999; 173:703–9.

[27] Kaplan P, Helms C, Dussault R, et al. Osseous trauma. In: Musculoskeletal MRI. Philadelphia: WB Saunders; 2001. p. 164–5.

[28] Anderson K, Strickland S, Warren R. Hip and groin injuries in athletes. Am J Sports Med 2001;29:521–33.

[29] Verrall G, Slavotinek J, Barnes P, et al. Diagnostic and prognostic value of clinical findings in 83 athletes with posterior thigh injury: comparison of clinical findings with magnetic resonance imaging documentation of hamstring muscle strain. Am J Sports Med 2003;31(6):969–73.

[30] Koulouris G, Connell D. Evaluation of the hamstring muscle complex following acute injury. Skeletal Radiol 2003;32(10):582–9.

[31] Fricker P. Management of groin pain in athletes. Br J Sports Med 1997;31:97–101.

[32] Kingzett-Taylor A, Tirman P, Feller J, et al. Tendinosis and tears of the gluteus medius and minimus muscles as a cause of hip pain: MR imaging findings. AJR Am J Roentgenol 1999;173:1123–6.

[33] May D, Disler D, Jones E, et al. Abnormal signal intensity in skeletal muscle at MR imaging: patterns, pearls, and pitfalls. Radiographics 2000;20:S295–315.
[34] Grossman M, Dusey S, Nadler S, et al. Meralgia paresthetica: diagnosis and treatment. J Am Acad Orthop Surg 2001;9(5):336–44.
[35] Akita K, Niga S, Yamato Y, et al. Anatomic basis of chronic groin pain with special reference to sports hernia. Surg Radiol Anat 1999;21(1):1–5.
[36] Lynch S, Renstrom P. Groin injuries in sport: treatment strategies. Sports Med 1999;28(2):137–44.
[37] Hackney R. The sports hernia: a cause of chronic groin pain. Br J Sports Med 1993;27(1):58–62.
[38] Simonet W, Saylor H, Sim L. Abdominal wall muscle tears in hockey players. Int J Sports Med 1995; 16(2):126–8.
[39] Gilmore J. Groin pain in the soccer athlete: fact, fiction, and treatment. Clin Sports Med 1998;17(4): 787–94.
[40] Susmallian S, Ezri T, Ellis M, et al. Laparoscopic repair of "sportsman's hernia" in soccer players as treatment of chronic inguinal pain. Med Sci Monit 2004;10(2):CR52–4.
[41] Lacroix V, Kinnear D, Mulder D, et al. Lower abdominal pain syndrome in national hockey league players: a report of 11 cases. Clin J Sports Med 1998;8(1):5–9.
[42] O'Connell M, Powell T, McCaffery N, et al. Symphyseal cleft injection in the diagnosis and treatment of osteitis pubis in athletes. AJR Am J Roentgenol 2002;179:955–9.
[43] Major N, Helms C. Pelvic stress injuries: the relationship between osteitis pubis (symphysis pubis stress injury) and sacroiliac abnormalities in athletes. Skeletal Radiol 1997;26:711–7.
[44] Verrall G, Slavotinek J, Fon G. Incidence of pubic bone marrow oedema in Australian rules football players: relation to groin pain. Br J Sports Med 2001;35:28–33.
[45] Brennan D, O'Connell M, Ryan M, et al. Secondary cleft sign as a marker of injury in athletes with groin pain: MR image appearance and interpretation. Radiol 2005;235:162–7.
[46] Gibbon W, Hession P. Diseases of the pubis and pubic symphysis: MR imaging appearances. AJR Am J Roentgenol 1997;169:849–53.
[47] Williams P, Thomas D, Downes E. Osteitis pubis and instability of the pubic symphysis: when nonoperative measures fail. Am J Sports Med 2000; 28:350–5.
[48] Cvitanic O, Henzie G, Skezas N, et al. MRI diagnosis of tears of the hip abductor tendons (gluteus medius and gluteus minimus). AJR Am J Roentgenol 2004;182:137–43.

ELSEVIER
SAUNDERS

Magn Reson Imaging Clin N Am
13 (2005) 743–755

MAGNETIC
RESONANCE
IMAGING CLINICS
of North America

# MR Imaging of Hip Infection and Inflammation

George Koulouris, MD*, William B. Morrison, MD

*Division of Musculoskeletal and General Diagnostic Imaging, Thomas Jefferson University Hospital, 111 South Street, Gibbon Building, Philadelphia, PA 19107, USA*

Musculoskeletal infections involving the hip may constitute a true radiologic and orthopedic emergency. Pyogenic organisms are most common; however, nonpyogenic arthropathy should remain a consideration, especially given the increase in immunosuppressed patients, such as seen in AIDS and organ transplantation. Infective processes of this region can be subclassified into those involving bone (osteomyelitis), the hip joint (septic arthritis), or the surrounding soft tissues (cellulitis, abscess, and septic bursitis); however, these often coexist, particularly in advanced cases, or cases arising from contiguous spread. Though not the first line modality in the investigation of inflammatory disorders of the hip MR imaging is highly sensitive in depicting early lesions of inflammatory and degenerative arthropathies and has particular advantage in assessing the state of the articular cartilage.

## Mechanism of infection

### *Hematogenous*

Hematogenous spread is the most common mode of infectious spread around the body, and at the hip this may cause septic arthritis, bursitis, myositis, or osteomyelitis. A rich anastomosing network of periarticular vessels form the ideal situation for hematogenous seeding of microbes which have a selective adherence to synovial tissue. This hypervascular nature of the synovial membrane is reflected in its normal vivid enhancement following contrast administration on MR imaging. Joint fluid is formed as a transudate from synovial capillaries, which is further elaborated by the synovial surface cells with hyaluronic acid. This material is an excellent growth medium for many pathogens. Elastases and collagenases released by the bacteria, as well as the recruited polymorphonuclear neutrophils and synovial cells rapidly destroy the critical ground substance and matrix components of articular cartilage. Even if the majority of cartilage is salvaged with the rapid institution of antibiotic therapy and joint washout, the insult sustained may be sufficient enough for the cartilage to lose its critical biomechanical properties. Thus, an early progression to secondary osteoarthritis is possible, even despite initial successful therapy.

### *Contiguous extension*

Contiguous extension of infection is common at the hip in paralyzed patients who develop decubitus ulcers over the ischia, sacrum and greater trochanters. Infection spreads from the ulcer base to the periarticular bursae, the underlying bones as well as the hip joint. Infection may also spread to contiguous structures from pathogens implanted or hematogenously deposited in the bone or joint. Infection tracking along the iliopsoas muscle and involving the iliopsoas bursa may extend into the hip joint, as the latter often acts as a conduit for infection entering or exiting the hip joint. This is accounted for by a communication between the hip joint and iliopsoas bursa in 15% of the population with normal hips [1]. Infection may also spread along fascial planes of the pelvis; communication with the iliopsoas bursa may result in spread of infection proximally into the pelvis. Infection of the sacrum, sacroiliac joint or ischium often spreads into the adjacent sciatic notch, resulting in severe

* Corresponding author.
*E-mail address:* drgeorgek@mbox.com.au (G. Koulouris).

1064-9689/05/$ - see front matter 
doi:10.1016/j.mric.2005.09.001

radicular pain. Infection may also extend along paraspinal muscles and fascia to the facet joints and even the discs.

*Direct implantation*

This mechanism of infection is usually the result of iatrogenic inoculation [2], specifically hip arthrography, arthrocentesis, or misplaced attempts at vascular catheter insertion. Septic arthritis caused by hip joint injection is exceedingly rare, with a frequency of 1:25,000 [3]. Other forms of penetrating trauma causing hip joint infection are also uncommon. It is possible that a septic process anterior to the hip joint (such as pyomyositis or fasciitis) may mimic septic arthritis. Hence, an attempt at aspirating a sterile joint to obtain a microbiological evaluation may end up in septic arthritis of the hip as the needle tip is contaminated by the extra-articular infection.

*Postoperative*

Any joint may become secondarily infected following arthrotomy, particularly after the introduction of foreign material (eg, a prosthesis). Acute postprocedural infections, such as those following joint arthroplasty, usually relate to direct contamination at the time of surgery. Delayed infection may be secondary to latent infection at the time of operation or hematogenous seeding. In this context, assessment is difficult because the prosthesis degrades the quality of CT and MR images by way of beam hardening and magnetic susceptibility artifact, respectively. Other complications that may occur in the postoperative patient may share imaging findings seen in infection, compounding the degree of diagnostic difficulty. Recent evidence suggests that many cases of prosthetic loosening, previously designated "aseptic loosening" may be due to a chronic low grade suppurative process, or "subclinical" infection, which may act alone or in combination with the osteolytic processes involved in the foreign body granulomatous response [4]. The cellular host response results in a high turnover state of the periprosthetic bone, which is of poor quality and inevitably undergoes mechanical failure [5].

## Imaging findings: infection

*Cellulitis*

Cellulitis is an acute infection of the skin and subcutaneous tissues characterized by inflammation, rarely requiring imaging for diagnosis, the diagnosis most often being clinical. MR imaging is helpful to exclude an underlying complication or diagnose a predisposing cause, such as myositis, abscess, sinus tract, fasciitis, or osteomyelitis. MR imaging is also useful for determining the extent of involvement of the infective process. Contrast enhancement is extremely useful for evaluation of inflammation and is recommended all MR imaging protocols used for diagnosis of infection or other inflammatory processes.

On MR imaging, manifestations of cellulitis include infiltration of the subcutaneous tissues with an increase in water content [6] secondary to the production of a serous exudate (Fig. 1). Fat is

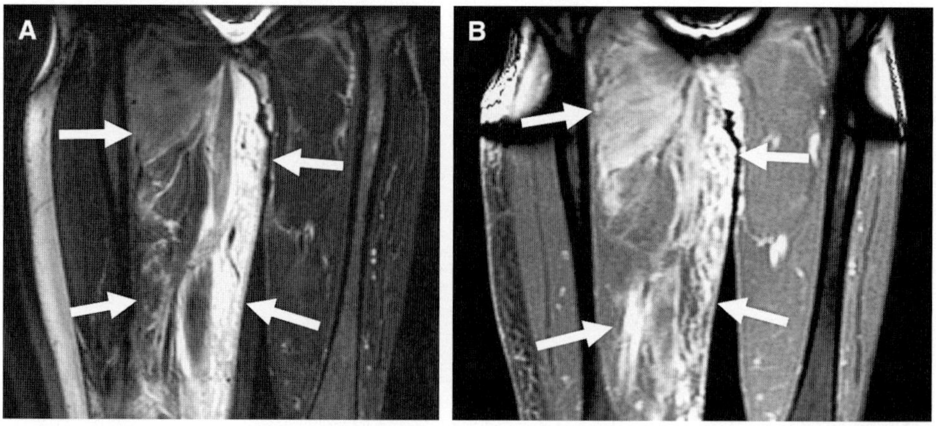


Fig. 1. Cellulitis and myositis; atypical organism (*Candida albicans*) in a patient with HIV. Coronal STIR (*A*) and post-contrast T1-weighted fat-suppressed fast multiplanar spoiled gradient echo (FMPSPGR) image (*B*) show diffuse edema and enhancement of the subcutaneous fat and adductor muscles (*arrows*) compatible with extensive infection.

metabolized within the inflammatory process. Hence, low T1 signal and high T2 signal is observed in the subcutaneous fat. Diffuse enhancement may be present after contrast administration, a factor that may distinguish noninfectious edema (eg, dependent edema) from cellulitis.

Infectious fasciitis is a true surgical emergency requiring immediate debridement and decompression as well as aggressive antibiotic therapy. Although MR imaging is very sensitive for the evaluation of fascial inflammation, fascial edema and even enhancement is not specific for clinically aggressive fascial infection. Additionally, fascial gas seen in aggressive cases may be difficult to see on routine MR imaging sequences, and delay in acquisition of the scan may preclude MR imaging as a sufficient diagnostic tool in this setting. CT may be more useful in this regard because of its wide availability, rapid acquisition, and high sensitivity for fascial gas. MR imaging remains useful for evaluating the extent of infection and presence of underlying abscess and osteomyelitis.

*Abscess*

An abscess is a localized collection of necrotic tissue, inflammatory cells, and neutrophils that is walled off by a highly vascular and typically irregular inflammatory pseudocapsule. A variable degree of surrounding soft tissue edema/cellulitis surrounds the process. Before liquefaction, an abscess is referred to as a phlegmon, an ill-defined inflammatory region of the subcutaneous or deep soft tissues without discrete fluid collection. With maturation, the infected tissue undergoes necrosis and liquefaction, thus becoming an abscess, with a peripheral hypercellular and hypervascular zone, particularly in the acute phase.

On MR imaging, the central cavity of an abscess is hypointense on T1-weighted images, but apart from asymmetric prominence of the soft tissues, the abscess may not be apparent, because the signal can be similar to that of adjacent muscle (Fig. 2). Most abscess collections are hyperintense on T2-weighted or short T1 inversion recovery (STIR) images with a variable surrounding degree

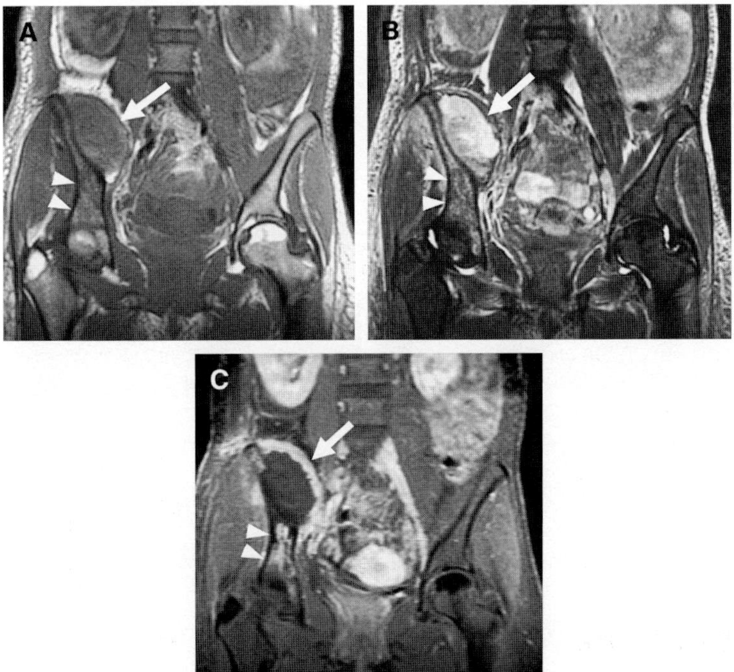


Fig. 2. Osteomyelitis and abscess in a patient with a history of fever and hip pain. Coronal T1-weighted SE (*A*), STIR (*B*), and postcontrast T1-weighted fat suppressed FMPSPGR (*C*) images show a rim-enhancing complex fluid collection (*arrow*) deep to the iliacus muscle, representing an abscess. Note signal abnormality (*arrowheads*) in the marrow of the iliac bone compared with the contralateral side, consistent with osteomyelitis.

of soft tissue edema. This edema may be quite intense and, again, the abscess cavity may blend with surrounding tissues. Fluid sensitive sequences tend to show heterogeneous signal within the abscess reflecting the necrotic tissue within. The margin, composed of hypervascular inflammatory tissue, demonstrates thick enhancement following contrast administration. The central portion remains hypointense, making the abscess cavity stand out on fat suppressed postcontrast images. The multiplanar capability of MR and soft tissue contrast make it the ideal modality in planning before surgery or percutaneous drainage. Heterotopic bone formation [7–9], as seen in spinal cord injury and following trauma, in its early stage of development may be confused with abscess formation, as these foci are also often T2 hyperintense and rim-enhance after gadolinium administration. Careful interpretation is warranted in the spinal cord injury patients, who are concomitantly at increased risk of decubitus ulcers and thus abscess formation. Gradient echo images, demonstrating blooming artifact, may be of assistance in differentiating between these two pathological processes by MR imaging.

### *Pyomyositis*

Muscle is relatively resistant to infection and as such, hematogenous pyomyositis is uncommon. However, the incidence is increased in the setting of AIDS [10] or iatrogenic immunosuppression (associated with solid organ transplantation, bone marrow transplantation, or chemotherapy) as well as intravenous drug abuse. The condition predominantly involves the lower extremities, particularly the thigh, and is multifocal in slightly less than half of cases. Secondary muscle infection may also occur related to contiguous spread from adjacent structures.

MR imaging is highly sensitive, with hyperintensity on T2-weighted or STIR images, which when diffuse (stage 1 disease) most commonly responds to conservative (antibiotic) therapy. On T1-weighted images the muscle may appear enlarged, but signal may appear relatively normal [11]. Perifascial infiltration may be seen on T1- and T2-weighted sequences. Postcontrast images show diffuse enhancement in the early stages and help separate this process from other entities such as diabetic myonecrosis. However, in later stages superimposed necrosis may also occur, and abscess formation can result in heterogeneous enhancement. With disease progression, more focal fluid collections are observed (stage 2). Postcontrast images demonstrate rim-enhancement of these small abscesses (Fig. 3). Stage 2 disease often requires more aggressive (surgical) intervention, depending on the patient's condition, size of the collections, and areas of necrosis that require debridement. Contrast-enhanced sequences can provide the surgeon with a roadmap, delineating areas requiring drainage and debridement [12]. Extension to adjacent structures resulting in septic arthritis or osteomyelitis or septicemia is considered stage 3 disease. Pyomyositis of the muscle

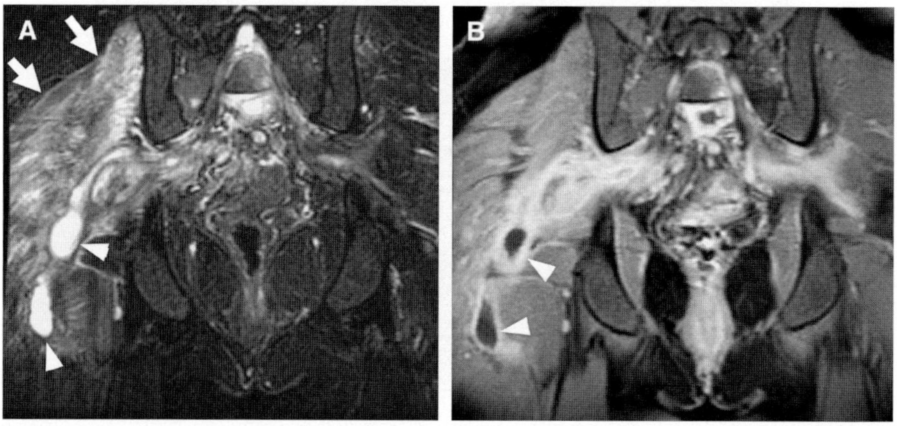


Fig. 3. Pyomyositis in a patient with history of intravenous drug abuse and sciatic pain. Coronal STIR (*A*) and postcontrast T1-weighted fat-suppressed FMPSPGR image (*B*) shows edema of the gluteus maximus muscle (*arrows*) with focal fluid collections (*arrowheads*) demonstrating rim-enhancement, representing intramuscular abscesses.

adjacent to the hip requires an accurate diagnosis, as it may be mistaken for septic arthritis of the hip [13].

Muscle edema on MR imaging is nonspecific, incorporating many differential diagnostic possibilities including injury, denervation, rhabdomyolysis, infarction and diabetic myonecrosis, polymyositis, and tumoral infiltration (sarcoma, lymphoma or metastatic disease). Hence, the value of clinical correlation is paramount.

### *Septic bursitis*

Hematogenous septic bursitis is rare; usually the cause is contiguous spread of infection, especially in paralyzed patients, or penetrating trauma. With respect to the hip, the greater trochanteric bursa is most frequently involved, related to trochanteric ulceration. Iliopsoas septic bursitis can be related to septic arthritis of the hip joint, decompressing through the hip capsule into the bursa. Because bursae are lined by synovium, the manifestations of bursal infection are similar to that seen in septic arthritis. Focal fluid signal corresponding to the bursal location with thick rim enhancement is characteristic (Fig. 4). However, this finding is not specific, and mechanical bursitis or inflammatory bursitis related to rheumatoid arthritis can appear identical. Obese patients often have fluid in the greater trochanteric bursa incidentally. In this situation, the finding is bilateral and symmetric. Paralyzed patients often develop heterotopic ossification at the hip bursae, which in early stages can appear similar to infection with fluid signal and rim enhancement [7,14].

### *Septic arthritis*

MR imaging is very sensitive for the detection of joint effusion, the hallmark feature of any type of arthritis. In septic arthritis, fluid is often complex [15,16], particularly in chronic infection. Complex effusion is also a characteristic of other noninfectious inflammatory arthropathies such as rheumatoid arthritis. Similar to septic bursitis, thick rim enhancement is seen (Fig. 5). In a study examining the distinguishing features between transient synovitis and septic arthritis [17], the presence of signal alteration of normal bone marrow on both contrast-enhanced fat suppressed T1- and T2-weighted imaging was a specific feature of septic arthropathy and excluded the diagnosis of transient synovitis, a condition common in children. Subchondral edema is common in septic arthritis and is related to hyperemia. However, when the edema or enhancement extends beyond the subchondral bone into the medullary cavity, osteomyelitis should be considered [18]. Bone erosions may also be seen at the femoral neck, although these are best assessed with CT. MR imaging can also assess the status of the articular cartilage, which is quickly eroded in septic arthritis.

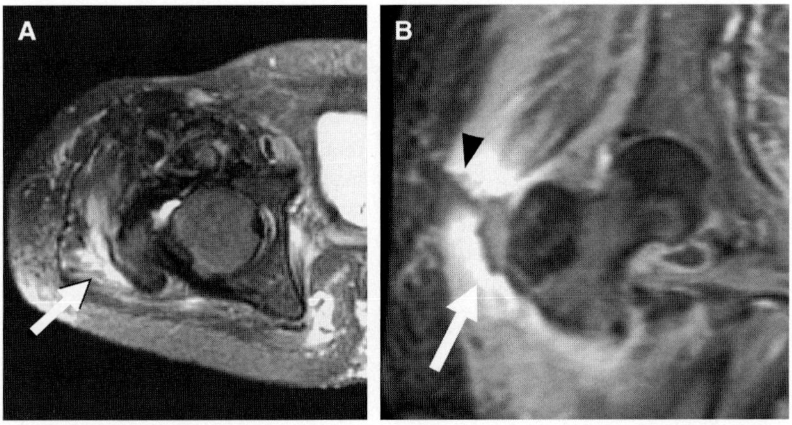


Fig. 4. Septic bursitis in a bedridden patient with hip pain and fever. (*A*) Axial fat-suppressed T2-weighted FSE image demonstrates a fluid collection (*arrow*) next to the greater trochanter. (*B*) Coronal postcontrast T1-weighted fat-suppressed FMPSPGR image shows thick rim enhancement (*arrow*) of the collection. These findings are nonspecific and can be seen with mechanical or noninfectious inflammatory bursitis; however, the clinical history along with a tract extending to the lateral soft tissues (*arrowhead*) raises the likelihood of infection.

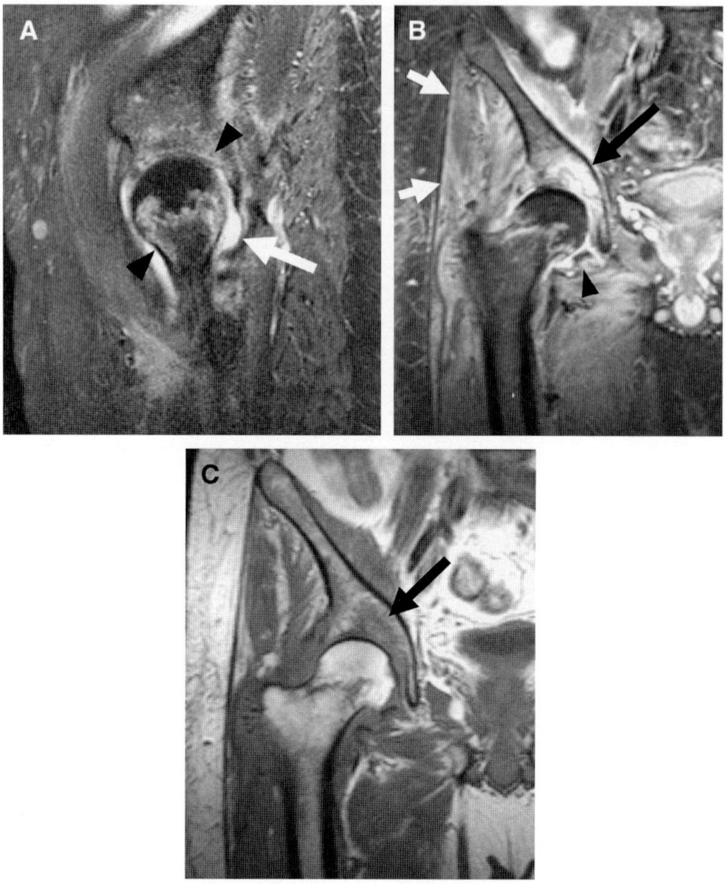


Fig. 5. Septic arthritis and osteomyelitis: hematogenous spread. (*A*) Sagittal T2-weighted fat-suppressed FSE image depicts a hip joint effusion (*arrow*) with subchondral edema in the femoral neck and acetabulum (*arrowheads*). (*B*) Coronal postcontrast T1-weighted fat suppressed FMPSPGR image demonstrates thick rim enhancement of the hip joint (*arrowhead*) consistent with septic arthritis. This finding can be seen in other synovial proliferative processes; however, inflammation of the surrounding periarticular soft tissues (*white arrows*) raises the probability of infection. Note enhancement extending into the acetabulum (*black arrow*), representing osteomyelitis. (*C*) Coronal T1-weighted SE image shows replacement of marrow fat signal in the acetabulum (*arrow*), consistent with osteomyelitis.

*Osteomyelitis*

MR imaging demonstrates marrow and cortical involvement, as well as having the added advantage of detecting joint fluid (and thus possible concomitant septic arthritis) and adjacent soft tissue extension. Sensitivity and specificity of MR imaging are 90% to 100% [19,20]. Osteomyelitis is characterized by marrow hypointensity on T1-weighted images, with edema and enhancement (see Figs. 2 and 5). However, marrow of the pelvis and proximal femurs has a high proportion of red marrow, which is slightly hypointense to fat on T1-weighted images, with mild hyperintensity on fat-suppressed T2-weighted or STIR images; unlike infection, hematopoietic marrow is symmetrically distributed, retains some fat signal, and enhances weakly or not at all. These imaging features must also be correlated with the clinical findings, because cellular infiltration from tumor, as well as trauma and infarction, may produce similar T1 and T2 marrow signal abnormalities. Periosteal reaction of the femoral shaft, characterized by a linear pattern of edema and enhancement along the cortex, may be seen with proximal femoral infection; however, periostitis is not seen in flat bones such as the pelvic bones, nor around joints. Therefore, periostitis is not commonly seen in infection around the hip unless the proximal femoral shaft is involved. Bone destruction may be seen in late stages of disease, with loss of the low signal cortical line.

MR imaging is very helpful in defining extent of osseous involvement before surgical debridement. Usually the margin of infected bone is well demonstrated on all sequences, although extent may appear more prominent on STIR or fat-suppressed T2-weighted images compared with T1-weighted images, due to high sensitivity of these sequences for reactive hyperemia of the surrounding bone. Soft tissue extent may also be demonstrated, including sinus tracts, septic arthritis, and periarticular abscesses.

Despite the poor spatial resolution of STIR, it is extremely sensitive to fluid. Thus, the absence of any STIR signal abnormality, or pathological contrast enhancement on fat-suppressed T1-weighted images, effectively excludes the diagnosis of osteomyelitis. MR imaging may distinguish between a primary soft tissue infection with secondary osteomyelitis or vice versa. In the former, a soft tissue mass, cortical disruption, and abnormal signal intensity strongly favors a primary extra osseous process. The absence of T2 signal abnormality (or thin hyperintensity limited to the subchondral bone) virtually excludes superimposed osteomyelitis. Occasionally, reactive edema can extend into the medullary bone beyond the subchondral location; there is evidence that the brighter the T2 signal abnormality, the more likely the edema is secondary to osteomyelitis rather than reactive hyperemia [21]. However, the MR image must still be considered suspicious for osteomyelitis in this situation.

MR imaging has the additional advantage of diagnosing active infection in areas complicated by trauma or prior surgery. Noncontrast MR imaging is unable to distinguish acute infarction from infection [22], because both demonstrate diffuse marrow edema. However, infarcted bone will not show enhancement following contrast administration, whereas infection enhances brightly. In the setting of sickle cell disease, the two are difficult to distinguish, because areas of infarction are often surrounded by reactive hyperemic zones, with enhancement and even periosteal reaction if the proximal femoral shaft is involved.

Chronic osteomyelitis (Fig. 6), commonly seen in paralyzed patients, can present with atypical patterns on MR imaging. It is often characterized by a mixed pattern of lysis, sclerosis, and cortical thickening. The sclerosis may be low signal on both T1-and T2-weighted images, with granulation tissue representing active infection demonstrating hyperintensity on T2-weighted images and enhancement on contrast-enhanced images. Sequestrum formation (intraosseous foci of hypointensity on all sequences, surrounded by enhancing inflammatory tissue) is important to recognize when present, because these avascular fragments of necrotic bone serve as a nidus for continuing infection and require debridement. Other features, such as cortical thickening may also be present with a low signal intensity rim being frequent (93%). A sinus tract, if present, is usually T2-hyperintense, and is well easily visualized, as are abscess cavities, serving as a useful preoperative plan before surgical excision. Differential possibilities for chronic osteomyelitis include bone neoplasms, in particular lymphoma.

### *Debilitated patients*

Patients with spinal cord injury, neuromuscular abnormalities and general debility as well as those with a predisposition to soft tissue infection (such as diabetes) and those with penetrating trauma, may all present with soft tissue defects/ulceration, the extent of which varies from a superficial location to as deep as the hip joint (gas, septic arthritis) and bones (osteomyelitis). Granulation tissue typically lines the cavity which is usually hypervascular and thus enhances post contrast, a finding not necessarily implying that the tissues are infected. The strength of MR imaging is its ability to visualize bone marrow abnormalities and accurately localize abnormalities to individual muscle/soft tissue compartments. The importance of accurate anatomical delineation of these abnormalities, combined with discrimination of infected and necrotic tissues, provides an invaluable tool to the treating clinician, particularly when surgery is contemplated [23].

## Infection of the postoperative hip

Assessment of suspected infection in the postoperative hip is difficult, especially because the request is usually made for patients who undergo total hip arthroplasty. Although the MR imaging findings of infection (Fig. 7) are similar to those of a nonoperated hip, image quality is poorer secondary to metallic susceptibility artifact. Metallic artifact can be reduced by a number of alterations to the protocol, including:

- using a higher bandwidth;
- using STIR instead of fat-saturated T2-weighted sequences;

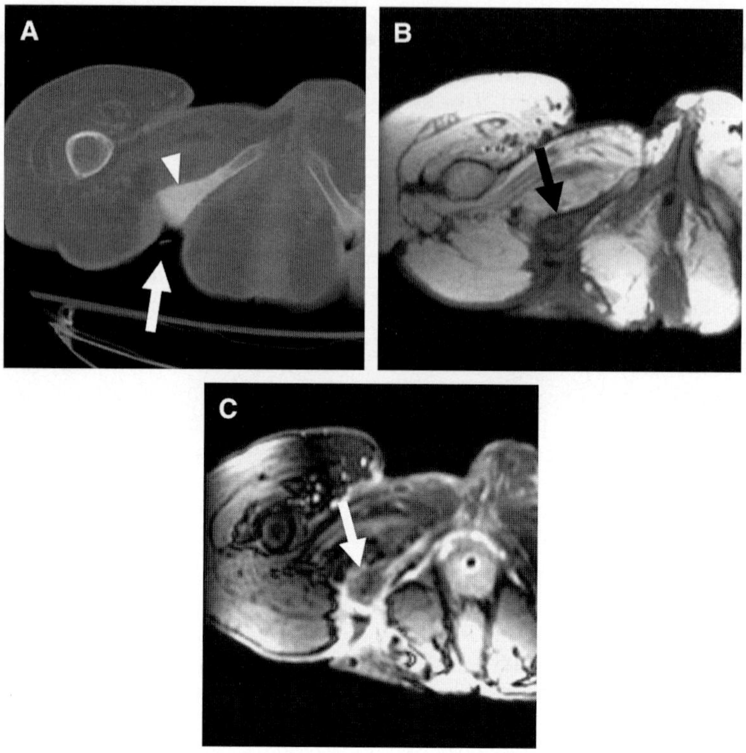


Fig. 6. Chronic osteomyelitis in a paralyzed patient with chronic ulceration. (*A*) Axial CT image shows a chronic decubitus ulcer (*arrow*) in this paralyzed patient. Note sclerosis of the adjacent ischium (*arrowhead*) representing chronic osteomyelitis. (*B*) Axial T1-weighted SE image shows low signal in the ischium (*arrow*) with replacement of marrow fat. (*C*) Axial postcontrast T1-weighted fat-suppressed FMPSPGR image demonstrates enhancement of the sclerotic bone (*arrow*), suggesting active inflammation.

- using fast-spin echo (FSE) instead of spin echo (SE) sequences [24];
- avoiding gradient echo sequences;
- lowering echo time (TE);
- using a large field of view and increasing the matrix; and
- performing pre- and postcontrast T1-weighted non–fat-saturated sequences.

Multidetector CT has also reduced beam hardening artifact and has been used increasingly for evaluation of hip prostheses, especially for the evaluation of periprosthetic bone changes such as osteolysis. Despite the artifact on MR imaging, it remains very useful for evaluation of the periprosthetic soft tissues (particularly for abscesses) and the adjacent marrow (for osteomyelitis). Using the metal artifact reduction techniques above, satisfactory images can be acquired with most prosthesis types.

Culture of hip aspirate remains necessary to diagnose infection [25], and image guidance plays an important role. Negative aspiration, however, does not exclude the presence of infection [26,27], and false positives (usually secondary to skin contamination) also may occur; however, differentiating between the two may difficult. Arthrography along with aspiration is the standard method for evaluation of a suspected hip prosthesis infection, but MR imaging can play a role in evaluating location and size of fluid collections around the prosthesis, and differentiation infection originating in the joint versus one arising in the soft tissues that may be missed on fluoroscopically guided aspiration.

## Imaging findings: inflammation

### *Rheumatoid arthritis*

Rheumatoid arthritis is the most common noninfectious inflammatory arthritis, affecting females more often than males at a ratio of 2 or

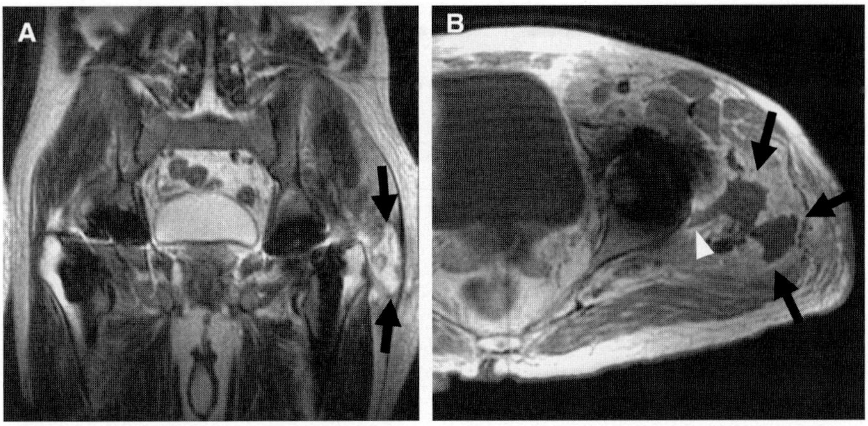


Fig. 7. Infected hip arthroplasty in a patient with fever and inability to bear weight on the left side. (*A*) Coronal T2-weighted FSE image without fat suppression shows artifact from bilateral total hip arthroplasties. Complex fluid collection is noted adjacent to the greater trochanter on the left (*arrows*). (*B*) Axial postcontrast T1-weighted FSE image without fat suppression indicates that the fluid collection communicates with the prosthetic hip joint via a thin tract (*arrowhead*). The collection itself shows thick rim enhancement (*arrows*) and the findings are compatible with infection of the prosthetic hip.

3 to 1. Typically, adult-type rheumatoid arthritis is recognized at a young age, usually in the 20s to 40s. Symptoms at presentation classically include joint stiffness, especially in the morning, with pain and swelling that is most commonly polyarticular and symmetric [28]. Often the symptoms are insidious with slow progression over months until treatment is sought [29]. During this period, intermittent arthralgias may occur in one or few joints (monarticular or pauciarticular) and involvement can be asymmetric. Systemic manifestations include fatigue and weight loss. Some patients have rapid progression of disease causing severe debilitation, but in many patients the disease becomes quiescent for long periods, with occasional flare-ups. Although most patients (~85%) have positive rheumatoid factor, a small subset are factor negative but fulfill other criteria characteristic of rheumatoid arthritis rather than the seronegative spondyloarthropathies. These patients may subsequently turn rheumatoid factor–positive.

The basic pathology of rheumatoid arthritis is inflammation and proliferation of synovium (called "pannus"), which leads to the various radiological appearances. Rheumatoid arthritis can affect any synovial structure, including bursae and tendon sheaths. Rheumatoid nodules occur in approximately 15% of all rheumatoid patients but are uncommon at the pelvis and hip. Bilateral involvement is very common at the hips, and severity is often symmetric (Fig. 8). This distribution is very helpful in confirming the diagnosis. Therefore, MR evaluation for synovitis at the hip should include sequences of the whole pelvis. This is also helpful for evaluation of periarticular disease such as bursitis, as well as the sacroiliac joints.

In patients with known rheumatoid arthritis, magnetic resonance imaging is useful for evaluation of effusion, erosions and synovial pannus formation as well as evaluation of the underlying cartilage [30]. Tracking changes in these characteristics over time can provide an objective measure of improvement or progression of disease. In patients with hip pain without a primary diagnosis, identification of mass-like pannus formation in the hip joint, particularly with bilateral involvement, can make the diagnosis.

As above, synovial proliferation in rheumatoid arthritis is classically seen on MR imaging as a mass-like prominence of tissue within the joint, low signal on T1-weighted images and hyperintense on T2-weighted or STIR sequences. Pannus may be homogeneous or heterogeneous. Occasionally pannus hemorrhages, forming areas of low signal hemosiderin. On postcontrast images, pannus markedly enhances, similar to other synovial inflammatory or hyperemic processes; this finding itself is nonspecific, whereas the mass-like morphology and symmetry of the process is more useful as a discriminatory feature. Due to the inflammatory nature of the synovial process, the

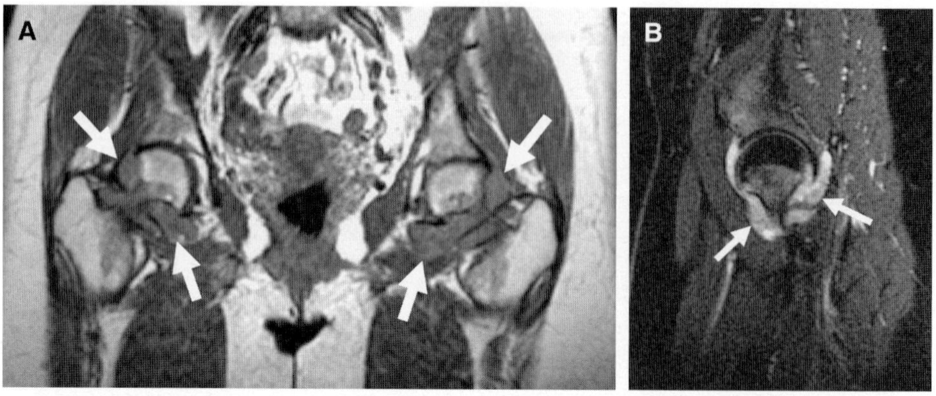


Fig. 8. Rheumatoid arthritis: early involvement of the hips. (*A*) Coronal T1-weighted image demonstrates masslike synovial proliferation symmetrically involving the hip joints bilaterally (*arrows*). Note erosion at the femoral necks. (*B*) Sagittal T2-weighted fat-suppressed image of the left hip shows complex ("dirty") fluid (*arrows*) in the joint representing synovial pannus.

underlying bone may become hyperemic, showing marrow edema and enhancement. This appearance can be confused for septic arthritis. Pannus often erodes into bone at the femoral neck and acetabulum, seen initially as focal areas of edema, followed by discrete erosions. Pannus may also extend from the joint from recesses along facial planes. Effusion is almost universal, but extent varies. In fact, when the joint is distended with pannus the synovium can exclude fluid with little actual aspirable effusion. In the setting of effusion, minor amounts of synovial proliferation is seen on MR imaging as "dirty fluid," or complex signal on T2-weighted or STIR images.

Subchondral cysts are very common at involved joints, and as above, pannus may erode into the central aspect of the acetabulum, simulating a cyst on radiographs and CT. Intraosseous pannus can be differentiated from cystic change on MR imaging because pannus will have signal lower than fluid on T2-weighted images, and enhances brightly; cysts should have fluid signal and demonstrate no more than marginal enhancement. Cysts may become so large that the articular surface becomes flattened, simulating collapse from avascular necrosis.

Involved hip joints generally demonstrate uniform cartilage loss; joint narrowing is classically concentric (diffuse) or central, with axial migration of the femoral head. With more advanced disease, the iliopectineal line bows inward and the central acetabulum thins [31], an appearance called 'protrusio acetabulae' (Fig. 9).

Development of advanced secondary osteoarthritis is common after the cartilage is destroyed, because the hips are weight-bearing joints. The end-stage hip may be so degenerated that it is difficult to determine the source of the initial insult without clinical information or evaluation of other joints. Large osteophytes form at the femoral head–neck junction, especially laterally. Cysts become very prominent and subchondral edema and enhancement is observed on MR images.

Involvement of the greater trochanteric bursa or iliopsoas bursa often occurs, and is seen as

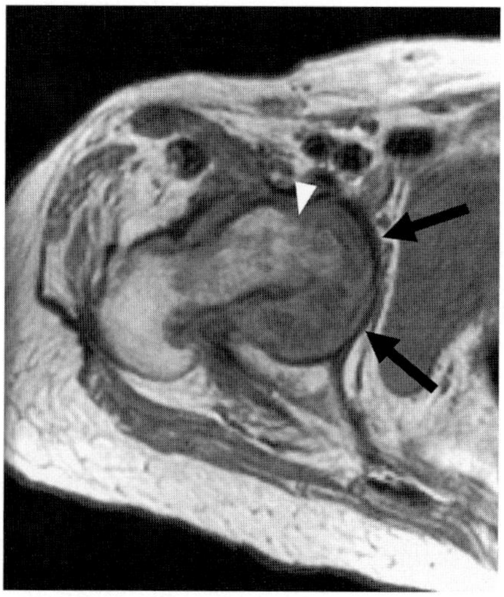

Fig. 9. Rheumatoid arthritis: late involvement. Axial intermediate-weighted FSE image shows marked erosion of the femoral head (*arrowhead*) and acetabulum with protrusio (*arrows*).

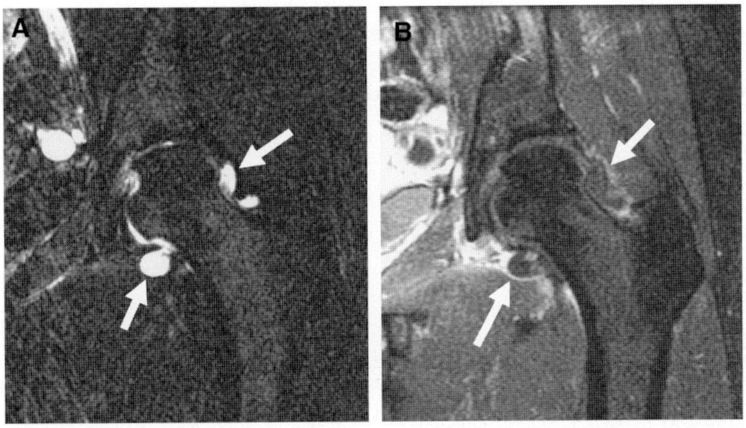

Fig. 10. Nonspecific synovial proliferation. Coronal STIR (*A*) and postcontrast T1-weighted fat suppressed FMPSPGR (*B*) images show a moderate joint effusion (*arrows*) with mild synovial enhancement. This is nonspecific and could represent infection as well as inflammatory arthritis (eg, rheumatoid arthritis), noninflammatory synovial proliferative processes (eg, synovial osteochondromatosis, pigmented villonodular synovitis), injury, or reactive hyperemia from an adjacent process (eg, osteoid osteoma). Clinical context is essential; aspiration may be necessary if there is concern for infection. The etiology in this case was not determined.

complex fluid signal in the distended bursa, with intense enhancement on postcontrast imaging.

*Differential diagnosis*

Joint effusion and synovial proliferation (Fig. 10) have a wide differential. Distribution and extent of synovial pannus are important in considering the differential diagnosis for hip inflammatory disease. Active rheumatoid arthritis involving the hips typically has mass-like synovial proliferation, with bilateral involvement. These characteristics help exclude other monarticular entities such as infection, synovial chondromatosis, and pigmented villonodular synovitis. Ankylosing spondylitis can also have a symmetric distribution in the hips, but the sacroiliac joints should be evaluated as well, which should be affected if the hips are involved, whereas rheumatoid arthritis rarely involves the sacroiliac joints. Gout, Reiter disease and psoriatic arthritis can also be in the differential for inflammatory arthritis, but are quite uncommon at the hip. Hemophiliacs in the early stages of articular disease can also

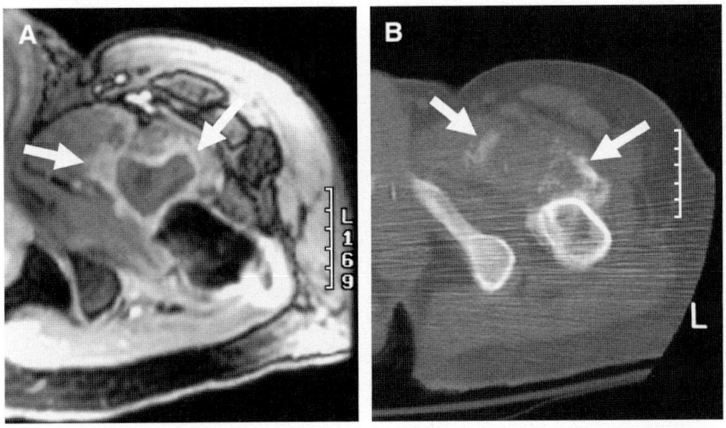

Fig. 11. Heterotopic ossification mimicking abscess on MRI: paralyzed patient. (*A*) Axial postcontrast T1-weighted fat suppressed FMPSPGR image shows thick rim enhancement in the region of the iliopsoas bursa (*arrows*), raising concern for abscess formation or septic bursitis. (*B*) Axial CT image demonstrates linear calcification around the rim of this focus (*arrows*), compatible with early heterotopic ossification rather than abscess.

demonstrate synovial proliferation which is generally bilateral in weight-bearing joints such as the hips, and can be considered with appropriate history. Similarly, aggressive or advanced degenerative arthritis can also show synovial proliferation. The end stage of osteoarthritis often presents on MR imaging with joint effusion and synovial enhancement that can simulate an inflammatory arthropathy. However, identification of large osteophytes disproportionate to the extent of effusion or synovitis should raise suspicion of degeneration as the primary condition. That being said, arthritic joints can become superinfected, and severe osteoarthritis is often seen in late stages of rheumatoid arthritis, so the clinical context must always be considered when generating a differential diagnosis.

In paralyzed patients, heterotopic ossification in the early stages can simulate abscess, with focal fluid signal and rim-enhancement (Fig. 11). The correct diagnosis can be suspected by margins of low signal representing zonal calcification, as well as typical location, around the hips, especially in the region of the iliopsoas or greater trochanteric bursa. Confirmation of rim calcification typical of heterotopic bone can be made by comparison with CT scan or radiographs. In mature heterotopic ossification, the focus will demonstrate corticomedullary differentiation, with internal fatty marrow signal, and at this stage differentiation from infection is straightforward. In paralyzed patients there is often coexistence of early and late forms of heterotopic ossification, so this can be another clue leading to the correct interpretation.

## Summary

With its superior anatomical resolution and high sensitivity in depicting pathological processes of the joint, bone marrow and surrounding soft tissue structures, MR imaging is the ideal modality for demonstrating the manifestations and sequelae of the infective and inflammatory conditions common to the hip. Though the imaging features of these conditions may overlap, combining the clinical history and results and other imaging modalities yields a higher degree of specificity, ultimately enhancing the confidence of the radiological interpretation.

## References

[1] Moran KM, Finkbeiner AA. Iliopsoas abscess following catheterization of the femoral artery: diagnostic and treatment strategies. Am J Orthop 1997;26:446–8.

[2] Nallamshetty L, Buchowski JM, Nazarian LA, et al. Septic arthritis of the hip following cortisone injection: case report and review of the literature. Clin Imaging 2003;27:225–8.

[3] Freiberger RH. Introducing arthrography. In: Freiberger RH, Kaye JJ, editors. Arthrography. Norwalk (CT): Appleton-Century Croft; 1979. p. 1.

[4] Savarino L, Baldini N, Tarabusi C, et al. Diagnosis of infection after total hip replacement. Biomed Mater Res 2004;70B:139–45.

[5] Takagi M, Santavirta S, Ida H, et al. High-turnover periprosthetic bone remodeling and immature bone formation around loose cemented total hip joints. J Bone Miner Res 2001;16:79–88.

[6] Beltran J. MR imaging of soft-tissue infection. Magn Reson Imaging Clin N Am 1995;3:743–51.

[7] Ledermann HP, Schweitzer ME, Morrison WB. Pelvic heterotopic ossification: MR imaging characteristics. Radiology 2002;222:189–95.

[8] Parikh J, Hyare H, Saifuddin A. The imaging features of post-traumatic myositis ossificans, with emphasis on MRI. Clin Radiol 2002;57:1058–66.

[9] Kransdorf MJ, Meis JM, Jelinek JS. Myositis ossificans: MR appearance with radiologic-pathologic correlation. AJR 1991;157:1243–8.

[10] Rodgers WB, Yodlowski ML, Mintzer CM. Pyomyositis in patients who have the human immunodeficiency virus. Case report and review of the literature. J Bone Joint Surg Am 1993;75:588–92.

[11] Struk DW, Munk PL, Lee MJ, et al. Imaging of soft tissue infections. Radiol Clin North Am 2001;39:277–303.

[12] Rahmouni A, Chosidow O, Mathieu D, et al. MR imaging in acute infectious cellulitis. Radiology 1994;192:493–6.

[13] King RJ, Laugharne D, Kerslake RW, et al. Primary obturator pyomyositis: a diagnostic challenge. J Bone Joint Surg Br 2003;85:895–8.

[14] Haritides J, Christodoulou P, Tsakonas A. Tuberculous trochanteric bursitis. Chir Organi Mov 2004;89:177–80.

[15] Brower AC. Septic arthritis. Radiol Clin North Am 1996;34:293–309.

[16] Resnick D, Niwayama G. Osteomyelitis, septic arthritis and soft tissue infection. In: Resnick D, Niwayama G, editors. Diagnosis of bone and joint disorders, Volume 3. 4th edition. Philadelphia: WB Saunders; 2002. p. 2419–35.

[17] Lee SK, Suh KJ, Kim YW, et al. Septic arthritis versus transient synovitis at MR imaging: preliminary assessment with signal intensity alterations in bone marrow. Radiology 1999;211:459–65.

[18] Greenspan A, Tehranzadeh J. Imaging of infectious arthritis. Radiol Clin North Am 2001;39:267–76.

[19] Morrison WB, Schweitzer ME, Bock GW, et al. Diagnosis of osteomyelitis: utility of fat-suppressed

contrast-enhanced MR imaging. Radiology 1993; 189:251–7.

[20] Kaiser S, Jorulf H, Hirsch G. Clinical value of imaging techniques in childhood osteomyelitis. Acta Radiol 1998;39:523–31.

[21] Craig JG, Amin MR, Wu K, et al. Osteomyelitis of diabetic foot: MR imaging pathologic correlation. Radiology 1997;203:849–55.

[22] Gylys-Morin VM. MR imaging of pediatric musculoskeletal iflammatory and infectious disorders. MRI Clin N Am 1998;6:537–59.

[23] Huang AB, Schweitzer ME, Hume E, et al. Osteomyelitis of the pelvis/hips in paralyzed patients: accuracy and clinical utility of MRI. J Comput Assist Tomogr 1998;22:437–43.

[24] White LM, Kim JK, Mehta M, et al. Complications of total hip arthroplasty: MR imaging-initial experience. Radiology 2000;215:254–62.

[25] Kraemer WJ, Saplys R, Waddell JP. Bone scan, gallium scan and hip aspiration in the diagnosis of infected total hip joint arthroplasty. J Arthroplasty 1993;8:611–6.

[26] Tehranzedeh J, Gubernick I, Blaha D. Propsective study of sequential technetium 99m phosphate and gallium imaging. Clin Nucl Med 1988;13: 229–36.

[27] Maus TP, Berquist TH, Bender CE, et al. Arthrographic study of painful study of painful total hip arthroplasty: refined criteria. Radiology 1987;162: 721–7.

[28] Kaarela K. Prognostic factors and diagnostic criteria in early rheumatoid arthritis. Scand J Rheumatol Suppl 1985;57:1–54.

[29] Molenaar ET, Voskuyl AE, Dinant HJ, et al. Progression of radiologic damage in patients with rheumatoid arthritis in clinical remission. Arthritis Rheum 2004;50:36–42.

[30] Peterfy CG. New developments in imaging in rheumatoid arthritis. Curr Opin Rheumatol 2003;15: 288–95.

[31] Damron TA, Heiner JP. Rapidly progressive protrusio acetabuli in patients with rheumatoid arthritis. Clin Orthop Relat Res 1993;289: 186–94.

ELSEVIER
SAUNDERS

Magn Reson Imaging Clin N Am
13 (2005) 757–774

MAGNETIC RESONANCE IMAGING CLINICS of North America

# MR Imaging of Tumors and Tumor-Like Lesions of the Hip

Laura W. Bancroft, MD*, Jeffrey J. Peterson, MD, Mark J. Kransdorf, MD

*Department of Radiology, Mayo Clinic College of Medicine, 4500 San Pablo Boulevard, Jacksonville, FL 32224, USA*

Multiple tumors and tumor-like conditions have a predilection for the hip (Box 1). Because of the sometimes characteristic imaging features, certain tumors and synovial-based processes may be diagnosed through a combination of radiographs, CT, and MR imaging. In this article, we first focus on the demographics, clinical behavior, and imaging findings of some of the more common malignant soft tissue and osseous tumors of the hip, such as the sarcomas. Subsequently, we review several benign osseous tumors of the hip, such as osteoid osteoma, osteochondroma, and enchondroma. Finally, this article concludes with an overview of tumor-like and synovial-based processes that can be characterized with the assistance of MR imaging.

## General comments on tumor imaging

### *Initial evaluation*

The imaging evaluation of a suspected hip mass begins with conventional radiographs. Although radiographs are frequently unrewarding, they can provide invaluable information when they are positive. Radiographs may reveal calcifications in soft tissue tumors that can be suggestive and sometimes characteristic of a specific diagnosis. For example, they may reveal the phleboliths within a hemangioma, the osteocartilaginous masses of synovial osteochondromatosis, or the peripherally more mature ossification of myositis ossificans. Radiographs can also provide an excellent method to assess osseous involvement of a soft tissue tumor, such as remodeling, periosteal reaction, or overt destruction.

Radiographs are the initial step in the assessment of osseous lesions. Critical analysis of a lesion's margin and any associated periosteal reaction remains the most accurate method of establishing a lesion's biologic potential. Certain tumors produce a matrix that can be identified when calcified or ossified. In such cases, radiographs are especially useful in establishing a tissue-specific diagnosis. Pathologic fractures through osseous tumors can also be depicted by radiography.

### *MR imaging*

MR imaging has emerged as the preferred modality for evaluating osseous and soft tissue masses of the hip by providing information for diagnosis and staging. A detailed review of imaging techniques is beyond the scope of this review, but some fundamentals should be emphasized. Lesions should be imaged in at least two orthogonal planes using conventional T1-weighted and fluid-sensitive MR pulse sequences in at least one of these planes. We find that standard spin-echo images, when possible, are most useful in establishing a specific diagnosis. It is the most reproducible technique and the one most often referenced in the tumor imaging literature. The main disadvantage of spin-echo imaging remains the relatively long acquisition times for double-echo T2-weighted sequences [1], and in cases in

* Corresponding author.
*E-mail address:* bancroft.laura@mayo.edu (L.W. Bancroft).

1064-9689/05/$ - see front matter 
doi:10.1016/j.mric.2005.08.003

mri.theclinics.com

**Box 1. Common tumors and tumor-like lesions of the hip**

*Malignant*

- Sarcoma
  - Undifferentiated pleomorphic sarcoma
  - Liposarcoma
  - Leiomyosarcoma
  - Synovial sarcoma
  - Chondrosarcoma (osseous and soft tissue)

*Benign*

- Osteoid osteoma
- Osteochondroma
- Enchondroma
- Chondroblastoma
- Intraosseous lipoma

*Tumor-like*

- Synovial-based
  - Pigmented villonodular synovitis
  - Synovial chondromatosis
  - Paralabral cysts
  - Distended bursae (trochanteric, iliopsoas, obturator)
- Metastatic calcification
- Fibrous dysplasia

which this is a problem, we substitute non–fat-suppressed fast T2-weighted images. Typically, we obtain axial T1- and T2-weighted spin-echo images and choose an additional imaging plane or planes, depending on the size and location of the mass.

Gradient-echo imaging techniques may be a useful adjunct in demonstrating hemosiderin because of hemosiderin's greater magnetic susceptibility; in general, susceptibility artifacts related to metallic material, hemorrhage, and air are accentuated on gradient-echo images [2]. Short tau inversion recovery (STIR) imaging produces fat suppression and enhances the identification of abnormal tissue with increased water content, which is useful to confirm subtle areas of soft tissue abnormality [3]. This technique increases lesion conspicuity [3,4], which is usually not a significant limitation in tumor imaging. STIR imaging typically has a lower signal-to-noise ratio than spin-echo imaging and is also more susceptible to degradation by motion [1,3]. Lesions are generally well seen on standard imaging, and, in our opinion, STIR imaging tends to reduce the variations in signal intensities identified on conventional spin-echo MR imaging, which are most helpful in tissue characterization.

Fat suppression on T2-weighted images is useful to increase lesion-to-background signal intensity differences for high signal intensity lesions that are located within the marrow or fatty soft tissue [1]. Fat suppression imaging is also useful in decreasing or eliminating the MR signal from fat, allowing increased conspicuity of lesions containing paramagnetic substances (eg, methemoglobin) on T1-weighted images and in identifying contrast enhancement. As with STIR techniques, fat-suppressed T2-weighted imaging decreases variations in tumor signal intensities; therefore, we do not use STIR and fat-suppressed imaging in place of conventional T2-weighted images.

In general, a small field of view is preferred; however, the field of view must be large enough to evaluate the lesion and allow appropriate staging. When the hip is being evaluated, it is not usually necessary to obtain images of the contralateral side for comparison unless no lesion is detected on initial sequences. It is useful to place a marker over the area of clinical concern to ensure that it is appropriately imaged. This becomes important in evaluation of lesions like subcutaneous lipoma or lipomatosis in which the lesion may not be appreciated as distinct from the adjacent adipose tissue.

Contrast enhancement is often not required; however, we find it especially useful in the detection of underlying tumors in the presence of hematoma. In such cases, contrast-enhanced imaging may reveal a small tumor nodule that may be inapparent within hemorrhage on conventional MR imaging [5,6]. Gadolinium-enhanced imaging may also be useful to differentiate solid from cystic (or necrotic) lesions and to identify cystic or necrotic areas within solid tumors—a distinction that may be difficult or impossible to make on conventional T2-weighted images.

## Malignant tumors

Malignant musculoskeletal tumors of the hip are not uncommon. Although there are a number of lesions that may occur in the lower extremity, there are certain lesions that are statistically more common and have a predilection for this location. It is difficult to determine the true prevalence of malignant tumors of the hip. Osseous lesions are usually not classified beyond the bone of origin;

for example, one cannot separate an innominate bone lesion of the pubis from a lesion of the acetabulum. The hip is not rigidly defined in the soft tissues, and lesions in this region are often coded as occurring in the proximal thigh, the buttocks, or the flank. Additionally, prevalence data are usually acquired from large referral populations; consequently, these data incorporate a significant referral bias. With these limitations in mind, descriptions of the most common osseous and soft tissue malignancies of the hip that we have encountered follow.

*Undifferentiated pleomorphic sarcoma*

Undifferentiated pleomorphic sarcoma, previously termed *malignant fibrous histiocytoma* (MFH) is the most common soft tissue sarcoma in adults, comprising 20% to 30% of all soft tissue sarcomas. Not surprisingly, it is also the most common soft tissue mass of the hip. There is a male predilection (1.5–2:1), with a peak incidence in the fifth and sixth decades, although the lesion occurs in patients of all ages [7]. Two thirds of lesions are deep intramuscular in location. Patients typically present with a painless but enlarging soft tissue mass.

Radiographs of patients with MFH typically reveal an indeterminate soft tissue mass, with mineralization detected in 5% to 20% of cases [8]. Deep intramuscular lesions may cause extrinsic erosion of adjacent long bones, a feature not commonly seen in other soft tissue sarcomas, with the exception of synovial sarcoma [9]. MR imaging typically demonstrates a large, lobulated, well-circumscribed mass with intermediate signal intensity on T1-weighted images and high signal intensity on conventional T2-weighted images. Lesions are usually heterogeneous on all pulse sequences, reflecting the variable histologic patterns within the tumor [9]. Nonnecrotic areas of the tumor usually demonstrate marked enhancement. Lesions are often large and lobulated, frequently with a relatively well-defined margin reflecting a surrounding pseudocapsule (of compressed normal tissue) [9]. Occasionally, lesions may show intermediate signal intensity on T2-weighted images.

*Liposarcoma*

Liposarcoma is the second most common soft tissue sarcoma and also the second most common soft tissue hip malignancy [7]. Most patients present in the fifth or sixth decade of life, with rare involvement in children [7]. Most patients present with a painless soft tissue mass; however, pain is reported in 10% to 15% of cases [10]. The imaging appearance and prognosis of liposarcoma vary with histologic subtype and degree of differentiation. There are four histologic subtypes (well-differentiated, myxoid, pleomorphic, and dedifferentiated).

Well-differentiated liposarcoma is the most common liposarcoma and is similar to lipoma grossly and histologically. It is a low-grade tumor with a tendency to recur locally but no propensity to metastasize. The terms *well-differentiated liposarcoma* and *atypical lipoma* are sometimes used interchangeably. In accordance with the recommendation of the World Health Organization, however, we use the term *atypical lipoma* only for subcutaneous extremity lesions, reserving the term *well-differentiated liposarcoma* for lesions with similar histologic findings in all remaining sites [11]. The dedifferentiated liposarcoma is an interesting variant of the well-differentiated liposarcoma, being defined as a bimorphic neoplasm in which a histologically different high-grade sarcoma is juxtaposed to the well-differentiated liposarcoma. Dedifferentiated liposarcoma is unusual outside the retroperitoneum but is being reported with increasing frequency [12–15].

The myxoid subtype is a low to intermediate grade lesion. Myxoid liposarcoma may have hypervascular areas, and tumors with these hypervascular areas show a more aggressive biologic behavior. Such tumors were previously termed *round cell liposarcoma* and are considered to be a high-grade sarcoma. Myxoid liposarcoma is more common in the extremities, especially the thigh, and may be seen around the hip. Pleomorphic liposarcoma, which is also a high-grade lesion, is the least common type and represents 10% to 15% of all liposarcomas [15].

The imaging appearance of liposarcoma reflects its gross morphology. Radiographs typically identify a nonspecific soft tissue mass. Fatty components may be seen, and calcification is infrequent, being reported in less than 10% of cases. MR imaging of well-differentiated liposarcoma reveals a heterogeneous lipomatous mass, resembling a lipoma, usually containing more than 75% adipose tissue (Fig. 1). The nonadipose component demonstrates septae and swirled or irregular nodular areas with nonspecific signal intensities [16–18]. Variable contrast enhancement patterns have been described for the nonadipose component [16]. Myxoid and pleomorphic liposarcomas usually contain significantly less fat,

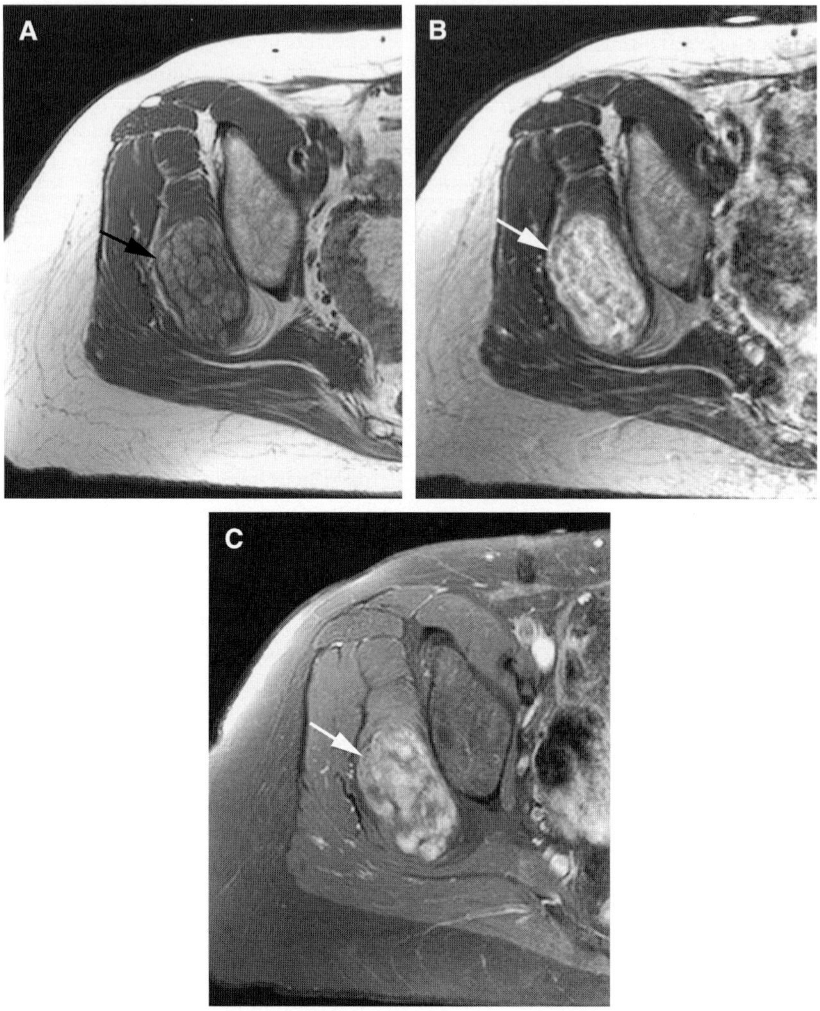


Fig. 1. A 79-year-old woman with well-differentiated liposarcoma in the buttocks. Axial T1-weighted (*A*) and T2-weighted (*B*) spin-echo MR images show a heterogeneous mass (*arrow*) with extensive "dirty" fat and nonspecific non-adipose tissue. (*C*) Axial enhanced, fat-suppressed, T1-weighted, spin-echo MR image shows extensive enhancement (*arrow*).

and only approximately three quarters of these tumors demonstrate fat radiologically. Approximately 20% of myxoid liposarcomas may demonstrate signal characteristics simulating those of a cyst [18]. Dedifferentiated liposarcoma is seen as a bimorphic neoplasm containing areas of well-differentiated liposarcoma with a juxtaposed nonlipomatous mass [13].

### *Leiomyosarcoma*

Leiomyosarcoma is a malignant tumor of smooth muscle differentiation. It accounts for approximately 9% of soft tissue sarcomas and is the third most common hip region malignancy after MFH and liposarcoma [7]. Leiomyosarcomas tend to occur in middle-aged to older adults with a median age in the fifth and sixth decades and are rare in children. Peripheral soft tissue lesions have a male predilection, whereas retroperitoneal tumors are more common in female patients. Overall, male and female patients are equally affected [19]. The prognosis is guarded, with an overall median 5-year survival rate of 35% and a median survival rate of 43 months.

Leiomyosarcoma may rarely arise in association with a vessel. Such lesions are four to five times more common in veins and are thought to be quite rare; however, it has recently been suggested that a vascular origin for leiomyosarcoma may be more common than previously reported. It is difficult to determine how frequently this occurs; however, Weiss and Goldblum [20] note that at least one third of cases of leiomyosarcoma arise from or involve a vessel.

Radiographs usually demonstrate a nonspecific soft tissue mass. Calcification is uncommon, as is invasion of the underlying osseous structures. MR imaging demonstrates a nonfatty mass, frequently with areas of necrosis (Fig. 2). Superficial lesions may be smaller and more homogeneous.

*Synovial sarcoma*

Synovial sarcoma accounts for approximately 5% of all malignant soft tissue tumors about the hip. Although it is not one of the most common lesions, it has a striking predilection for young adults and is one of the most common hip lesions in this age group. Patients often present with a palpable soft tissue mass. Metastases are present in 25% of patients at the time of diagnosis, with lung metastases most common, followed by lymph node and bone lesions. Local recurrence or metastases is seen in 80% of patients [21]. The prognosis is guarded, because the median survival

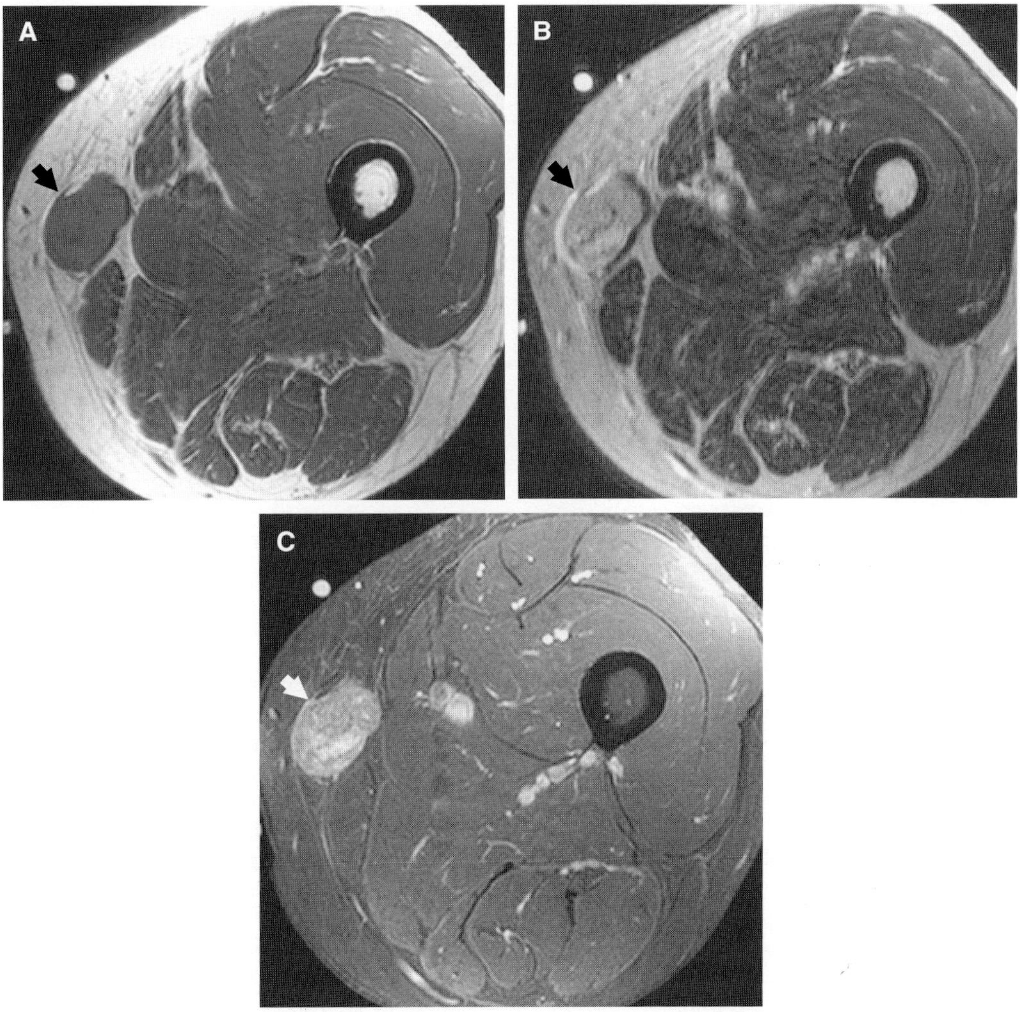


Fig. 2. A 52-year-old man presented with slowly growing leiomyosarcoma of the saphenous vein. Axial T1-weighted (*A*) and T2-weighted (*B*) spin-echo MR images show a mass (*arrow*) in the subcutaneous adipose tissue of the medial thigh. The lesion shows intermediate signal intensity of both imaging sequences. (*C*) Axial fat-suppressed, enhanced, T1-weighted, spin-echo MR image shows mildly intense heterogeneous enhancement (*arrow*).

after diagnosis is 33 months, with a 5-year survival rate of 27% to 55%. Young patients, small tumors, and lesions with extensive calcification have a better prognosis [22].

Radiographs may be normal in 50% of patients with synovial sarcoma. A soft tissue mass is seen in the remainder, with calcification seen in up to one third of all lesions. Adjacent osseous involvement has been reported in 10% to 20% of cases. On MR imaging, the lesion demonstrates heterogeneous signal intensity, with an intensity approximately equal to that of muscle on T1-weighted images and increased signal intensity on T2-weighted sequences. Evidence of prior hemorrhage may be seen within the lesion in up to 40% of cases, with fluid-fluid levels seen in 10% to 25% [23]. Heterogeneous enhancement may be seen on postgadolinium images. It must be emphasized that although lesions are typically heterogeneous, small lesions may appear to be quite "innocent."

### *Chondrosarcoma of bone*

Chondrosarcoma of bone is a malignant tumor that produces cartilage matrix. Although the lesion is common, other lesions of bone may be statistically more common; however, chondrosarcoma frequently shows a characteristic imaging appearance. Lesions that occur de novo are termed *primary,* whereas those that arise in preexisting benign cartilage lesions are termed *secondary*. Primary chondrosarcoma of bone comprises approximately 25% of all primary malignant osseous neoplasms.

The conventional intramedullary chondrosarcoma is the most frequent type and has also been referred to as central chondrosarcoma. Patients with conventional chondrosarcoma most commonly present in the fourth and fifth decades of life. There is a male predilection of 1.5 to 2.0:1. Clinical symptoms are nonspecific, with pain being the most frequent and occurring in most patients [24]. A palpable soft tissue mass or fullness has been described in a significant number of patients. Pathologic fractures are also common at initial presentation [24].

Osseous chondrosarcoma has a predilection for the pelvis and is most common in the region of the triradiate cartilage. Although benign enchondromas of the long bone are quite common, solitary enchondromas are extraordinarily rare in the pelvis [24], and pelvic cartilage lesions should be assumed to be malignant until proven otherwise. Radiographs of conventional chondrosarcoma typically reveal a mixed lytic and sclerotic appearance characteristic of a mineralized chondroid "ring and arc" matrix pattern of calcification (Fig. 3) [24,25]. There is frequently associated flocculent calcification, and this characteristic chondroid calcification usually permits confident radiographic diagnosis of a cartilaginous lesion.

Although radiographs are frequently diagnostic, CT allows optimal detection and characterization of matrix mineralization, particularly when it is subtle or in complex areas of anatomy. Areas of matrix mineralization are seen in 94% of long bone chondrosarcomas on CT [25]. MR imaging provides the best method for depiction of the extent of marrow involvement by conventional intramedullary chondrosarcoma [24–27]. The nonmineralized components of chondrosarcoma reveal high signal intensity on T2- weighted MR images, again, a reflection of the high water content of hyaline cartilage. The cartilaginous lobules may be surrounded by low signal intensity septae. Areas of matrix mineralization are common in intramedullary chondrosarcoma and show low signal intensity on all MR pulse sequences [25]. This often creates marked heterogeneity on T2-weighted MR images. The detection and, in particular, the characterization of matrix mineralization are superiorly achieved by radiography and CT, however. Areas of low signal intensity on T2-weighted MR images, although corresponding to matrix mineralization, are nonspecific and have numerous other potential causes, including fibrous tissue with high collagen content and other types of calcification.

Clear cell chondrosarcoma is a rare variant comprising only 1% to 2% of all chondrosarcomas. Despite this overall rarity, it has an unusual predilection for the proximal femur, with 55% to 60% of lesions occurring in this location. There is also a marked predilection for epiphyseal involvement, although metaphyseal extension is common. Patients are most typically affected in the third to fifth decade of life. Men are affected twice as often as women [24,28,29]. The lesion grows slowly and is less aggressive than higher grade conventional chondrosarcoma, with a resultant improvement in prognosis. Symptoms include localized pain and decreased range of motion of the adjacent joint. Pathologic fracture is the cause for initial clinical presentation in approximately 25% of cases [24].

Radiographs reveal a predominantly lytic lesion with a narrow or wide zone of transition. In up to 20% of cases, a peripheral rind of sclerosis

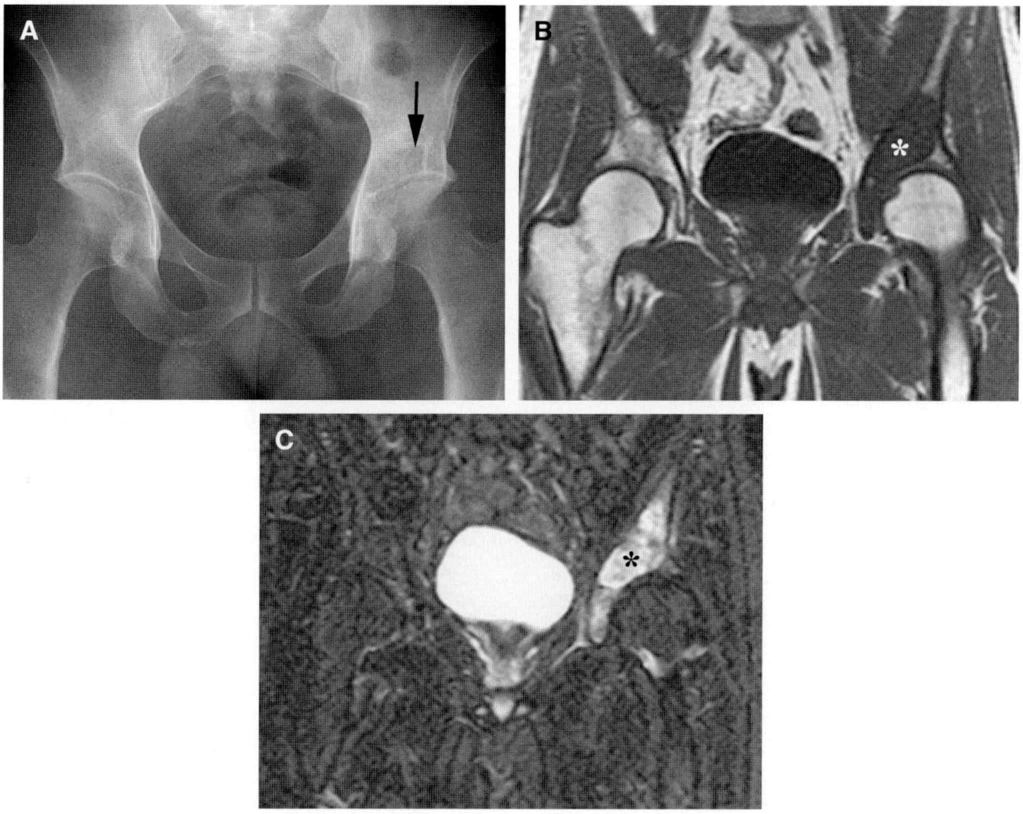


Fig. 3. A 47-year-old man with low-grade chondrosarcoma presented with hip pain. (*A*) Anteroposterior radiograph of the pelvis shows a poorly defined lytic lesion (*arrow*) in the left acetabulum with loss of the definition of the acetabular roof and mineralized matrix. Coronal (*B*) T1-weighted and (*C*) T2-weighted images through the pelvis define the extent of the marrow-replacing lesion (*) in the left superior acetabulum, which primarily follows the signal characteristics of cartilage.

simulating a benign lesion is apparent. In approximately one third of cases, mild expansile remodeling of bone may be seen, particularly in larger lesions, although soft tissue extension is unusual (less than 10% of cases) [24,28,29]. As with other chondroid lesions, CT can better demonstrate matrix mineralization, cortical destruction, or soft tissue extension as compared with radiography. The nonmineralized areas typically have low attenuation on CT.

MR imaging of clear cell chondrosarcoma typically shows homogeneous intermediate signal intensity on T1-weighted sequences and heterogeneous high signal intensity on T2-weighted sequences [28,29]. One author has reported heterogeneous low to intermediate signal intensity on T2-weighted images, which may correspond to lesions with histologic marked mineralization or osseous metaplasia [29]. These lesions show heterogeneous enhancement after administration of intravenous gadolinium.

**Benign tumors**

Although not infrequent, benign bone tumors are three times less frequent than malignant tumors of the bone in series of cases undergoing biopsy [30]. Most benign bone tumors involving the hip can be subdivided into three major categories: osteogenic, chondrogenic, and fibro-osseous lesions. Osteogenic lesions are least common and include osteoid osteoma and osteoblastoma. Chondrogenic lesions are more common and include osteochondroma, enchondroma, and chondroblastoma. Fibro-osseous lesions are also common and include intraosseous lipomas, liposclerosing myxofibrous tumor (LSMFT), and fibrous dysplasia. Giant cell tumor of bone, which does not fit well into any of these categories, is another benign lesion that can occur about the hip and is included in this section.

*Osteoid osteoma*

Osteoid osteoma occurs frequently in the hip. Sixty percent of all osteoid osteomas occur in the lower extremity, and 29% occur in the proximal femur [31]. Osteoid osteoma is a benign osteogenic lesion that occurs mainly in adolescents and young adults. The clinical hallmark is local pain, which is typically worse at night and relieved by aspirin or other nonsteroidal anti-inflammatory agents. The clinical and radiologic features of osteoid osteoma are typically characteristic; however, occasionally, the presentation can be unclear, which may lead to significant delay in diagnosis.

Osteoid osteomas can be subdivided into cortical, cancellous, and subperiosteal based on location [32]. Cortical lesions are most common, located within the cortex of affected long bones. Cancellous lesions are less common, located more centrally in the bone. Cancellous lesions tend to be intra-articular and are most commonly found about the hip joint [32]. Because of their intra-articular location, cancellous osteoid osteomas tend to be associated with joint effusions and synovitis. The least common type of osteoid osteoma is the subperiosteal type located along the surface of the bone. Subperiosteal osteoid osteomas are also most commonly found in the femoral neck [32]. Recent reports have postulated that many osteoid osteomas classified as cortical may in fact be subperiosteal osteoid osteomas with abundant surrounding reactive sclerosis and that subperiosteal osteomas may not be as uncommon as previously reported [33].

Although radiographic and CT imaging features are typically characteristic, the MR imaging findings of osteoid osteomas can be subtle or misleading. Lesions are typically surrounded by extensive edema-like signal within the adjacent marrow that may be misinterpreted for bone contusion or edema resulting from avascular necrosis of the femoral head or transient osteoporosis of the hip. This abnormal surrounding marrow signal is often most prominent on STIR or T2-weighted images with fat saturation. One of the keys to diagnosis is to identify the nidus of the lesion. Unfortunately, the nidus can be quite small within a large area of surrounding reactive marrow signal, and if the slice thickness or slice spacing is too great, the lesion may not be well appreciated. Typically, the nidus is seen on MR imaging as a small (less than 1.5 cm) focus of predominantly low signal on T1- and T2-weighted images surrounded by a reactive edema-like signal (Fig. 4). In more chronic cases, the nidus may be surrounded by dense fusiform reactive sclerosis; in such a case, the nidus demonstrates increased signal in relation to the low signal surrounding sclerotic bone and cortex. Imaging after administration of intravenous gadolinium typically demonstrates enhancement of the vascular nidus of the lesion. It is often helpful to confirm cases of suspected osteoid osteoma found on MR imaging with high-resolution CT to characterize the lesion

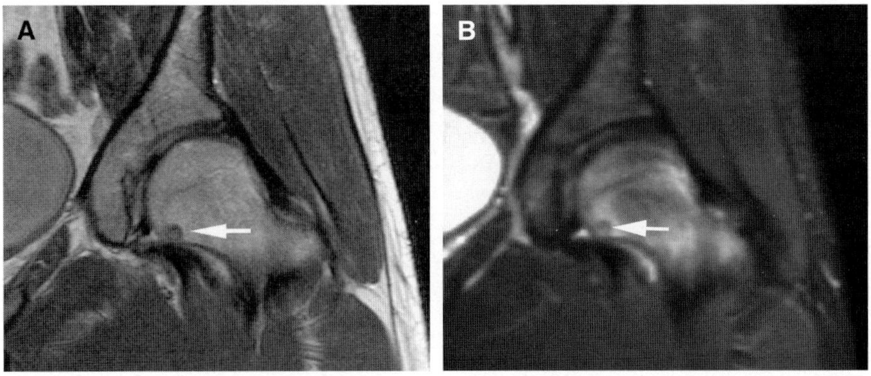


Fig. 4. A 17-year-old male patient with osteoid osteoma. The patient presented with hip pain, which was worse at night and relieved by nonsteroidal anti-inflammatory medications. T1-weighted (*A*) and T2-weighted (*B*) coronal MR images depict an osteoid osteoma (*arrow*) involving the inferomedial aspect of the left femoral head, with extensive surrounding marrow edema.

more definitively. The preferred treatment of osteoid osteoma is percutaneous image-guided radiofrequency ablation.

### *Osteochondroma*

Osteochondroma is a common benign skeletal lesion that not infrequently occurs about the hip. Approximately 9% of all osteochondromas occur in the proximal femur [31]. Osteochondromas present with well-defined osseous excrescences that grow in continuity with the underlying cortex and medullary cavity of the host bone. Lesions are juxta-articular in location and typically involve the metaphysis of the affected bone. Osteochondromas are thought to arise from ectopic growth plate cartilage that is displaced to the metaphyseal region. The ectopic growth plate cartilage forms a cartilaginous cap over the exostosis, and this provides the source of growth of the osseous excrescence [34]. Osteochondromas may be pedunculated with an elongated stalk or sessile with a broad-based attachment of the underlying bone. Pedunculated osteochondromas typically point away from the adjacent joint related to growth in the underlying host bone, which causes the lesion to lag behind and direct away from the adjacent joint. Lesions are often seen as incidental findings but can be symptomatic and related to compression or frictional forces on adjacent structures [34].

Ninety percent of osteochondromas are solitary lesions, whereas 10% of cases have multiple lesions. Multiple lesions are usually associated with hereditary multiple exostosis (HME) or familial osteochondromatosis, which is an autosomal dominant disorder characterized by numerous osteochondromas. Osteochondromas typically have a benign course, with less than 1% of solitary osteochondromas undergoing malignant degeneration to chondrosarcoma. Malignant transformation is more common in patients with HME or familial osteochondromatosis and is seen in up to 15% of such cases [34]. There are a number of findings that would suggest malignant transformation. Growth of lesions typically arrests after puberty, so growth in adult patients or rapid growth in younger patients is worrisome. Onset of increased pain associated with the lesion also should raise suspicion. Imaging findings that would suggest malignant change include development of destructive changes within the lesion or focal thickening of the cartilaginous cap greater than 1.5 cm [35].

Although the diagnosis of osteochondroma is typically made radiographically, MR imaging can be quite useful in characterizing symptomatic lesions. MR imaging can accurately demonstrate the thickness of the cartilaginous cap and define the anatomic relation of the lesion to surrounding structures. The hallmark of lesions on all imaging studies is corticomedullary continuity with the underlying host bone, and this can be precisely depicted with MR imaging. The cartilaginous cap can be well demonstrated draped over the lesion and is seen as low signal intensity on T1-weighted images and as high signal intensity on fluid-sensitive sequences. Lesions may occasionally be associated with bursal formation related to frictional forces with surrounding tissues, which can also be easily seen with MR imaging.

### *Enchondroma*

Enchondroma is a cartilaginous lesion that is frequently seen as an incidental finding about the hip joint. Enchondroma is a benign tumor composed of rests of hyaline cartilage that are ectopically located in the medullary canal [35]. Enchondromas are most commonly seen in adults, although they can be seen in nearly any age group [31]. Men and women are equally affected. Lesions are most commonly seen in the hands and long bones. Lesions are found in the proximal femur in approximately 8% of cases [31]. Enchondromas are usually incidental findings, and most are asymptomatic. Pain at presentation should suggest a complication of the enchondroma, such as pathologic fracture or, in rare cases, malignant transformation. Pathologic fracture through the lesion is not uncommon, especially in those lesions that are large or eccentric in location. Malignant transformation of enchondromas is distinctly unusual and is seen in less than 1% of cases.

Lesions are typically centered in the intramedullary canal but may occasionally be eccentrically located within the bone [35]. Enchondromas typically demonstrate a lobulated pattern of growth with variable margins, depending on location and rate of growth. MR imaging features of enchondromas are characteristic (Fig. 5). Lesions demonstrate a well-circumscribed margin that is multilobulated, relating to the numerous lobules of hyaline cartilage that make up the tumor. The hyaline cartilage components of the tumor are seen as low signal intensity on T1-weighted images and as high signal intensity on

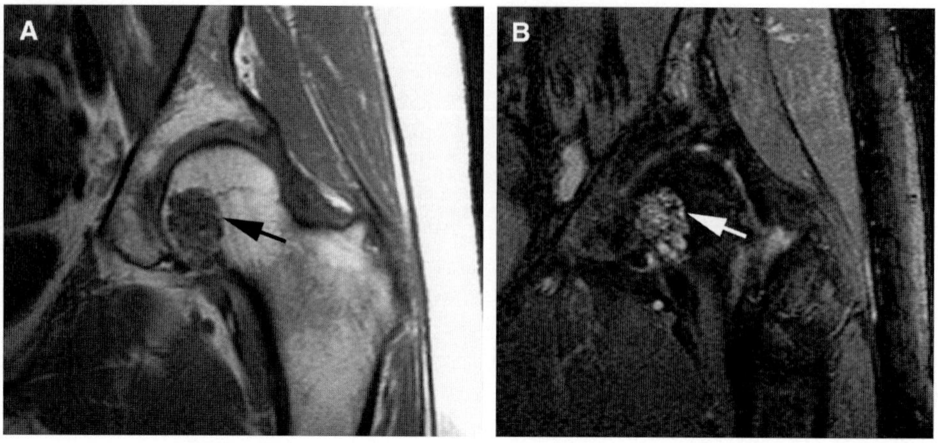


Fig. 5. A 62-year old woman with enchondroma. Incidental enchondroma was noted in the left femoral head during imaging for indication of pelvic pain. Coronal (*A*) T1-weighted and (*B*) T2-weighted images demonstrate a lobulated tumor (*arrow*) in the medial femoral head that is primarily isointense to hyaline cartilage, with areas of signal voids corresponding to chondroid calcification.

T2-weighted images. Chondroid matrix and mineralization are frequently present within the lesion and are depicted on MR imaging as punctate foci of signal voids on all sequences. Intervening areas of preserved marrow fat are often seen extending between the lobules of hyaline cartilage at the margins of the lesion. This is best seen on T1-weighted images and gives a characteristic appearance of the lesion that allows confident diagnosis of a cartilage lesion. Postgadolinium imaging reveals heterogeneous septal and peripheral enhancement of the lesions.

The main differential consideration for an enchondroma is a chondrosarcoma. Unfortunately, these two lesions can be quite difficult to differentiate radiographically and histologically. MR imaging, with its multiplanar capability, can be quite useful to evaluate an equivocal lesion seen on radiographs. Helpful distinguishing features favoring chondrosarcoma rather than enchondroma include frank soft tissue extension of the lesion and endosteal scalloping greater than two thirds the width of the cortex associated with the lesion.

### *Chondroblastoma*

Chondroblastoma is one of the most common benign tumors involving the hip and the most common benign tumor to occur entirely in the capital epiphysis of the proximal femur [30]. The femoral head accounts for 9.3% of all chondroblastomas [36]. Lesions may also occur in the greater trochanter and acetabulum. Chondroblastomas predominantly occur in children and young adults. The peak age for lesions is in the second decade of life, with approximately half of all cases occurring in this age group. Approximately 90% of cases occur in individuals between the ages of 5 and 25 years. Men and boys are typically affected two to three times more commonly than girls and women. Pain associated with the lesion is the most common complaint and is nearly universal [31]. The lesion arises from the epiphyseal growth plate cartilage and extends into the epiphysis.

MR imaging typically demonstrates lesions as having low to intermediate signal intensity on T1-weighted images and intermediate to high signal intensity on T2-weighted images. Chondroblastomas are typically oval or round in shape and small. Approximately 80% are 1 to 4 cm in diameter. Lesions are typically associated with extensive surrounding marrow edema in the epiphysis and surrounding soft tissues. An associated joint effusion is often seen in the involved joint in approximately 30% of cases. Approximately half of all lesions are associated with a thick solid periosteal reaction along the shaft of the involved long bone. After administration of contrast, lesions, and often the surrounding edematous changes, depict significant enhancement.

### *Intraosseous lipoma*

Intraosseous lipoma has been previously reported to be an uncommon lesion; however, with the proliferation of MR imaging, these lesions have been increasingly recognized and the true incidence seems to be much higher than previously thought [37]. Lesions are almost always asymptomatic, which contributes to the underestimation of the incidence of these lesions. Although lesions can occur in nearly any bone in the body, they are commonly found in the intertrochanteric and subtrochanteric regions about the hip. Lesions can be subdivided into three types [38]. Stage 1 lesions are predominantly solid and contain viable lipocytes. Stage 2 lesions represent a transition between stage 1 and 3 lesions and depict a combination of viable lipocytes and an area of fat necrosis that may demonstrate cyst formation or calcification. Stage 3 lesions are advanced lesions that demonstrate extensive involutional change, such that fat may not be appreciated. Cyst formation and calcification may be present. It is thought that there is a progression of lesions from stage 1 to stage 3 related to ischemia and infarction. It has been postulated that this may occur related to lipocyte growth and multiplication in the rigid confines of the bony architecture, which leads to ischemia, cell death, and fat necrosis [37].

MR imaging is ideal for depicting intraosseous lipomas. Lesions are commonly well defined, often with sclerotic margins (Fig. 6). Similar to subcutaneous lipomas, however, a certain subset of lesions demonstrates ill-defined margins and is difficult to differentiate from surrounding marrow fat. As expected, imaging features parallel the histologic stage of the lesion [37]. Stage 1 lesions are predominantly viable lipocytes and thus have mainly high signal intensity on T1- and T2-weighted images and demonstrate suppression on fat-saturated or inversion recovery sequences. Stage 2 lesions depict varying stages of fat necrosis within the lesion ranging from stranding of the fat to small focal areas of calcification or cyst formation (see Fig. 6). Stage 3 lesions are predominantly necrotic fat and thus demonstrate extensive cyst formation with low signal on T1-weighted images and high signal on T2-weighted images. Foci of dystrophic calcification are also common in stage 3 lesions, seen as foci of low signal on T1- and T2-weighted images. Stage 3 lesions more commonly demonstrate well-defined sclerotic margins [37].

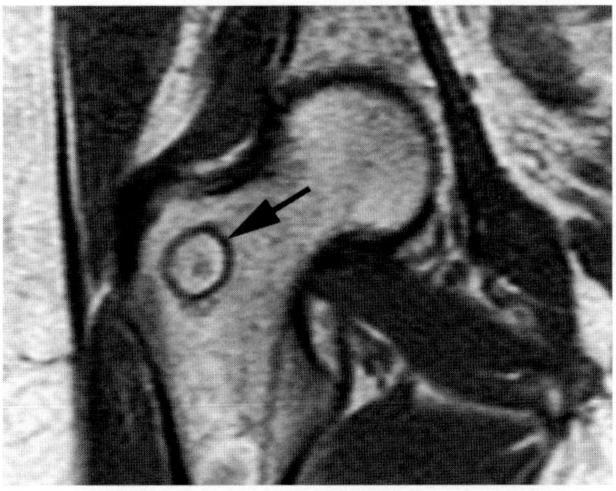

Fig. 6. Intraosseous lipoma. An older gentleman presented with contralateral hip pain and an incidental intraosseous lipoma (*arrow*) involving the intertrochanteric region of the right proximal femur. The lesion is well defined with a sclerotic margin, with stranding of the fat centrally compatible with mild internal fat necrosis on a T1-weighted coronal image of the right hip.

## Tumor-like conditions

Although tumors of the hip are not uncommon, tumor-like processes are far more commonly encountered in clinical practice. These include synovial-based tumor-like processes, such as pigmented villonodular synovitis (PVNS) and synovial chondromatosis. Various soft tissue and osseous lesions could be misinterpreted as true tumors if the radiologist is unaware of underlying pathophysiology. Finally, MR imaging can serve to exclude underlying tumors when radiographs display aggressive features of tumor-like processes.

### *Pigmented villonodular synovitis*

PVNS is a diffuse, proliferative, synovial-based disorder that most often affects the knee. The hip joint is the second most commonly affected joint; in a large series from the Mayo Clinic, almost 20% of cases involved the hip [39]. Patients usually present in their third or fourth decade, and there is a female predominance. Patients can present with mechanical pain, swelling, or decreased range of motion [39]. Grossly, proliferation and hemosiderin deposition give the synovium the appearance of a red shaggy beard.

Radiographically, PVNS of the hip may present with normal radiographs, large and multiple osseous lucencies, arthrosis, osteonecrosis of the femoral head, or joint destruction with acetabular protrusion [40]. Well-defined erosions with thin sclerotic borders can be present in up to 50% of all cases of PVNS, being more common in joints with tight capsules, such as the hip. Osseous erosions are typically multiple and occur on both sides of the joint. MR imaging is the imaging modality of choice for diagnosis. MR imaging demonstrates a diffuse heterogeneous process that involves the synovium. Nodules are typically isointense to hypointense relative to skeletal muscle on T1-weighted and conventional T2-weighted images (Fig. 7). There may be scattered areas of high T1-weighted signal, correlating to areas of high lipid-laden macrophage content. Uncommonly, lesions may be cystic, or there may be adjacent osseous edema-like signal changes. Gradient-echo imaging may be helpful in eliciting "blooming" artifact attributable to the paramagnetic effect of hemosiderin in the soft tissues. Treatment consists of complete synovectomy and prosthetic replacement of the hip [39].

### *Synovial chondromatosis*

Synovial chondromatosis is an uncommon, benign, synovial-based process that occurs in a large joint, such as the knee, hip, elbow, or shoulder. This process can also affect tendon sheaths, bursae, or surrounding soft tissues, however [41]. Patients typically present in the fourth or fifth decade, and men are afflicted two to four times more frequently than women [42]. Multiple small metaplastic cartilaginous or osteocartilaginous nodules are attached to the synovial membrane of the joint, such as the hip. Nodules can then become detached within the hip joint, becoming loose bodies.

Patients without mineralized loose bodies may present with normal radiographs, a nonspecific periarticular soft tissue mass, widened joint space, osseous erosions, or early osteoarthrosis [42]. In a series of 15 patients with synovial chondromatosis of the hip, radiographs demonstrated ossified or calcified juxta-articular bodies in 80% of patients, osseous erosions in 53%, osteophytes in 47%, juxta-articular osteopenia in 33%, and joint space narrowing in 33% [43]. MR imaging depicted synovial thickening in 87% of these patients, osseous erosion in 73%, intra-articular bodies in 73%, and an extra-articular herniation sac in 40% (Fig. 8) [44]. The signal characteristics of the intra-articular bodies depend on their composition. If the bodies are unmineralized, they follow cartilage on all sequences. If the bodies are ossified, they have signal characteristics similar to bone marrow signal centrally and hypointense cortical signal peripherally. Uniformly calcified bodies are present as signal voids. Of note, extracapsular extension of synovial osteochondromatosis in the hip has been documented along the iliopsoas and obturator externus fat plane [43].

### *Paralabral cysts*

Paralabral cysts are cystic foci adjacent to the acetabular labra that are associated with labral

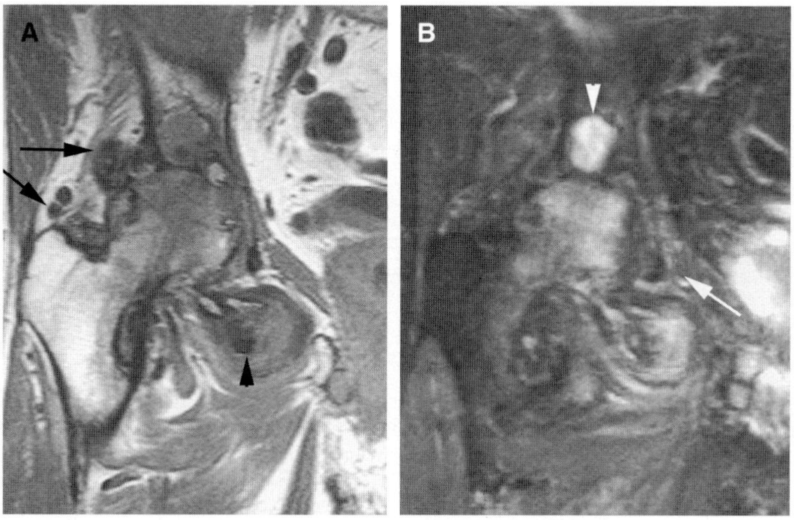


Fig. 7. A 78-year-old man with PVNS of the right hip. Coronal (*A*) T1-weighted and (*B*) T2-weighted images demonstrate multiple intra-articular and periarticular low-density nodular foci (*black arrows*) involving the right hip and obturator externus bursa (*black arrowhead*). Also note the subchondral cysts (*white arrowhead*) and edema-like marrow signal (*white arrow*) involving both sides of the hip joint.

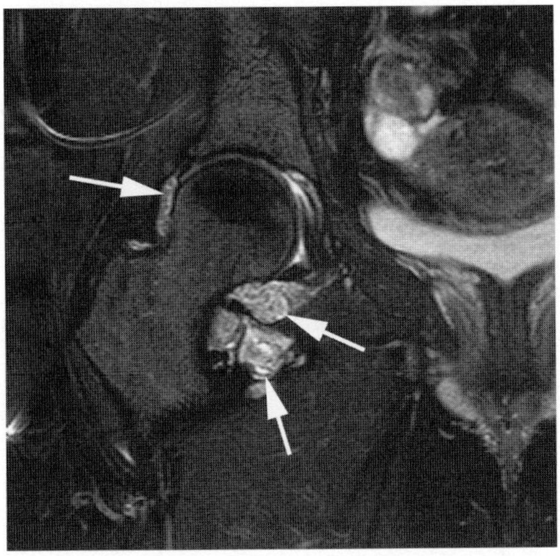

Fig. 8. A 42-year-old woman with synovial chondromatosis of the right hip. Coronal fast spin-echo, T2-weighted, fat-suppressed image through the right hip demonstrates multiple small filling defects (*arrows*) within the hip joint that are isointense to cartilage.

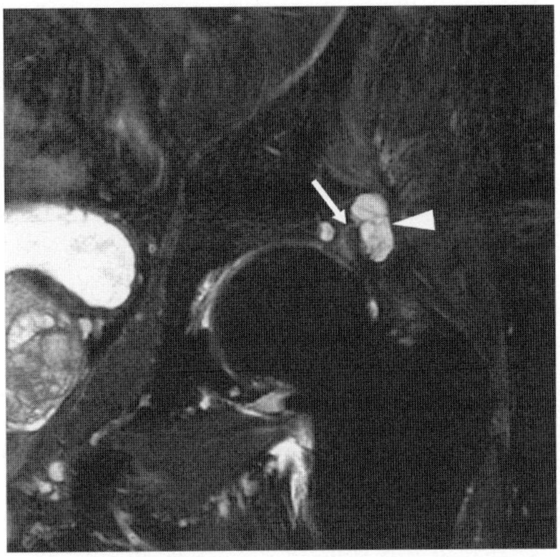

Fig. 9. An 82-year-old man with a paralabral cyst and associated labral tear. Coronal fast spin-echo, T2-weighted, fat-suppressed image through the left hip delineates a cystic focus (*arrowhead*) lateral to the superior labral tear (*arrow*). Also present are degenerative chondromalacia and subchondral cyst formation.

tears. The cause of these cysts is currently believed to be synovial fluid that is forced through the labral defects via a one-way valve mechanism. Paralabral cysts have been reported in patients with a history of trauma, hip dysplasia, and degenerative arthrosis. Patients often clinically present with acute exacerbation of hip pain, sharp mechanical pain, or clicking [43]. Pathology specimens reveal myxoid degeneration and mucoid debris within the cysts, sometimes with identifiable synovial tissue [45].

MR imaging is quite sensitive for the detection of paralabral cysts. Imaging can depict round or ovoid cystic masses ranging in size from a few millimeters to up to 3 cm and with intermediate to low signal intensity on T1-weighted images and high signal on T2-weighted images (Fig. 9) [46]. The paralabral cysts almost always are adjacent to a labral tear or an abnormal labrum. These cysts occur in the anterosuperior [47,48] or

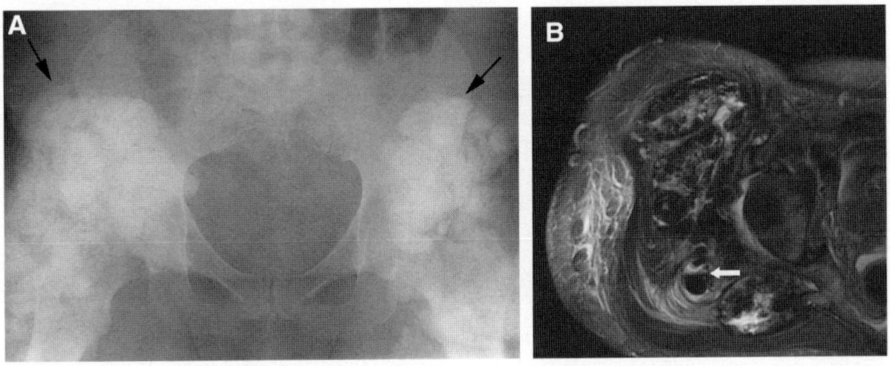


Fig. 10. A 34-year-old man with metastatic calcific deposits around the hips. The patient is on hemodialysis for renal failure. (*A*) Anteroposterior view of the pelvis demonstrates large tumor-like metastatic calcific deposits (*arrows*) around the hips. (*B*) Axial fast spin-echo, T2-weighted, fat-suppressed image through the right hemipelvis demonstrates multiple primarily low signal intensity masses throughout the gluteal and quadriceps muscles. Notice the fluid-fluid level in one of the cystic spaces (*arrow*), corresponding to dependent milk-of-calcium within the cyst.

posterosuperior portion of the labrum [45]. MR arthrography can increase the sensitivity and accuracy for the detection of the associated labral tears.

*Distended bursae*

Distended bursae around the hip can sometimes be confused with soft tissue tumors. Of the 15 synovial-lined bursae about the hip, the more commonly imaged include the trochanteric, iliopsoas, and obturator bursae. The three bursae comprising the trochanteric bursa complex have been elucidated in the literature through cadaveric and clinical studies [49]. This bursal complex is discussed in this issue in the article on the iliopsoas tendon. The iliopsoas bursa is commonly identified on MR imaging because it communicates with the hip joint in up to 15% of normal patients and has an even higher incidence in patients with hip pathologic findings. A distended obturator externus bursa (see Fig. 7B) is thought to be formed by the protrusion of the posterior hip joint between the ischiofemoral capsular ligament and the zona orbicularis and is evident deep to the obturator externus tendon and posteroinferior to the hip joint on MR imaging [50].

*Metastatic calcification*

Metastatic calcification related to a disturbance in calcium or phosphorus metabolism can be caused by hyperparathyroidism, hypoparathyroidism, renal osteodystrophy, hypervitaminosis D, milk-alkali syndrome, sarcoidosis, metastases, myeloma, or leukemia [51]. The term *tumoral calcinosis* is reserved for the idiopathic condition in which these causes are excluded.

These metastatic calcifications typically present as large periarticular calcified masses around large joints, such as the hip, shoulder, or elbow. Layering milk-of-calcium within cystic spaces can be detected on horizontal beam radiographs or CT or MR images [52]. MR imaging can demonstrate signal voids layering within the dependent portion of the cysts (corresponding to the calcium) and nondependent fluid-like signal (Fig. 10). MR imaging is also useful in defining the extent of involvement throughout the muscles and other soft tissue planes.

*Fibrous dysplasia*

Fibrous dysplasia is a common benign disorder that predominantly affects adolescents and young adults. Rather than a true neoplasm, fibrous dysplasia is a developmental anomaly in which

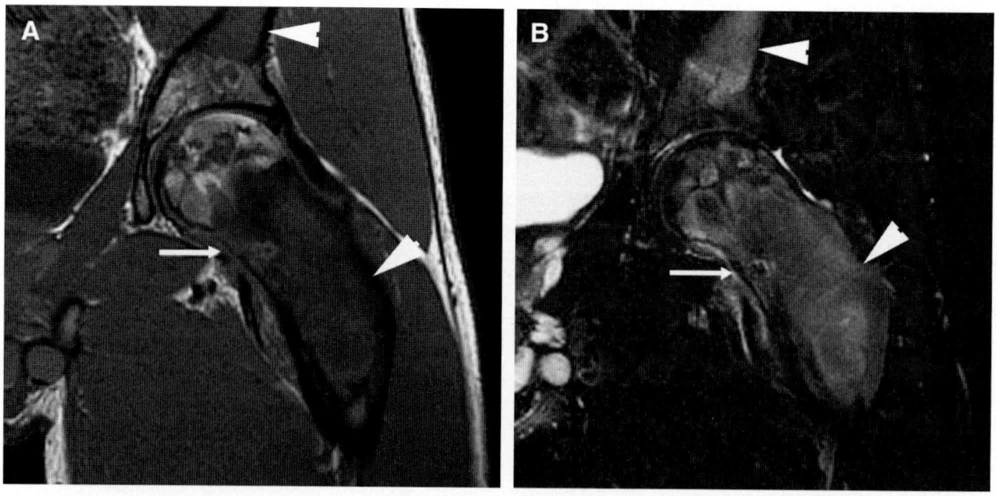


Fig. 11. A 17-year-old boy with polyostotic fibrous dysplasia and pathologic fracture. The patient is a cross-country runner with hip pain. (*A*) T1-weighted coronal image demonstrates foci of abnormal signal isointense to skeletal muscle in the superior acetabulum and proximal femur (*arrowheads*), with peripheral areas of lower signal intensity. There is focal loss of the medial femoral neck hypointense cortex, corresponding to a nondisplaced incomplete fracture (*arrow*). (*B*) Fast spin-echo, T2-weighted, fat-suppressed coronal image displays increased and slightly heterogeneous signal intensity as well as hypointense rinds about the lesions (*arrowheads*). Note the subtle hypointense fracture line (*arrow*) through the medial femoral neck, with surrounding fluid signal.

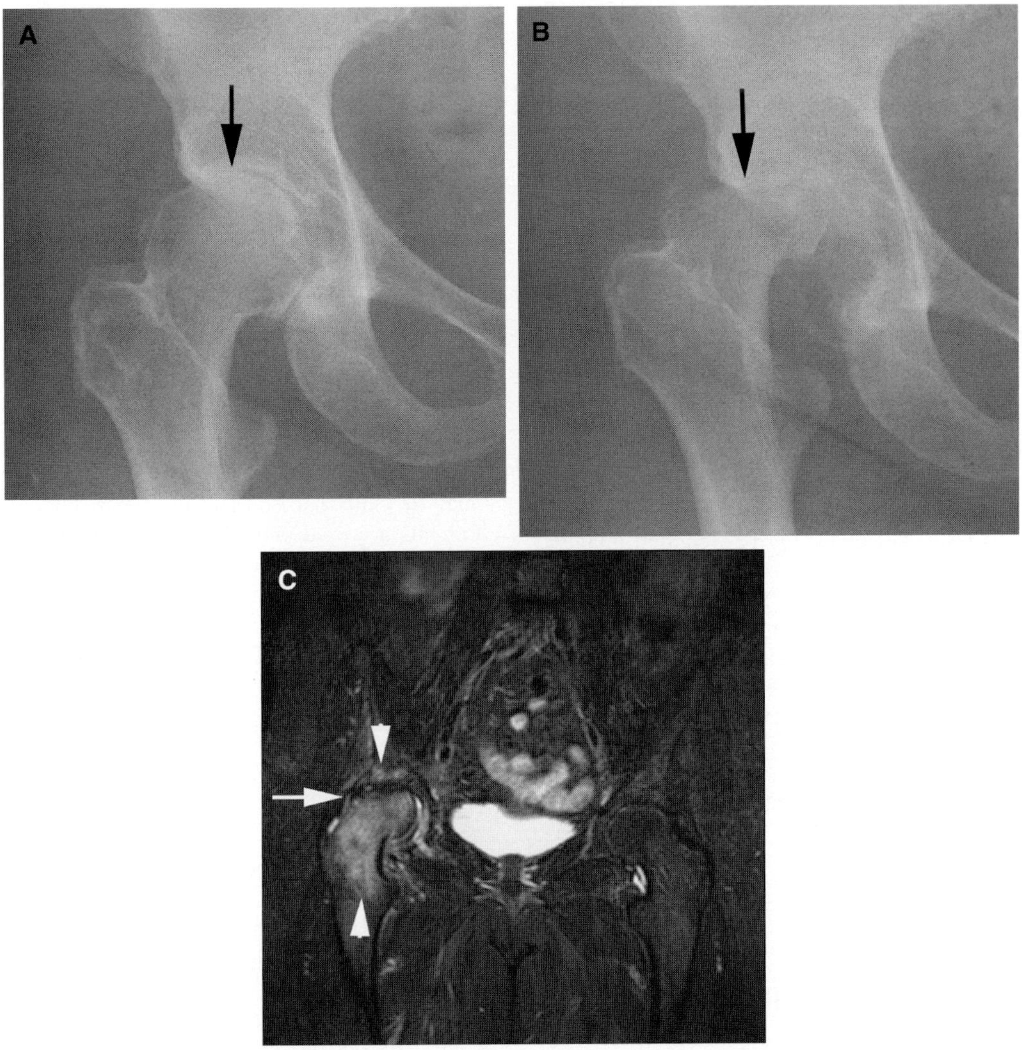


Fig. 12. Rapidly progressive osteoarthritis of the hip. (*A*) A 74-year-old woman presented with right hip pain. A baseline anteroposterior right hip radiograph demonstrates narrowing of the superior hip joint (*arrow*) but an intact femoral head. (*B*) Anteroposterior right hip radiograph obtained 4 months later depicts the rapid destruction of the right femoral head and obliteration of the joint space (*arrow*). (*C*) Coronal T1-weighted image through the pelvis of a 68-year-old woman with rapidly progressive osteoarthritis of the hip depicts the amputated appearance of the superior femoral head (*arrow*) and increased signal intensity throughout the proximal femur and acetabulum (*arrowheads*). No osseous or soft tissue mass is identified.

the normal medullary space is replaced by fibro-osseous tissue [53]. Lesions may be monostotic, involving a single bone, or polyostotic. Polyostotic disease can occur as part of the McCune-Albright or Mazabraud syndromes. Monostotic lesions are six times more common than polyostotic lesions [53]. Approximately 18% of lesions affect the femur, with preferential involvement of the femoral neck. Most patients are asymptomatic, although pain may be associated with the lesions and deformity may occur, resulting in gait disorders. Complications include aneurysmal bone cyst formation, pathologic fracture (Fig. 11), and malignant degeneration. Malignancy occurs in less than 1% of cases in the form of osteosarcoma, fibrosarcoma, MFH, or, rarely, chondrosarcoma [53].

Lesions are well defined, intramedullary, and associated with expansile remodeling, and they usually have a ground-glass appearance. Fibrous dysplasia can also present as a radiolucent or sclerotic lesion, however. Lesions typically involve the metaphysis and diaphysis of the bone. Shepard's crook deformity is a commonly seen bowing deformity with varus angulation in cases of fibrous dysplasia involving the proximal femur [53]. Radiography is superior to other modalities for the diagnosis of fibrous dysplasia. MR imaging can be quite variable in cases of fibrous dysplasia and typically does not add any additional information to that obtained from radiographs. Variations in the cellular constituents of fibrous dysplasia account for the variable appearance on MR imaging [53]. Lesions typically have signal intensity similar to that of skeletal muscle on T1-weighted images and variable signal intensity on T2-weighted images (see Fig. 11). Approximately one third of all lesions demonstrate signal intensity less than that of fat on T2-weighted images, whereas two thirds of cases demonstrate signal intensity greater than that of fat [53]. Hypointense rinds can be appreciated in up to 77% of cases [54]. Less common MR imaging findings include internal septations, hypointense bony trabeculae, cystic changes, soft tissue extension, and pathologic fracture (see Fig. 11) [54]. After contrast administration, 75% of lesions demonstrate central enhancement, whereas peripheral enhancement is seen in 25% [54].

### *Liposclerosing myxofibrous tumor*

LSMFT is a benign fibro-osseous lesion that has also been referred to as "polymorphic fibrocystic disease of bone" and "polymorphic fibro-osseous lesion of bone." Lesions are characterized by complex mixtures of histologic elements that may include lipoma, fibroxanthoma, myxoma, myxofibroma, fat necrosis, ischemic ossification, cyst formation, and fibrous dysplasia–like features [55]. Lesions have a characteristic skeletal distribution, are most commonly found in the femur, and are typically seen proximally in the intertrochanteric region. In a study of 39 lesions, 33 (85%) were located in the femur, and of these lesions, 30 (91%) were located in the intertrochanteric region [55]. The significance of these lesions is that they have a slightly higher incidence of malignant transformation than usual benign fibro-osseous lesions and therefore require surveillance.

The MR imaging features of LSMFT are characteristic. Lesions present as a well-defined geographic lesion with low signal intensity margins corresponding to sclerotic margins seen on radiographs. These findings are compatible with their indolent pattern of growth [55]. T1-weighted images demonstrate the lesion to be fairly homogeneous with signal intensity similar to that of skeletal muscle. T2-weighted images depict the lesion as slightly more heterogeneous, with signal intensity similar to or greater than that of fat on non–fat-suppressed sequences. Fat-suppressed fluid-sensitive sequences depict the lesion as having heterogeneous high signal intensity.

### *Rapidly progressive osteoarthritis of the hip*

Rapidly progressive osteoarthritis of the hip (Fig. 12) is an unusual form of osteoarthrosis characterized by rapid chondrolysis, in which there is greater than 2 mm of cartilage loss or 50% of joint space narrowing within 1 year [56]. Patients are predominantly female, with an average age of 60 to 70 years, and present with rapid destruction of the hip joint within months of the onset of hip pain [56,57]. Treatment is usually total joint replacement.

## Summary

In conclusion, a wide variety of tumors and tumor-like conditions have a predilection for the hip. The imaging evaluation of these lesions begins with radiographs. Radiographs can depict the extent of disease; any characteristic calcifications; and osseous changes, such as remodeling, periosteal reaction, or destruction. MR imaging has emerged as the preferred imaging modality of choice for evaluating osseous and soft tissue masses of the hip by providing information for diagnosis and staging. The MR imaging signal characteristics and enhancement patterns of malignant and benign hip tumors permit specific diagnoses in some cases. Synovial-based tumor-like processes of the hip can be characterized by MR signal characteristics, such as the hemosiderin within PVNS or the cartilage within synovial chondromatosis. Finally, MR imaging can serve to exclude underlying osseous or soft tissue tumors when radiographs display aggressive features of tumor-like processes.

## References

[1] Rubin DA, Kneeland JB. MR imaging of the musculoskeletal system: technical considerations for enhancing image quality and diagnostic yield. AJR Am J Roentgenol 1994;163:1155–63.

[2] Mirowitz SA. Fast scanning and fat-suppression MR imaging of musculoskeletal disorders. AJR Am J Roentgenol 1993;161:1147–57.
[3] Shuman WP, Baron RL, Peters MJ, et al. Comparison of STIR and spin-echo MR imaging at 1.5 T in 90 lesions of the chest, liver and pelvis. AJR Am J Roentgenol 1989;152:853–9.
[4] Dwyer AJ, Frank JA, Sank VJ, et al. Short-T1 inversion-recovery pulse sequence: analysis and initial experience in cancer imaging. Radiology 1988;168: 827–36.
[5] Harkens KL, Moore TE, Yuh WTC, et al. Gadolinium-enhanced MRI of soft-tissue masses. Australas Radiol 1993;37:30–4.
[6] Seeger LL, Widoff BE, Bassett LW, et al. Preoperative evaluation of osteosarcoma: value of gadopentetate dimeglumine-enhanced MR imaging. AJR Am J Roentgenol 1991;157:347–51.
[7] Kransdorf MJ. Malignant soft tissue tumors in a large referral population: distribution of diagnosis by age, sex, and location. AJR Am J Roentgenol 1995;164:129–34.
[8] Bhagavan BS, Dorfman HD. The significance of bone and cartilage formation in malignant fibrous histiocytoma of soft tissue. Cancer 1982;49:480–8.
[9] Murphey MD, Gross TM, Rosenthal HG. Musculoskeletal malignant fibrous histiocytoma: Radiologic-pathologic correlation. Radiographics 1994; 14:807–26.
[10] Rezel PA, Soule EH, Coventry MB. Liposarcoma of the extremities and limb girdles. A study of two hundred twenty-two cases. J Bone Joint Surg Am 1966; 48:229–44.
[11] Weiss SW. Lipomatous tumors. In: Weiss SW, Brooks JSJ, editors. Soft tissue tumors. Baltimore (MD): Williams & Wilkins; 1996. p. 207–51.
[12] Ippolito V, Brien EW, Menendez LR, et al. Case report 797. "Dedifferentiated" lipoma-like liposarcoma of soft-tissue with focal transformation to high-grade "sclerosing" osteosarcoma. Skeletal Radiol 1993;22:604–8.
[13] Kransdorf MJ, Meis JM, Jelinek JS. Dedifferentiated liposarcoma of the extremities: imaging findings in four patients. AJR Am J Roentgenol 1993;161: 127–30.
[14] Weiss SW, Rao VK. Well-differentiated liposarcoma (atypical lipoma) of deep soft tissues of the extremities, retroperitoneum, and miscellaneous sites: a follow-up study of 92 cases with analysis of the incidence of "dedifferentiation." Am J Surg Pathol 1992;16:1051–8.
[15] Weiss SW, Goldblum JR. Liposarcoma. In: Weiss SW, Goldblum JR, editors. Enzinger and Weiss's soft tissue tumors. 4th edition. St. Louis (MO): CV Mosby Company; 2001. p. 641–93.
[16] Arkun R, Memis A, Akalin T, et al. Liposarcoma of soft tissue: MRI findings with pathologic correlation. Skeletal Radiol 1997;26:167–72.
[17] Munk PL, Lee MJ, Janzen DL, et al. Lipoma and liposarcoma: evaluation using CT and MR imaging. AJR Am J Roentgenol 1997;169:589–94.
[18] Jelinek JS, Kransdorf MJ, Shmookler BM, et al. Liposarcoma of the extremities: MR and CT findings of the histologic subtypes. Radiology 1993; 186:455–9.
[19] Wile AG, Evans HL, Romsdahl MM. Leiomyosarcoma of soft tissue: a clinicopathologic study. Cancer 1981;48:1022–32.
[20] Weiss SW, Goldblum JR. Leiomyosarcoma. In: Weiss SW, Goldblum JR, editors. Enzinger and Weiss's soft tissue tumors. 4th edition. St. Louis (MO): CV Mosby; 2001. p. 727–48.
[21] Ryan JR, Baker LH, Benjamin RS. The natural history of metastatic synovial sarcoma. The experience of the Southwest Oncology Group. Clin Orthop 1982;164:257–60.
[22] Wright PH, Sim FH, Soule EH, et al. Synovial sarcoma. J Bone Joint Surg Am 1982;64:112–22.
[23] Jones BC, Sundaram M, Kransdorf MJ. Synovial sarcoma: MR imaging findings in 34 patients. AJR Am J Roentgenol 1993;161:827–30.
[24] Murphey MD, Walker EA, Wilson AJ, et al. Imaging of primary chondrosarcoma: radiologic-pathologic correlation. Radiographics 2003;23:1245–78.
[25] Murphey MD, Flemming DJ, Boyea SR, et al. Enchondroma versus chondrosarcoma in the appendicular skeleton: differentiating features. Radiographics 1998;18:1213–38.
[26] Janzen L, Logan PM, O'Connell JX, et al. Intramedullary chondroid tumors of bone: correlation of abnormal peritumoral marrow and soft-tissue MRI signal with rumor type. Skeletal Radiol 1997;26: 100–6.
[27] Varma DGK, Ayala AG, Carrascco SG, et al. Chondrosarcoma: MR imaging with pathologic correlation. Radiographics 1992;12:687–704.
[28] Mirra JM. Intramedullary cartilage and chondroid-producing tumors. In: Mirra JM, editor. Bone tumors: clinical, radiologic, and pathologic correlations. Philadelphia: Lea & Febiger; 1989. p. 439–535.
[29] Kaim AH, Hugli R, Bonel HM, et al. Chondroblastoma and clear-cell chondrosarcoma: radiological and MRI characteristics with histopathological correlation. Skeletal Radiol 2002;31:88–95.
[30] McBryde AM. Benign (intracapsular) tumors of the hip. Curr Pract Orthop Surg 1977;7:154–78.
[31] Wold LE, McLeod RA, Sim FH, et al. Atlas of orthopedic pathology. Philadelphia: WB Saunders; 1990.
[32] Kransdorf MJ, Stull MA, Gilkey FW, et al. From the archives of the AFIP: osteoid osteoma. Radiographics 1991;11:671–95.
[33] Kayser F, Resnick D, Haghighi P, et al. Evidence of the subperiosteal origin of osteoid osteomas in tubular bones: analysis by CT and MR imaging. AJR Am J Roentgenol 1998;3:609–14.

[34] Karasick D, Schweitzer ME, Eschelman DJ. Symptomatic osteochondromas: imaging features. AJR Am J Roentgenol 1997;168:1507–12.
[35] Greenfield GB, Arrington JA. Imaging of bone tumors. A multimodality approach. Philadelphia: JB Lippincott; 1995.
[36] McBryde A, Goldner JL. Chondroblastoma of bone. Am Surg 1970;36:94–108.
[37] Propech T, Bullard MA, Lin J, et al. Radiologic-pathologic correlation of intraosseous lipomas. AJR Am J Roentgenol 2000;175:673–8.
[38] Milgram JW. Intraosseous lipomas: radiologic and pathologic manifestations. Radiology 1988;167: 155–60.
[39] Schwartz HS, Unni KK, Pritchard DJ. Pigmented villonodular synovitis: a retrospective review of affected large joints. Clin Orthop 1989;247:243–55.
[40] Cotton A, Flipo RM, Chastanet P, et al. Pigmented villonodular synovitis of the hip: review of radiographic features in 58 patients. Skeletal Radiol 1995;24:1–6.
[41] Enzinger FM, Weiss SW. Benign tumors and tumor-like lesions of synovial tissue. In: Weiss SW, Goldblum JR, editors. Cartilaginous soft tissue tumors. St. Louis (MO): Mosby; 2001. p. 1366–8.
[42] Llauger J, Palmer J, Roson N, et al. Nonseptic monoarthritis: imaging features with clinical and histopathologic correlation. Radiographics 2000; 20(Suppl):S263–78.
[43] Robinson P, White LM, Kandel R, et al. Primary synovial osteochondromatosis of the hip: extracapsular patterns of spread. Skeletal Radiol 2004;33:210–5.
[44] Kim SH, Hong SJ, Park JS, et al. Idiopathic synovial osteochondromatosis of the hip: radiographic and MR appearances in 15 patients. Korean J Radiol 2002;3:254–9.
[45] Magee T, Hinson G. Association of paralabral cysts with acetabular disorders. AJR Am J Roentgenol 2000;174:1381–4.
[46] Schnarkowski P, Steinbach LS, Tirman PFJ, et al. Magnetic resonance imaging of labral cysts of the hip. Skeletal Radiol 1996;25:733–7.
[47] Petersilge C, Haque MA, Petersilge WJ, et al. Acetabular labral tears: evaluation with MR arthrography. Radiology 1996;200:231–5.
[48] Czerny C, Hofmann S, Neuhold A, et al. Lesions of the acetabular labrum: accuracy of MR imaging and MR arthrography in detection and staging. Radiology 1996;200:225–30.
[49] Pfirrmann CWA, Chung CB, Theumann NH, et al. Greater trochanter of the hip: attachment of the abductor mechanism and a complex of three bursae—MR imaging and MR bursography in cadavers and MR imaging in asymptomatic volunteers. Radiology 2001;221:469–77.
[50] Robinson P, White LM, Agur A, et al. Obturator externus bursa: anatomic origin and MR imaging features of pathologic involvement. Radiology 2003;228:230–4.
[51] Resnick D. Soft tissue disorders. In: Resnick D, editor. Diagnosis of bone and joint disorders. 4th edition. Philadelphia: WB Saunders; 2002. p. 4635–6.
[52] Gordon LF, Arger PH, Dalinka MK, et al. Computed tomography in soft tissue calcification layering. Comput Assist Tomogr 1984;8:71–3.
[53] Fitzpatrick KA, Taljanovic M, Speer DP, et al. Imaging findings of fibrous dysplasia with histopathologic and intraoperative correlation. AJR Am J Roentgenol 2004;182:1389–98.
[54] Jee W, Choi K, Choe B, et al. Fibrous dysplasia: MR imaging characteristics with radiopathologic correlation. AJR Am J Roentgenol 1996;167: 1523–7.
[55] Kransdorf MJ, Murphey MD, Sweet DE. Liposclerosing myxofibrous tumor: a radiologic-pathologic-distinct fibro-osseous lesion of bone with a marked predilection of the intertrochanteric region of the femur. Radiology 1999;212:693–8.
[56] Boutry N, Paul C, Leroy X, et al. Rapidly destructive osteoarthritis of the hip: MR imaging findings. AJR Am J Roentgenol 2002;179:657–63.
[57] Lawrance JAL, Athanasou NA. Rapidly destructive hip disease. Skeletal Radiol 1995;24:639–41.

ELSEVIER
SAUNDERS

Magn Reson Imaging Clin N Am
13 (2005) 775–782

MAGNETIC
RESONANCE
IMAGING CLINICS
of North America

# Morel-Lavallée Lesion: Review with Emphasis on MR Imaging

José M. Mellado, MD[a,*], Jenny T. Bencardino, MD[b]

[a] *Institut de Diagnostic per la Imatge, Hospital Universitari de Tarragona Joan XXIII, Carrer Doctor Mallafrè Guasch, 4, 43007 Tarragona, Spain*

[b] *Medical Arts Radiology Group, PC, and Department of Radiology, Huntington Hospital, North Shore Long Island Jewish Health System, 270 Park Avenue, Huntington, NY 11743, USA*

In 1863, the French surgeon Victor Auguste François Morel-Lavallée first described posttraumatic fluid collections dissecting subcutaneous fatty tissues [1]. These collections are particularly common in the trochanteric region and proximal thigh, where they have been termed Morel-Lavallée (ML) lesions [2]. Similar lesions in the hip, thigh, and other locations have been described in the literature under various different names, such as post-traumatic soft-tissue cyst [3], pseudocyst [4], pseudolipoma [5], ML extravasation [4], ML effusion [6,7], and ML hematoma [8]. Related posttraumatic entities that involve the subcutaneous tissues, such as ancient hematoma [9], organizing hematoma [10], and chronic expanding hematoma [11], may represent the end-stage process of many longstanding ML lesions [12].

ML lesions are well known to orthopedic surgeons but rarely have been discussed in the radiologic literature [6,12,13]. We briefly review the relevant anatomy, presumed etiology, histopathology, clinical diagnosis, imaging features, and treatment options of ML lesions in the hip region. We also wish to emphasize the role of MR imaging in the detection, characterization, and staging of ML lesions.

## Anatomic considerations

ML effusions may involve the subcutaneous tissues of the abdominal wall, the buttock, the lower lumbar spine, the scapular region, or the calf. ML lesions of the trochanteric region and proximal thigh are especially frequent and typically dissect perifascial planes adjacent to the fascia lata and iliotibial band [2].

In the thigh region, the superficial fascia represents the deepest portion of the cellular subcutaneous tissue. It occasionally separates into two or more layers, between which superficial vessels and nerves are found. The deep fascia—or fascia lata—covers the outer surface of the thigh muscles. The fascia lata is thicker in the upper and lateral part of the thigh, where it receives fibers from the gluteus maximus and where the tensor fascia lata muscle lies between its layers. These layers fuse downward, giving rise to a reinforcement of the fascia lata, the so-called iliotibial band.

In the anterolateral region of the thigh, the lateral circumflex artery provides perforating vessels to the rectus femoris, vastus lateralis, and tensor fascia lata muscles and septocutaneous vessels to the anterolateral skin of the thigh. Some perforators to the vastus lateralis also pierce the fascia lata and reach the anterolateral thigh skin [14].

The exposed nature of the trochanteric region and proximal thigh, the great extension and firm attachment of the anterolateral fascia lata and iliotibial band, the relative mobility of the regional skin, and the rich pattern of local dermic vascularization may account for the high frequency of ML effusions in this region [15–19].

## Clinical considerations

ML effusions typically result from tangential trauma, most commonly in the setting of high-speed

* Corresponding author. Current address: Servicio de Radiodiagnostico, Hospital Reina Sofia de Tudela, Carretera Tarazona, KM 4, 31500-Tudela, Navarra, Spain.

*E-mail address:* jmellado@comz.org (J.M. Mellado).


doi:10.1016/j.mric.2005.08.006

motor vehicle crashes. ML lesions of the trochanteric region and proximal thigh are particularly frequent in motorcycle accidents, usually in association with pelvic and acetabular fractures [2,15–19]. They also may occur after plastic surgery, especially when liposuction and abdominoplasty are combined [4].

ML effusions represent abnormal dissection of the virtual space comprised between the superficial and deep fasciae, a lesion pattern frequently referred to as closed degloving injury. As a consequence of violent trauma, excessive shearing or compressive forces may cause abrupt separation of the skin and subcutaneous fatty tissue from the underlying deep fascia. This separation causes disruption of perforating vessels that pierce the deep fascia, which results in draining of lymph or blood into the perifascial plane. Subsequently, debris from fat necrosis and blood clots may arise. Factors in the blood clotting cascade and blood breakdown products are said to be involved in a chronic inflammatory reaction, which may cause further bleeding and originate a peripheral capsule with granulation tissue, capillaries, and fibrosis. This reaction may account for the occasional slow growth and self-perpetuation of the process [9,14–17,19,20].

The classic description of ML lesions refers to fluctuant subcutaneous cystic structures lined by a fibrous capsule and filled with a sterile hemolymphatic or serohematic content [1]. Longstanding ML lesions also may present as firm subcutaneous pseudotumors, however [12]. Analysis of resected specimens in such cases has shown an encapsulated lesion, which contains a complex combination of recent hemorrhage, organized blood clots, debris, fibrin, and normal or necrotic fatty tissue. The peripheral capsule of such lesions consists of hyalinized, mostly hypocellular fibrous tissue and occasionally shows mild inflammatory infiltrates. Such histologic backgrounds closely resemble those of related entities, such as ancient hematoma [9], organizing hematoma [10], or chronic expanding hematoma [11].

ML lesions may be detected during the first hours to days after trauma. The clinical diagnosis of acute ML lesions is suspected when a soft, fluctuant area of skin is found in a region exposed to previous tangential trauma. In general, patients with ML lesions show evidence of soft tissue swelling, contour deformity, or palpable bulge. Decreased cutaneous sensation, abrasions, and local contusions can be encountered. The lesions may remain stable, progressively decrease in size, or show slow growth. When a lesion is extensive and severe, potential complications, such as infection and necrosis of the overlying skin, may occur [16–18].

The presence of ML lesions initially may be missed in up to one third of cases and may be detected months or years after trauma, when the acute lesions already have resolved [2,15,17,18,20]. In such instances, especially if local pain or slow growth is present, a clinical misdiagnosis of soft tissue tumor may occur, which warrants further imaging assessment [15,17,19].

## Diagnostic imaging

The use of diagnostic imaging for detecting, characterizing, or staging ML lesions rarely has been addressed in the literature [6, 9–13]. Plain radiography may reveal a nonspecific, noncalcified soft tissue mass [6,10]. The ultrasound appearance of ML lesion is that of a complex cystic mass, either anechoic or mildly hyperechoic [6,11,13]. On CT, ML lesions appear as well-defined, encapsulated fluid collections that occasionally show fluid-fluid levels [6,10,11,14]. MR imaging is better suited than other imaging modalities for evaluating ML lesions because of its superb soft tissue contrast [9,12,13].

## MR imaging features

ML lesions typically are found within the subcutaneous perifascial planes of the trochanteric region and anterolateral proximal thigh (Figs. 1–8). They may be bilateral, may reach variable, occasionally large dimensions, and usually manifest some mass effect, generating contour abnormalities or compressive deformities on adjacent muscle bellies. ML lesions are usually well defined and oval or fusiform in shape and may have tapering margins that fuse with adjacent fascial planes. ML lesions may show variable internal signal intensity, partial or complete septations, and fluid-fluid levels. They tend to be partially or completely surrounded by a peripheral rim, which appears hypointense on all pulse sequences and represents a fibrous capsule. This capsule may be absent, however, especially in the early stages [12,13].

Based on our observations of more than 20 cases of ML lesions studied with MR imaging with corresponding histopathology, we propose the following MR classification (Table 1).

Type I ML lesions exhibit fluid-like MR signal characteristics. When compared with skeletal

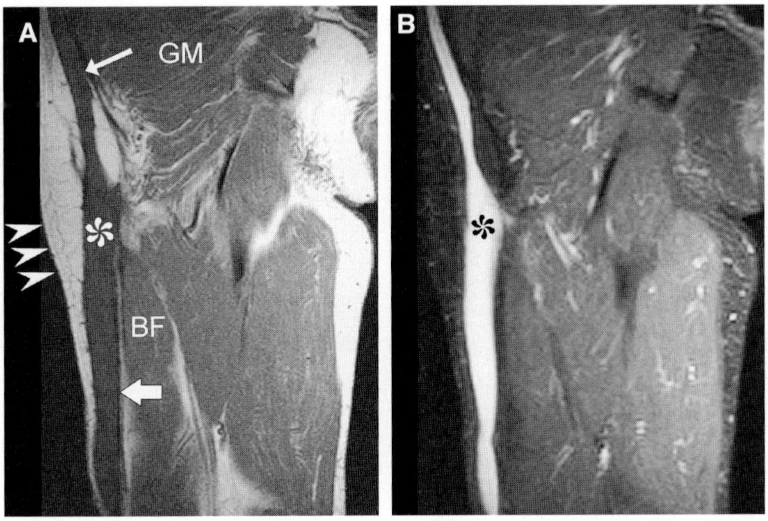


Fig. 1. Type I ML lesion: seroma. (*A*) Coronal T1-weighted MR image of the right thigh demonstrates a longstanding ML effusion (*), which dissects the virtual space between the subcutaneous fatty tissue (*arrowheads*), the fascia lata (*thin arrow*) and the iliotibial band (*thick arrow*). The fluid collection is homogeneously hypointense to skeletal muscle. (*B*) Coronal inversion recovery image shows a homogeneous, hyperintense effusion (*). Needle aspiration analysis was consistent with a serohematic effusion or seroma. BF, biceps femoris; GM, gluteus maximus. (*From* Mellado JM, Perez del Palomar L, Diaz L, et al. Long-standing Morel-Lavallee lesions of the trochanteric region and proximal thigh: MRI features in five patients. AJR Am J Roentgenol 2004;182(5):1294; with permission.)

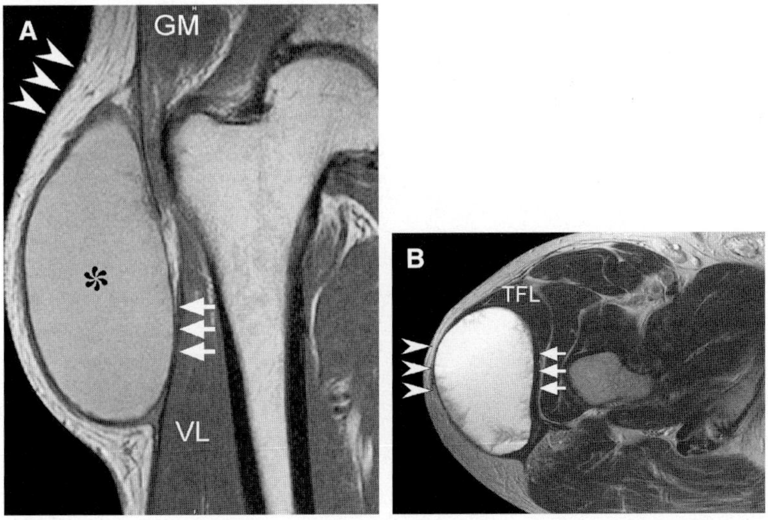


Fig. 2. Type II ML lesion: subacute hematoma. (*A*) Coronal T1-weighted MR image reveals a longstanding hyperintense ML lesion (*), which dissects the plane between the fascia lata (*arrows*) and the subcutaneous fatty tissue (*arrowheads*) of the right trochanteric region and proximal thigh. (*B*) Axial T2-weighted MR image demonstrates internal homogeneous hyperintensity and a thick capsule (*arrowheads*). The lesion is adjacent to the iliotibial band (*arrows*) and tensor fascia lata muscle. GM, gluteus maximus muscle; TFL, tensor fascia lata; VL, vastus lateralis. (*A*, *From* Mellado JM, Perez del Palomar L, Diaz L, et al. Long-standing Morel-Lavallee lesions of the trochanteric region and proximal thigh: MRI features in five patients. AJR Am J Roentgenol 2004;182(5):1292; with permission.)

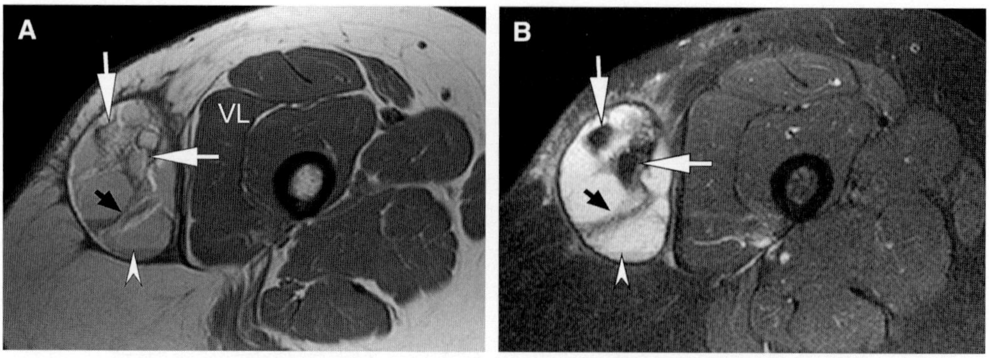


Fig. 3. Type II ML lesion: subacute hematoma. Axial T1-weighted (*A*), and inversion recovery (*B*) MR images reveal a longstanding encapsulated ML lesion within the subcutaneous perifascial plane of the anterolateral proximal thigh, adjacent to the vastus lateralis muscle, which shows characteristics of a subacute hematoma. Entrapped fatty globules (*white arrows*), fluid-fluid levels (*white arrowhead*), and internal septae (*black arrow*) are seen. VL, vastus lateralis.

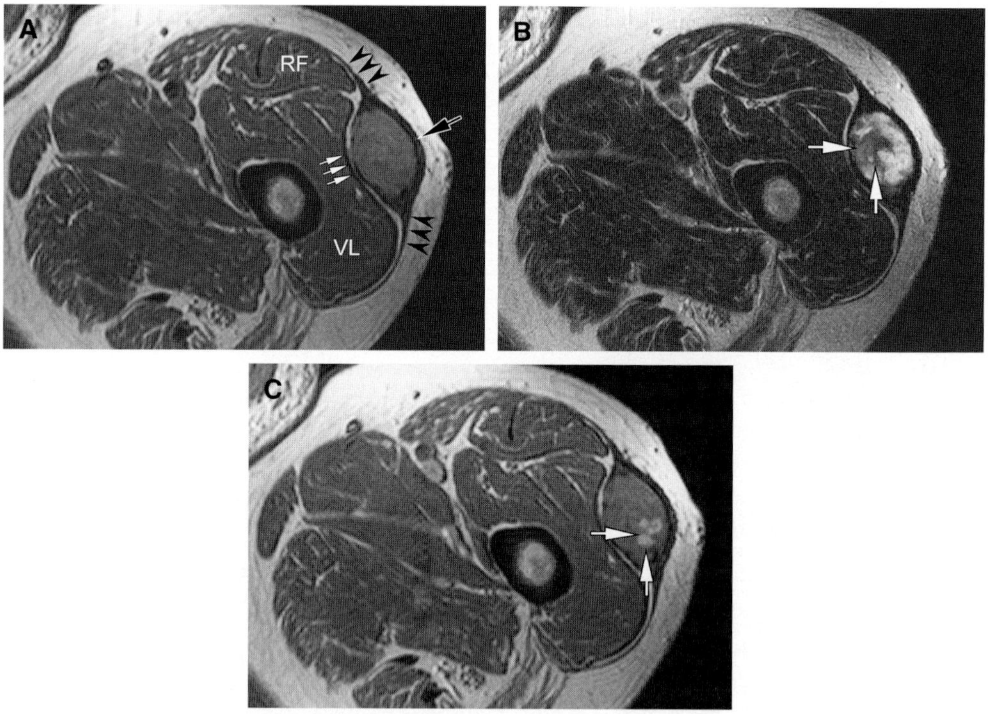


Fig. 4. Type III ML lesion: chronic organizing hematoma. (*A*) Axial T1-weighted MR image through the proximal aspect of the left thigh shows a longstanding ML lesion (*black arrow*) causing compression deformity on the adjacent vastus lateralis muscle (*white arrows*). The lesion is hyperintense to skeletal muscle, is surrounded by a thick hypointense capsule, and shows tapering margins that fuse with normal contiguous fascia lata (*black arrowheads*). (*B*) Axial T2-weighted MR image shows heterogeneous hyperintensity within the lesion, with areas of internal hypointensity (*arrows*). (*C*) Contrast-enhanced T1-weighted MR image shows a focus of internal enhancement (*arrows*) within the lesion. RF, rectus femoris; VL, vastus lateralis. (*From* Mellado JM, Perez del Palomar L, Diaz L, et al. Long-standing Morel-Lavallee lesions of the trochanteric region and proximal thigh: MRI features in five patients. AJR Am J Roentgenol 2004;182(5):1290; with permission.)

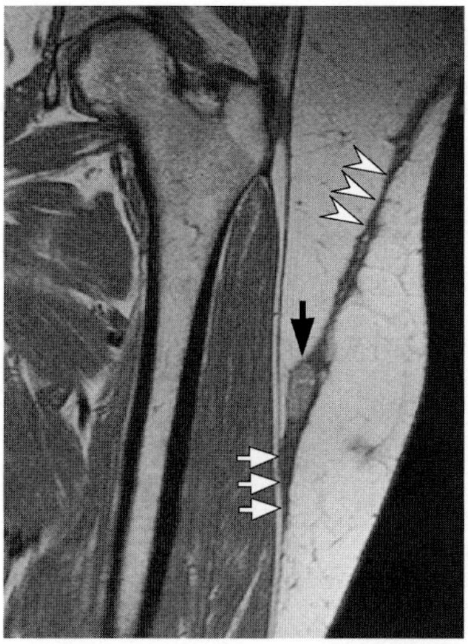

Fig. 5. Type IV ML lesion: closed laceration. Coronal T1-weighted MR image of the left thigh shows a longstanding ML lesion characterized by dissection of perifascial planes adjacent to the fascia lata (*white arrows*) associated with closed laceration of the subcutaneous fatty tissue (*white arrowheads*). A black arrow points to a small hyperintense oval globule, possibly a blood clot.

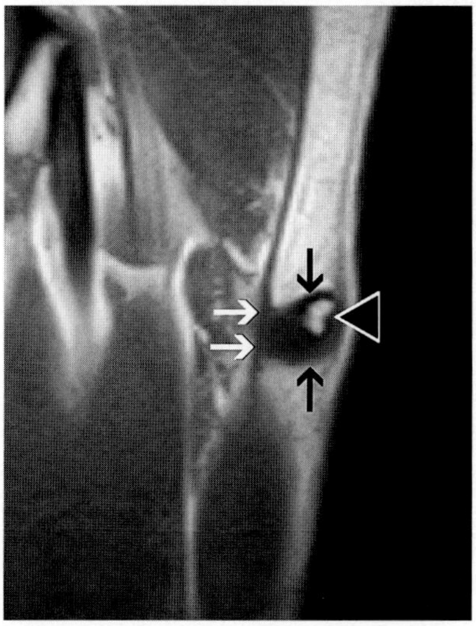

Fig. 6. Type V ML lesion: pseudonodular. Coronal T1-weighted MR image shows a small pseudonodular ML lesion (*black arrows*) within the subcutaneous region of the left thigh, abutting the perifascial planes (*white arrows*). Internal hypointensity is consistent with serous content. A small internal focus of high signal (*arrowhead*) suggests an entrapped fatty globule.

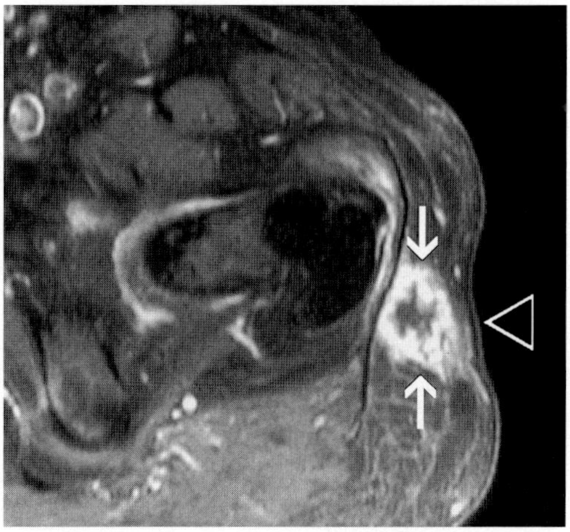

Fig. 7. Type V ML lesion: pseudonodular. Axial fat-suppressed, contrast-enhanced T1-weighted MR image shows a small pseudonodular longstanding ML lesion (*white arrows*) within the subcutaneous perifascial planes of the left hip. There is retraction of the overlying skin (*arrowhead*) and thick irregular peripheral enhancement.

muscle, these lesions are homogeneously hypointense on T1-weighted sequences and hyperintense on T2-weighted sequences [12]. This MR pattern typically reflects the existence of a serohematic effusion or seroma, which may be found in acute and chronic settings, may or not be encapsulated, and closely follows the classic description of ML lesions (see Fig. 1) [1].

Type II ML lesions exhibit predominantly homogeneous hyperintensity on T1- and T2-weighted MR imaging sequences (see Fig. 2) [12,13]. This MR pattern, particularly the T1 shortening, is probably related to the existence of methemoglobin, which is characteristic of subacute hematomas. Methemoglobin is first observed on the periphery of early subacute hematomas and progressively acquires a more homogeneous distribution [21]. The internal T1 shortening within the ML lesions also may reflect the existence of entrapped fatty tissue (see Fig. 3) [13].

Type III ML lesions demonstrate intermediate signal intensity on T1-weighted images and heterogeneous hyperintensity on T2-weighted sequences, with internal areas of T2 hypointensity. This MR pattern likely reflects the coexistence of hemosiderin deposition, granulation tissue, necrotic debris, fibrin, and blood clots, which are characteristic of chronic organizing hematoma (see Fig. 4). In this MR pattern, patchy internal and peripheral enhancement can be seen on post-contrast MR imaging [12].

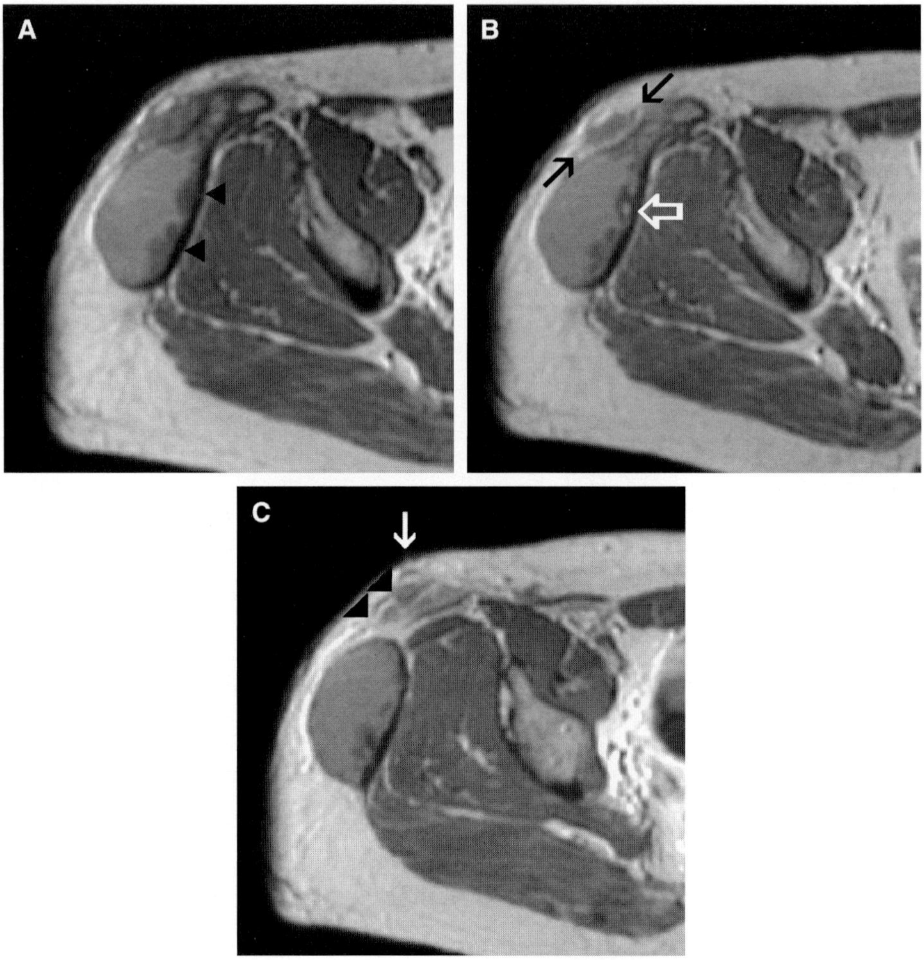


Fig. 8. Type VI ML lesion: infected. (*A*) Axial T1-weighted MR image of the right hip demonstrates a large subcutaneous perifascial effusion (*arrowheads*) causing mild compression deformity of the adjacent tensor fascia lata and gluteal muscles. A thick capsule with internal peripheral nodularity and subcutaneous fluid leakage is noted. (*B*) Axial contrast-enhanced T1-weighted MR image at the same level as that in panel *A* shows peripheral enhancement of the ML lesion (*open arrow*) and extravasated fluid (*black arrows*). (*C*) Axial contrast-enhanced T1-weighted MR image distal to *A* and *B* depicts sinus tract enhancement (*arrowheads*) leading to draining skin fistula (*arrow*) marked by vitamin E capsule. Fluid cultures grew *Staphylococcus aureus*.

Longstanding ML lesions also may present more atypical MR imaging features. Type IV ML lesions show a combination of perifascial dissection and closed fatty tissue laceration (see Fig. 5) with or without associated serous/hemorrhagic collection. Type V ML lesions have a perifascial pseudonodular appearance (see Fig. 6) and occasionally show irregular peripheral enhancement and skin retraction (see Fig. 7). Type VI lesions correspond to an infected ML lesion, which may present with a thick enhancing peripheral capsule and internal septations, inflammatory reaction of the adjacent fatty tissue and fascia, peripheral fluid leakage, and sinus tract formation (see Fig. 8).

## Differential diagnosis and treatment

The differential diagnosis of ML lesions includes other subcutaneous lesions of posttraumatic origin, such as fat necrosis and pseudolipoma, coagulopathy-related hematoma, and some soft tissue tumors.

Subcutaneous fat necrosis in children may present as a posttraumatic palpable lump [22].

Table 1
MR classification of Morel-Lavallée lesions

| | Type I | Type II | Type III | Type IV | Type V | Type VI |
|---|---|---|---|---|---|---|
| | Seroma | Subacute hematoma | Chronic organizing hematoma | Closed laceration | Pseudonodular | Infected |
| Morphology | Laminar | Oval | Oval | Linear | Round | Variable Sinus tract |
| Capsule | Occasional | Thin | Thick | Absent | Thin/thick | Thick |
| T1 signal | Hypointense | Hyperintense | Intermediate | Hypointense | Variable | Variable |
| T2 signal | Hyperintense | Hyperintense | Heterogeneous | Hyperintense | Variable | Variable |
| Enhancement | Absent | Variable | Internal/ peripheral | Variable | Internal/ peripheral | Internal/ peripheral |

The interval between trauma and lesion detection may be considerable [23]. The MR characteristics of fat necrosis vary depending on the age of injury. On MR imaging, subcutaneous fat necrosis may appear as small, well-defined linear spiculations, may show globular shape, or may adopt a laminar configuration [22–24]. Their MR signal characteristics are highly variable because they may appear hypo- or hyperintense on T1- and T2-weighted images [22,23]. Not infrequently, they present as high signal intensity areas in the subcutaneous fatty tissue, are surrounded by low signal septations, and resemble a bunch of grapes [25]. Fat necrosis occasionally may resemble a pseudonodular ML lesion (see Fig. 6) but belongs to the spectrum of histologic changes that may be found in ML lesions.

Posttraumatic pseudolipomas may develop at a site of prior blunt trauma or surgical procedure, often antedated by a soft tissue hematoma. Pseudolipomas also may arise from closed degloving injury [5]. Clinically, they present as subcutaneous masses with the consistency of normal adipose tissue. Characteristic MR imaging findings are nonencapsulated subcutaneous fatty masses without contrast enhancement [26].

Coagulopathy-related hematomas frequently are disproportionate to the degree of trauma or even may present without traumatic cause. Clinical distinction is usually based on history and laboratory tests. Finally, some soft tissue tumors may involve fascial or perifascial planes, particularly nodular fasciitis. In such cases, a prior traumatic event is typically missing, and the location of the mass is much less predictable.

In the acute traumatic setting, ML lesions require surgical intervention and débridement of necrotic tissue to avoid risk of infection. Conservative treatment also may be attempted. Once the serohematic effusion becomes encapsulated, simple percutaneous drainage may not be curative and typically is followed by repetitive recurrences. Although partial aponeurotic resection may be attempted [7], wide surgical excision is usually recommended [16].

## Summary

MR imaging is the diagnostic imaging modality of choice in the assessment of ML lesions in the hip region. Given their typical location, morphology, signal behavior, and enhancement pattern, ML lesions can be identified readily on MR examinations of the hip and proximal thigh. Correct preoperative MR diagnosis of ML lesions can be useful for treatment planning.

## References

[1] Morel-Lavallée VAF. [Décollements traumatiques de la peau et des couches sous-jacentes]. Arch Gen Med 1863;1:20–38, 172–200, 300–32 [in French].

[2] Letournel E, Judet R. Fractures of the acetabulum. 2nd edition. Berlin: Springer-Verlag; 1993.

[3] Sterling A, Butterfield WC, Bonner R Jr, et al. Posttraumatic cysts of soft tissue. J Trauma 1977;17: 392–6.

[4] Zecha PJ, Missotten FE. Pseudocyst formation after abdominoplasty: extravasations of Morel-Lavallee. Br J Plast Surg 1999;52(6):500–2.

[5] Ozyazgan I, Eskitascglu T. Development of pseudolipoma after an endoscopically confirmed closed degloving injury. Plast Reconstr Surg 2004;114(7): 1987–9.

[6] Parra JA, Fernandez MA, Encinas B, et al. Morel-Lavallée effusions in the thigh. Skeletal Radiol 1997;26(4):239–41.

[7] Ronceray J. Active drainage by partial aponeurotic resection of Morel-Lavallee effusions. Nouv Presse Med 1976;5(20):1305–6.

[8] Beaulieu S, De Parades V, Manaouil D, et al. Retro-sacral hematoma of Morel-Lavallee: a rare cause of perianal sepsis. Gastroenterol Clin Biol 2001;25(11): 1031–2.

[9] Mentzel T, Goodlad JR, Smith MA, et al. Ancient hematoma: a unifying concept for a post-traumatic lesion mimicking an aggressive soft tissue neoplasm. Mod Pathol 1997;10:334–40.

[10] Lovern RE, Bosse DA, Hartshorne MF, et al. Organizing hematoma of the thigh: multiple imaging techniques. Clin Nucl Med 1987;12(8):661–4.

[11] Nakano M, Kondoh T, Igarashi J, et al. A case of chronic expanding hematoma in the tensor fascia lata. Dermatol Online J 2001;7:6.

[12] Mellado JM, Perez del Palomar L, Diaz L, et al. Long-standing Morel-Lavallee lesions of the trochanteric region and proximal thigh: MRI features in five patients. AJR Am J Roentgenol 2004; 182(5):1289–94.

[13] Gilbert BC, Bui-Mansfield LT, Dejong S. MRI of a Morel-Lavallée lesion. AJR Am J Roentgenol 2004;182:1347–8.

[14] Gosain AK, Yan JG, Aydin MA, et al. The vascular supply of the extended tensor fasciae latae flap: how far can the skin paddle extend? Plast Reconstr Surg 2002;110:1655–61.

[15] Collinge C, Tornetta P III. Soft tissue injuries associated with pelvic fractures. Orthop Clin North Am 2004;35(4):451–6.

[16] Hak DJ, Olson SA, Matta JM. Diagnosis and management of closed internal degloving injuries associated with pelvic and acetabular fractures: the Morel-Lavallée lesion. J Trauma 1997;42:1046–51.

[17] Hudson DA, Knottenbelt JD, Krige JE. Closed degloving injuries: results following conservative surgery. Plast Reconstr Surg 1992;89(5):853–5.

[18] Kottmeier SA, Wilson SC, Born CT, et al. Surgical management of soft tissue lesions associated with pelvic ring injury. Clin Orthop Relat Res 1996;329: 46–53.

[19] Gregory P, Sanders R. The management of severe fractures of the lower extremities. Clin Orthop Relat Res 1995;318:95–105.

[20] Rempel JH. Missed closed degloving injuries: late presentation as a contour deformity. Plast Reconstr Surg 1998;101(4):1159–60.

[21] Bush CH. The magnetic resonance imaging of musculoskeletal hemorrhage. Skeletal Radiol 2000;29: 1–9.

[22] Tsai TS, Evans HA, Donnelly LF, et al. Fat necrosis after trauma: a benign cause of palpable lumps in children. AJR Am J Roentgenol 1997;169:1623–6.

[23] Chan LP, Gee R, Keogh C, et al. Imaging features of fat necrosis. AJR Am J Roentgenol 2003;181:955–9.

[24] Lopez JA, Saez F, Alejandro Larena J, et al. MR diagnosis and follow-up of subcutaneous fat necrosis. J Magn Reson Imaging 1997;7:929–32.

[25] Canteli B, Saez F, de los Rios A, et al. Fat necrosis. Skeletal Radiol 1996;25:305–7.

[26] Theumann N, Abdelmoumene A, Wintermark M, et al. Posttraumatic pseudolipoma: MRI appearances. Eur Radiol 2005;15(9):1876–80.

ELSEVIER
SAUNDERS

Magn Reson Imaging Clin N Am
13 (2005) 783–797

MAGNETIC RESONANCE IMAGING CLINICS of North America

# MR Imaging of Congenital/Developmental and Acquired Disorders of the Pediatric Hip and Pelvis

Johanne E. Dillon, MD[a,*], Susan A. Connolly, MD[b], Leonard P. Connolly, MD[c], Young-Jo Kim, MD, PhD[d], Diego Jaramillo, MD[e]

[a]*Department of Radiology, Massachusetts General Hospital, Ellison 237, 55 Fruit Street, Boston, MA 02114, USA*
[b]*Department of Radiology, Children's Hospital Boston, Main 2, 300 Longwood Avenue, Boston, MA 02115, USA*
[c]*Division of Nuclear Medicine, Children's Hospital Boston, Pavilion 2, 300 Longwood Avenue, Boston, MA 02115, USA*
[d]*Children's Hospital Boston, Hunnewell 225, 300 Longwood Avenue, Boston, MA 02115, USA*
[e]*Children's Hospital of Philadelphia, 34th Street and Civic Center Boulevard, Philadelphia, PA 19104, USA*

This article reviews the MR imaging appearances of important congenital and acquired disorders of the pediatric hip and pelvis. MR imaging provides an accurate method of evaluating the hip and pelvis, and although multidetector CT shares its multiplanar imaging capabilities, the soft tissue resolution of MR imaging is superior to CT and is indispensable for purposes of imaging cartilage. This article discusses the standard MR imaging techniques for the hip and pelvis that we use, accompanied by any nonstandard techniques pertinent to the specific disorder.

## Technical considerations

Children aged 6 years and younger frequently require sedation to optimize MR imaging. An institutional sedation program should be a collaborative effort among imaging specialists, clinical practitioners, anesthesiologists, and nursing personnel. Personnel trained in pediatric advanced life support, monitoring and resuscitative equipment, and an active quality assurance program are essential components of a sedation program. Guidelines, such as those advanced by the American Society of Anesthesiologists [1], American College of Radiology [2], Joint Commission on Accreditation of Health Care Organizations [3], and American Academy of Pediatrics [4], are useful in establishing a sedation program. Sedation protocols, particularly regarding the recommended medications and their dosages, vary from institution to institution. Commonly used sedatives include barbiturates (eg, pentobarbital sodium) and opiates (eg, fentanyl). During sedation, patient monitoring must be the primary responsibility of a designated health care practitioner. After the procedure, a patient must be monitored in a suitably equipped area until established discharge criteria are met.

MR imaging of the hip and pelvis is performed with a phased array coil. Higher resolution images are obtained with a local surface coil, such as the shoulder coil. The proximal femora and the pelvis in its entirety are included within the field of view. The standard imaging protocol includes coronal T1-weighted spin echo, coronal short tau inversion recovery, axial T2-weighted fast spin echo (FSE) fat-saturated (f/s), oblique sagittal FSE proton density (PD) f/s, and axial FSE PD images. Coronal three-dimensional spoiled gradient recall echo with f/s is added when a physeal (growth plate) growth arrest is suspected. The clinical question determines whether intravenous gadolinium is administered and followed by multiplanar T1-weighted f/s images. Additional protocols for

* Corresponding author.
*E-mail address:* jedillon@partners.org (J.E. Dillon).

1064-9689/05/$ - see front matter 
doi:10.1016/j.mric.2005.08.007

nonstandard studies are included in each specific section where appropriate.

## Congenital and developmental disorders

### *Proximal femoral focal deficiency*

Proximal femoral focal deficiency (PFFD) encompasses a spectrum from hypoplasia to aplasia of the proximal femur, including the femoral head, neck, and proximal diaphysis. PFFD is unilateral in approximately 90% of cases and is congenital but not usually heritable. The incidence of this disorder is approximately 1 case per 52,000 live births [5]. Affected children are usually identified during infancy with limb shortening. Although numerous classifications systems are used for PFFD, the most commonly used is the Aitken classification (types A–D). Acetabular dysplasia correlates with the extent of femoral head hypoplasia or deformity. The presence and location of the femoral head and neck, which defines the Aitken classification of PFFD [6], are also clinically relevant for surgical planning and family counseling regarding treatment options. In type A PFFD, for example, early on there is an apparent radiographic defect in the upper femur that only later in life, when the secondary center of the proximal femur ossifies, evidences a well-formed femoral head within the acetabulum. MR imaging is able to distinguish among bone, cartilage, and fibrous tissue (Fig. 1) [5].

A related disorder, called congenital shortening of the femur, consists of shortening and anterolateral bowing of the femur with a valgus deformity of the knee. Absence of the anterior cruciate ligament leads to instability of the knee, whereas hamstring shortening limits straight leg raising. Ipsilateral fibular hemimelia and foot deformities are seen in association with congenital shortening of the femur. In addition to evaluating the hip structures, MR imaging reveals the extent of involvement of the musculature and ligaments (Fig. 2) [7].

Preoperative planning for children who have PFFD and congenital shortening is complicated. MR imaging provides the most accurate determination of the type of PFFD, including prediction of leg length discrepancy at maturity, hip joint integrity, and stability of the femoral segment. If there is an associated fibular hemimelia with congenital shortening of the femur, MR imaging can demonstrate the extent of involvement of the rays of the foot and the presence of tarsal coalition. These factors determine which children are candidates for a leg lengthening procedure, fusion of the femur to the pelvis, fusion of the knee, rotationoplasty, or amputation [8]. Contrast-enhanced MR angiography is important for purposes of demonstrating vascular structures when considering amputation or limb-salvage surgery, which may require soft tissue resection and rotation of the femur or tibia in an attempt to improve function (Fig. 3).

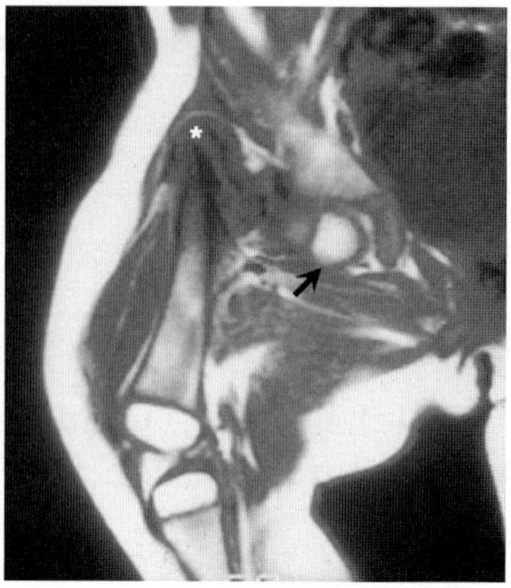


Fig. 1. Proximal focal femoral deficiency. Aitken type I. MR coronal T1-weighted image. The right femoral head demonstrates T1 high signal intensity and fatty marrow (*arrow*) and articulates with a well-formed acetabulum. A pseudoathrosis (*) formed in the T1 low signal intensity, fibrous tissue of the short proximal femur, which resulted in a subtrochanteric varus deformity.

### *Coxa vara*

Coxa vara is defined as an abnormally small angle, less than 120°, between the femoral neck and shaft. In the neonate this angle is normally approximately 150° and decreases during development. With progressive weight bearing during childhood, there is relatively greater growth of the lateral aspect of the proximal femoral physis, such that the angle decreases to approximately 120° to 130° in adults.

Coxa vara may be congenital and present a birth, developmental, or acquired secondary to other conditions. Congenital coxa vara is believed to be caused by a limb bud insult and typically demonstrates little progression after birth.

Developmental (infantile) coxa vara is likely secondary to abnormal proliferation of cartilage cells in the medial physis, which results in greater

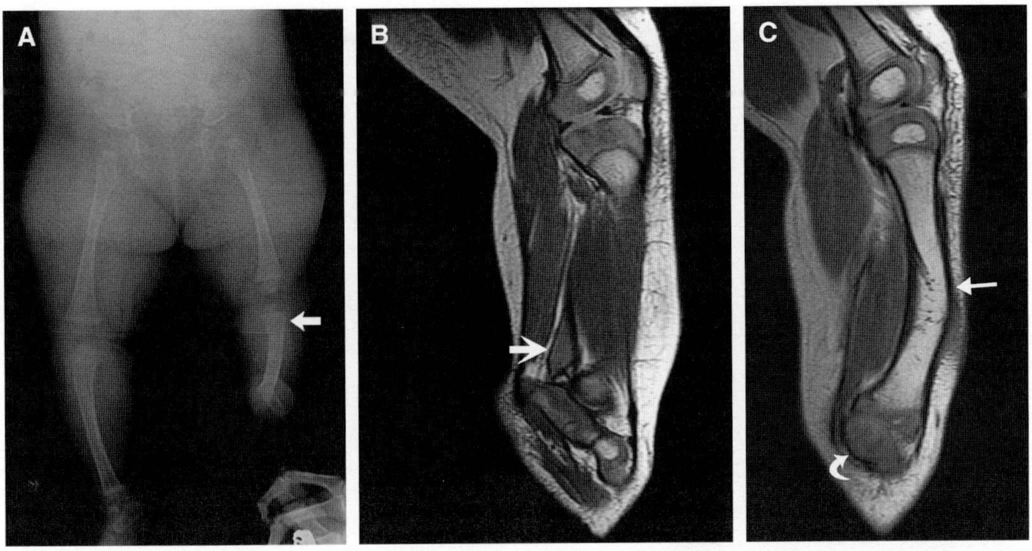


Fig. 2. (*A*) Radiograph of bilateral lower extremities in an infant with congenital shortening of the left femur. A short left femur with mild anterolateral bowing is seen in association with an apparent complete fibular hemimelia (*arrow*). (*B, C*) MR sagittal FSE PD images of the same patient demonstrate the presence of a cartilaginous distal fibula, which is intermediate in signal intensity on T1-weighted images (*arrow*). (*C*) The tibia is bowed anteriorly (*arrow*) and articulates directly with the calcaneus (*curved arrow*).

growth laterally. Children with developmental coxa vara usually present at approximately age 2 years with either a waddling gait or a painless limp. Compared with PFFD, which demonstrates subtrochanteric varus, developmental coxa vara is related to a true decrease in the neck-shaft angle, is more progressive, and occasionally is familial and bilateral. Bilateral involvement is reported in as many as 50% of cases [9].

Characteristic radiographic findings of developmental coxa vara include a decreased femoral neck-shaft angle, a wide and irregular vertically aligned physis, and a triangular metaphyseal bony fragment that is medial and inferior to the physis [10]. The nearly vertical orientation of the physis results in abnormal shearing forces that predispose to multiple epiphyseal slips. MR imaging using a three-dimensional spoiled gradient recall echo f/s sequence is particularly useful in demonstrating physeal changes (Fig. 4).

Acquired coxa vara is seen in association with generalized congenital conditions, such as osteogenesis imperfecta, fibrous dysplasia, spondyloepiphyseal dysplasia congenita, cleidocranial dysostosis, metaphyseal chondrodysplasia, and spondylometaphyseal dysplasia [9]. True coxa vara should not be mistaken for apparent coxa vara, in which the femoral neck-shaft angle is normal but femoral neck shortening and relative trochanteric overgrowth are present. The disturbed growth of the proximal femoral physis may be secondary to trauma, infection, or avascular necrosis (AVN) (Fig. 5) [10,11].

The primary role of MR imaging in the evaluation of children with coxa vara is in preoperative planning. MR imaging delineates the relationship of the acetabulum, femoral head, neck, and shaft and distinguishes between cartilaginous and bony components. Occasionally we are asked to evaluate a child with coxa vara and a painful hip; in that setting, MR imaging is ideal for assessing the marrow for the presence of edema, which may indicate abnormal mechanical stress. MR imaging also aids in the diagnosis of impingement by evaluating the relationship of the femoral neck-head complex, including the greater trochanter, to the acetabular labrum.

### *Developmental dysplasia of the hip*

Developmental dysplasia of the hip (DDH) encompasses a range of abnormalities of the femoral head-acetabular relationship and development. Normal acetabular development requires appropriate positioning of the femoral head within the acetabulum. The acetabular dysplasia

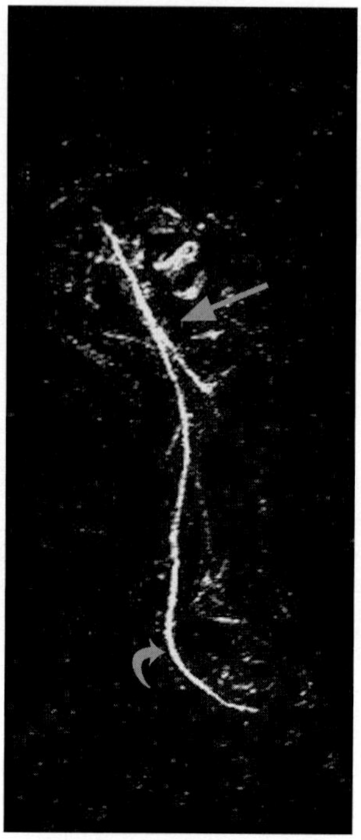

Fig. 3. Congenital shortening of the femur associated with ipsilateral fibular hemimelia that required management with a knee arthrodesis, foot amputation, and eventual fitting of a prosthesis (same patient as in Fig. 2). Surgical planning with contrast-enhanced MR angiography demonstrates two vessels (*arrow*) instead of three below the level of the popliteal artery. Distally, only the posterior arterial branch is seen reaching the hind foot (*curved arrow*).

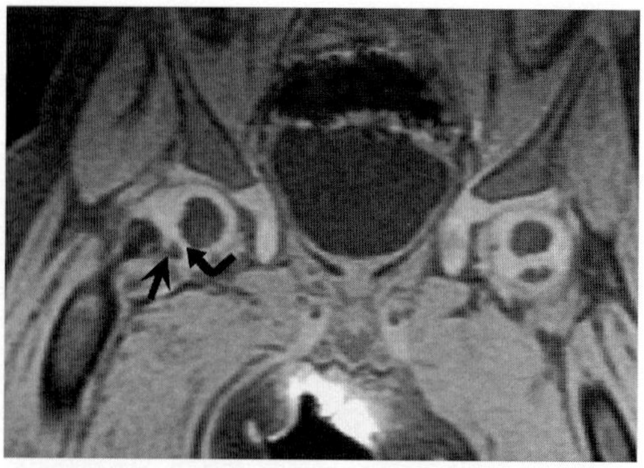

Fig. 4. A 10-month-old child with an unusual gait and developmental coxa vara. The nearly vertical orientation of the right proximal femoral physis (*curved arrow*), which is slightly wide and irregular, and the triangular metaphyseal fragment (*arrow*) are evident on the three-dimensional spoiled gradient recall echo f/s image of the pelvis.

seen in DDH has several causes. Teratologic dislocation, which is seen in approximately 2% of individuals with DDH, occurs during weeks 12 to 18 of gestation and is secondary to congenital neuromuscular disorders (eg, myelodysplasia and arthrogryposis). Approximately 98% of DDH occurs during the last month of gestation and may be secondary to mechanical or physiologic causes. Mechanical causes include oligohydramnios, constricting primigravida musculature, and breech presentation. Physiologic causes are related to maternal hormones, including estrogen, which is not metabolized by the fetal liver, and relaxin, a pregnancy hormone that contributes to ligamentous laxity [12]. DDH is far more common in female infants (9:1 girls versus boys) because girls are more sensitive to maternal estrogens. The prevalence of DDH varies from 1 in 100 births in clinically screened populations to 8 in 100 births in sonographically screened populations [6].

Sonography has replaced the routine use of plain radiographs in the initial diagnosis and subsequent follow-up of uncomplicated, nonteratologic DDH. In general, infants who are not diagnosed within 6 to 8 weeks of life or who do not respond to abduction splinting with a Pavlik harness by 8 to 12 weeks of life require further treatment, including prereduction traction, open

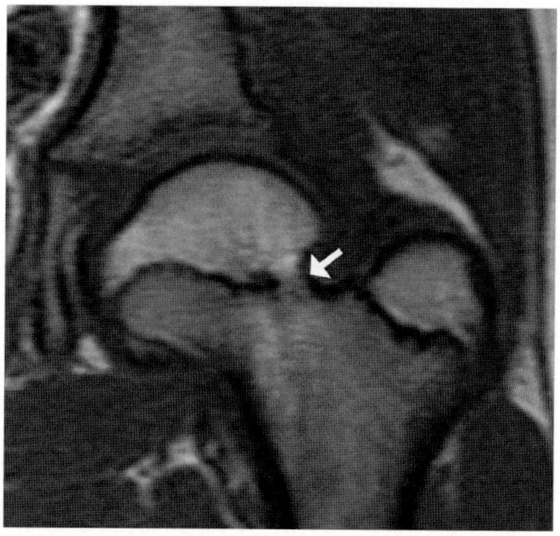

Fig. 5. MR coronal T1-weighted image of the left femur in a child with apparent coxa vara caused by a proximal femoral growth arrest (*arrow*). The patient required extracorporeal membrane oxygenation as a neonate because of a congenital diaphragmatic hernia.

reduction procedures, adductor tenotomy, and hip spica casting. Infants who have DDH that requires a closed reduction procedure have a higher incidence of AVN, with the reported incidence in some studies as high as 47% [13].

Given its multiplanar capabilities and superior visualization of the largely cartilaginous portions of the acetabulum and femoral epiphysis, MR imaging is uniquely suited for the evaluation of infants who do not respond to abduction harness bracing or who have complicated DDH (ie, teratologic dislocations that require closed reduction or surgery) (Fig. 6). MR imaging accurately demonstrates the most critical components of neonatal hip stability and obstacles to reduction, including the shape of the femoral epiphysis and acetabulum, degree of femoral and acetabular anteversion, labral position, joint capsule invagination by the iliopsoas tendon, fibro-fatty pulvinar, hypertrophy of the ligamentum teres, and position of the transverse acetabular ligament (Fig. 7) [6,14].

MR imaging after surgical reduction of DDH requires neither sedation nor additional restraints because all infants are placed in a spica abduction cast and the imaging time is kept to a minimum (usually less than 3 minutes). At our institution, this limited MR imaging examination has supplanted the use of CT in the postoperative evaluation of infants who have DDH [15].

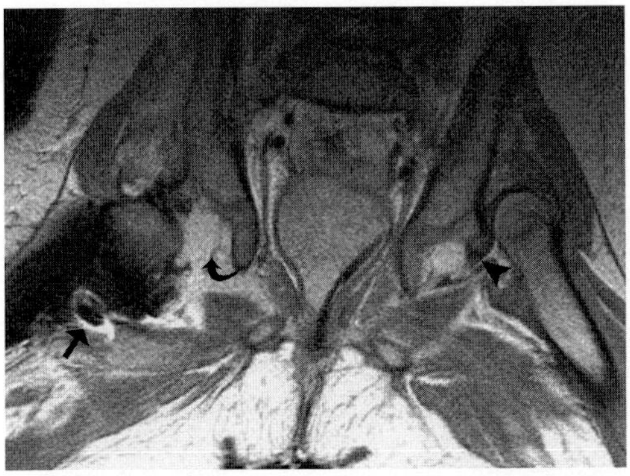

Fig. 6. MR coronal FSE PD image of the pelvis in an infant with arthrogryposis and teratologic dislocation of the hips that required a right femoral varus osteotomy. Note the hardware artifact (*arrow*). The femoral head remains laterally dislocated and prominent fibro-fatty pulvinar is present within the acetabulum (*curved arrow*). The unoperated left femoral head remains dislocated superior to the dysplastic left acetabulum. A redundant ligamentum teres is seen medially (*arrowhead*).

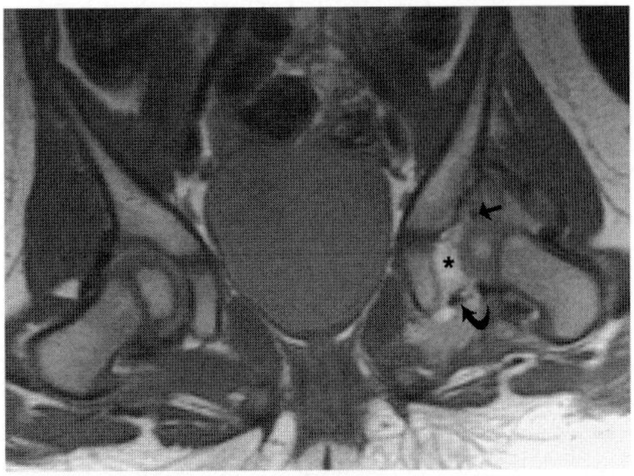

Fig. 7. Infant with developmental dysplasia of the left hip that required surgical reduction and spica casting. MR coronal FSE PD image demonstrated obstacles to reduction, including inversion of the acetabular labrum (*arrow*), pulvinar (*), and interposed iliopsoas tendon (*curved arrow*), any of which may prevent concentric reduction of the hip.

Depending on the size of the infant or child, MR imaging examinations are performed with either a phased array coil (cardiac) or a surface coil, such as the shoulder coil. Transverse FSE PD images can demonstrate concentric reduction of the femoral head and impediments to reduction.

Previous MR imaging literature supports the notion that excessive abduction impairs blood flow to the femoral epiphysis and may lead to ischemia [14,16]. In patients in whom there is a question of AVN secondary to ischemia during treatment-related abduction, the evaluation of femoral head perfusion can be achieved with scan times of less than 15 seconds per sequence with intravenous contrast-enhanced repeated FSE PD-weighted or three-dimensional T1-weighted spoiled gradient recall echo sequences (Fig. 8). MR imaging is particularly useful in complex cases that involve growth disturbances or problems related to reduction. In a recent retrospective study presented by Kim and colleagues [17], MR imaging with gadolinium was used as a predictor of AVN after closed reduction in 27 infants (28 hips) who were followed for 13 to 42 months for radiographic evidence of AVN as classified by Salter and colleagues [18]. Enhancement patterns of the femoral epiphysis on MR imaging after gadolinium administration were rated as either asymmetric or focally or globally decreased enhancement. Twenty-one percent of these infants (6 of 28 hips) developed significant AVN (Salter class 4 or 5). The hips, which showed a global decrease

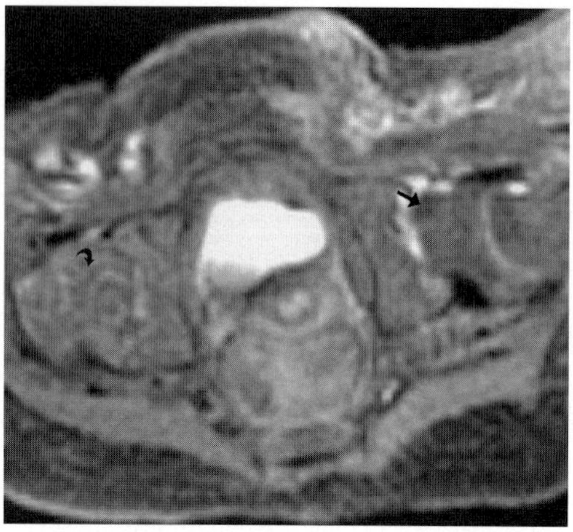

Fig. 8. Infant with left DDH after adductor tenotomy, reduction, and spica cast placement. A contrast-enhanced MR axial FSE PD f/s image shows global ischemia of the left femoral head (*arrow*). Note the normal enhancement of the right femoral epiphyseal cartilage, which has a striated or linear pattern of enhancement because of the cartilage canals (*curved arrow*).

in perfusion, were ten times more likely to develop AVN (Fig. 9). These data suggest that this group of patients may benefit from changing the hip position in the spica cast to improve perfusion to the femoral epiphysis.

In patients in whom there has been a late diagnosis of DDH or in patients who are refractory to treatment, MR imaging and CT with three-dimensional imaging capabilities are important in the preoperative assessment of femoral head deformity, acetabular dysplasia, and femoral head coverage by the bony acetabulum [7]. Osteoarthritis is a potential complication of DDH. The deficient acetabular coverage leads to anterolateral positioning of the femoral head, which produces abnormal chronic stress on the acetabular rim [19]. In untreated DDH, an enlarged acetabular labrum contributes to femoral head containment. If chronic stress is unrelieved, the acetabular labrum undergoes myxoid degeneration with possible adjacent ganglion formation, acetabular labral separation, and acetabular rim fragmentation (Fig. 10). Hip pain and accelerated progressive osteoarthritis have been associated with acetabular labral damage. The normal labrum acts as buffer and protects the hip joint articular cartilage. Repetitive, uneven stress across the joint cartilage by the femoral head produces chondral injury and osteoarthritis [20].

Direct MR arthrography with radial sequences is more sensitive and specific than other imaging techniques for detecting acetabular labral abnormalities. The technique of radial sequence MR arthrography as described by Kubo and colleagues [21] allows an examination of the relationship between acetabular labral abnormalities and femoral head morphology. The radial sequence displays the entire acetabular rim. At 10° intervals, sequential radial slices are obtained perpendicular to

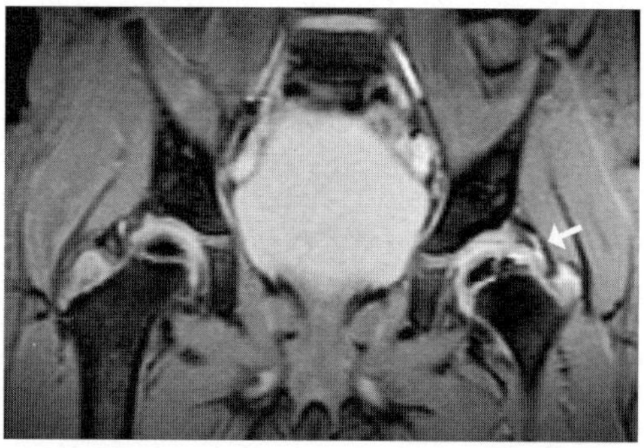

Fig. 9. In the same patient as in Fig. 8, 1 year after surgical treatment for DDH, the coronal MPGR image shows a small, fragmented left femoral head (*arrow*) with broadening and shortening of the femoral neck, consistent with AVN.

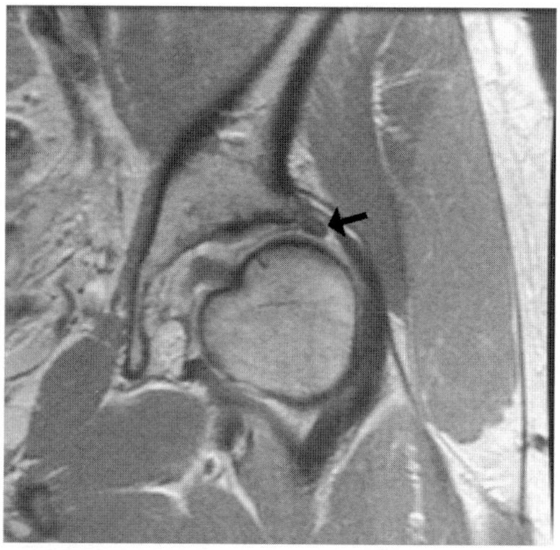

Fig. 10. A 20-year-old woman with left hip pain and a dysplastic left hip. Coronal FSE PD MR image of the left hip shows features of hip dysplasia with deficient acetabular coverage, superior joint space narrowing, and an enlarged globular labrum (*arrow*). The intrasubstance high signal seen within the labrum suggests myxoid degeneration.

a tangent to the acetabular rim (Fig. 11), which is intended to overcome partial volume effects and improve depiction of the labral anatomy (Fig. 12). A standard mixture of 0.1 mL gadolinium-DTPA$^{-2}$ (Gd-DTPA$^{-2}$), 10 mL normal saline, 5 mL nonionic iodinated contrast material, and 5 mL of 0.1% bupivicaine is used to obtain a dilute concentration of gadolinium in a 20-mL syringe. A 22-gauge needle is used to inject 8 to 10 mL of this mixture into the hip joint using fluoroscopic guidance. MR arthrographic sequences include coronal, sagittal, oblique axial (oriented along the axis of the femoral neck inclined toward the femoral head), and radial sequence T1-weighted spin echo f/s and coronal short tau inversion recovery images.

Newer MR imaging techniques, such as delayed gadolinium-enhanced MR imaging of cartilage (dGEMRIC), have been applied to evaluating patients with hip dysplasia and early changes of osteoarthritis and have shown a correlation between the dGEMRIC index and the severity of dysplasia, even in the absence of plain film findings of joint space narrowing, and the dGEMRIC index and pain [22].

Cartilage is composed of water, cells, and glycosaminoglycans, a proteoglycan. The negatively charged carboxyl and sulfate groups on glycosaminoglycans are the basis for the dGEMRIC technique. The negatively charged MR contrast agent Gd-DTPA$^{-2}$ is used as an MR imaging probe to measure the charge density of cartilage by using the fact that Gd-DTPA$^{-2}$ can better penetrate cartilage with low concentrations of glycosaminoglycans (ie, arthritic cartilage), whereas Gd-DTPA$^{-2}$ penetrates less in normal cartilage because of the higher concentration of similarly charged glycosaminoglycans [23]. At our institution, we use a double dose (0.4 mL/kg) of Gd-DTPA$^{-2}$, which is injected intravenously. After injection and before scanning, the patient walks for 30 minutes. A multislice FSE sequence is obtained and accompanied by four coronal T1 maps of both hips using saturation recovery technique, an echo time of 14 msec, repetition times of 300, 500, 750, 1000, 1500, and 2000 msec, a slice thickness of 4 mm, and a 1-mm interslice gap. A T1 map is generated by fitting a saturation recovery curve to the varying image intensity as the repetition time is varied. The dGEMRIC index is calculated as the average of the T1 values of the acetabular and femoral head cartilage in the weight-bearing zone of the four coronal slices. In the group of patients with hip dysplasia studied by Kim and colleagues [17], radiographic measures of joint space narrowing did not correlate with the severity of dysplasia; however, there was a strong correlation between the severity of dysplasia and the dGEMRIC index, in which the dGEMRIC index was lower in the severe

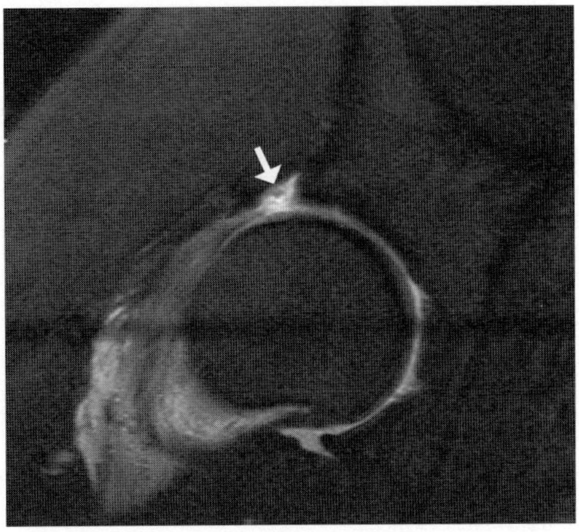

Fig. 12. A 19-year-old woman with hip pain and right hip dysplasia. In direct MR arthrography with a radial sequence, T1-weighted f/s image demonstrates fraying of the superoanterior labrum (*arrow*) at the 2 o'clock position.

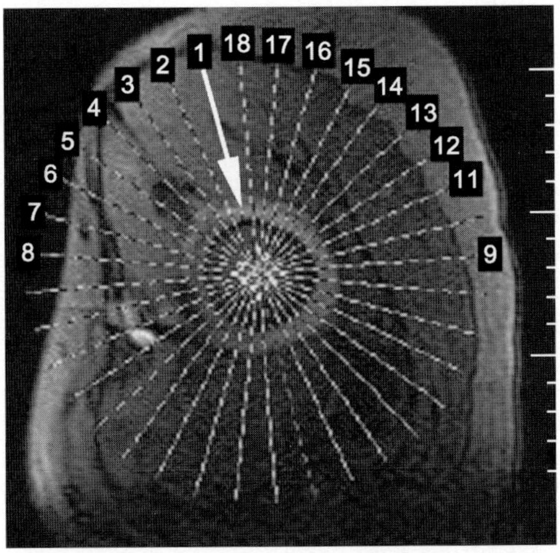


Fig. 11. En face view of the right acetabulum is used as the scout view to proscribe radial slices when performing radial MR arthrography imaging. The radial slices are centered through the right femoral head at 10° intervals and provide a sequential display of the entire acetabular labrum. Note image 1 (*arrow*) is through the superior acetabulum (the 12 o'clock position).

dysplasia group (ie, hips with more severe dysplasia had more arthritis on MR imaging) (Fig. 13). MR imaging has become the primary imaging modality in the pretreatment evaluation of complicated DDH and in the evaluation of postsurgical reduction and long-term sequelae of partially or untreated DDH.

## Acquired disorders

### *Transient synovitis and septic arthritis*

Transient synovitis is a leading cause of hip pain in children. Its cause is unknown. Trauma and viral infections have been implicated because no organisms are found on joint aspiration. This disorder is typically seen between the ages of 2 and 10 years. Boys are affected more commonly than girls. Signs and symptoms of transient synovitis include a low-grade fever, hip pain, refusal to walk, restricted motion, and muscle spasm [24]. No specific treatment is advocated.

Septic arthritis is principally monoarticular in the pediatric population, and the hip is the most frequent site of infection. Organisms enter the joint by hematogenous seeding of the synovium, spread from adjacent acute osteomyelitis of intra-articular bone or by direct puncture wounds. The most common pathogens are gram-positive cocci and coliforms in neonates. *Haemophilus influenzae* type B, once a common cause in this age group, currently accounts for a minority of cases since the development of a vaccine [25]. *Staphylococcus aureus* and group A streptococci are the most common pathogens in infants and children. The peak incidence of septic arthritis occurs in the early part of the first decade [26]. Prompt diagnosis helps lower the risk of complications secondary to destruction of epiphyseal and articular cartilage and AVN. Arthrocentesis is required for the definitive diagnosis of septic arthritis.

MR imaging shows a joint effusion and evidence of synovial inflammation in transient synovitis and septic arthritis [27]. The degree of synovial enhancement, which can be demonstrated with intravenous gadolinium on T1-weighted images, is a nonspecific finding and does not distinguish septic arthritis from toxic synovitis. Hypertrophied synovium is not well differentiated from joint fluid on either T2-weighted or short tau inversion recovery images [28]. Although inflammatory changes may be seen without intravenous gadolinium enhancement on T1-weighted images, they are far more evident after gadolinium enhancement. Bone marrow signal alterations, defined as low signal intensity on T1-weighted images and high signal intensity on T2-weighted images that enhance after contrast administration, when limited to the periarticular subchondral bone suggests the diagnosis of septic arthritis. The bone marrow signal alterations in septic arthritis probably represent reactive bone marrow edema. When septic arthritis is associated with osteomyelitis, the bone marrow signal alterations are generally more extensive and not limited to the adjacent periarticular subchondral bone [29]. Potential complications of a joint effusion, whether from toxic synovitis or septic arthritis, include hip dislocation and vascular tamponade, which may lead to AVN (Fig. 14).

### *Legg-Calvé-Perthes disease*

Legg-Calvé-Perthes disease (LCP) is an idiopathic AVN of the immature capital femoral epiphysis. Proposed mechanisms include vascular tamponade as the result of a joint effusion from any cause and increased viscosity or trauma to the intraepiphyseal vessels. These conditions may cause varying degrees of ischemia, which may lead to

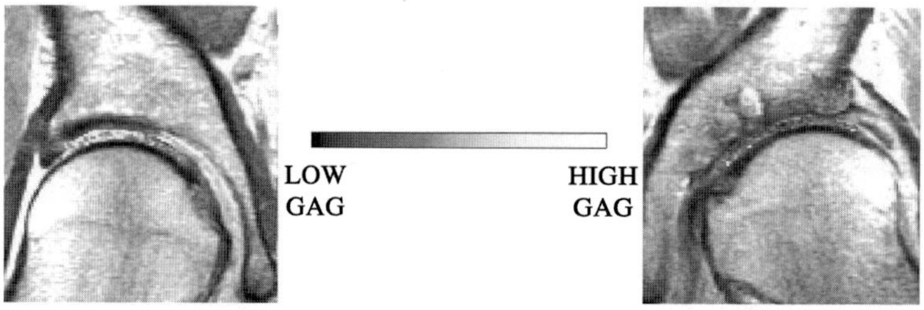


Fig. 13. Adult patient with a painful dysplastic left hip and a normal right hip. The dGEMRIC scan shows a low glycosaminoglycan (GAC) content on the left relative to the normal right hip. Low glycosaminoglycan content, or a low dGEMRIC index, indicates a relatively high concentration of Gd-DTPA$^{-2}$, which is seen in degraded cartilage.

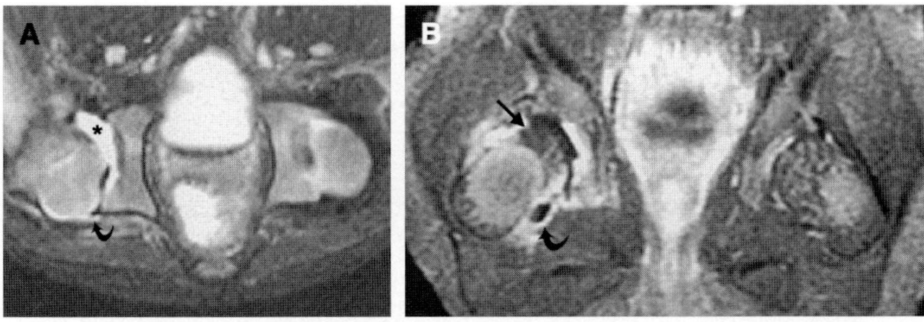


Fig. 14. Hip subluxation and AVN in an infant with a septic right hip. (*A*) Axial T2-weighted f/s MR image of the right hip shows a hip effusion (*) and posterior subluxation of the femoral head (*curved arrow*). (*B*) Coronal T1-weighted f/s image after gadolinium administration shows enhancement of the synovium (*curved arrow*) and lack of enhancement in the lateral aspect of the right femoral head (*arrow*).

AVN if prolonged or repeated [30]. Despite extensive study, the cause of LCP remains elusive. Most patients are white boys between the ages of 5 and 8 years. Almost 90% of LCP is unilateral. Clinically, children who have LCP typically present with limping. Hip, thigh, or knee pain may be present.

The age at presentation is the most significant prognostic indicator. Children who are older than age 8 are more likely to develop a disability. Various radiographic grading systems, including systems based on the work of Caterall, have been used to determine the need for early intervention and prognosis. The Catterall Classification divides LCP into four groups, which depend on the extent of epiphyseal involvement. In group I, only the anterior epiphysis is involved and there is no evidence of collapse or sequestration. Metaphyseal changes may be seen at later stages. In group II, there is more extensive involvement, with collapse and sequestration followed by absorption and regeneration. In group III, all but a small portion of the epiphysis is sequestered, broadening of the femoral neck is common, and changes in the metaphysis are more generalized than in group II. In group IV, the entire epiphysis is involved and total collapse may be seen with epiphyseal changes [6].

Multiple studies have shown that there is poor inter- and intraobserver reliability in recognizing the radiographic features of the head at risk for AVN [31]. De Sanctis and Rondinella [26] described a classification based on MR imaging with two main groups, A and B, which depend on the extent of epiphyseal involvement. In group A, less than 50% of the epiphysis is involved; in group B, there is more than 50% epiphyseal involvement. There are also six classes that depend on the extent of physeal involvement and lateral extrusion. This classification system also has been used as a prognostic tool and provides guidelines for interventions [26].

MR imaging is useful in cases of suspected LCP when radiographs are unrevealing, because it is highly sensitive for the detection of early ischemia. MR imaging signal changes that indicate marrow edema are early signs of LCP, including diffuse low signal on T1-weighted images and high signal on T2-weighted images, which typically occur in the affected femoral head. Dynamic MR imaging enhancement with the use of intravenous gadolinium also aids in early detection of LCP because the absence of marrow enhancement confirms the diagnosis. MR imaging can demonstrate the presence and extent of infarction of the femoral head and shows involvement of the physis [6]. Reversible ischemia cannot be predicted based on the routine musculoskeletal imaging protocols. Experimentally, in the pig model of transient and long-term femoral ischemia, Jaramillo and colleagues [32] applied diffusion-weighted MR imaging techniques that have been shown to be sensitive to brain ischemia. They hypothesized that the use of diffusion-weighted imaging could predict the course of ischemia and showed that in early ischemia there was an initial restriction in diffusion, or decrease in apparent diffusion coefficient, which was followed by an increase in diffusion if ischemia persisted. Further experimental studies are needed to show if this shift from restricted to increased diffusion heralds the transition from reversible ischemia to infarction (Fig. 15) [32].

In addition to facilitating early diagnosis, MR imaging is able to identify children who are at

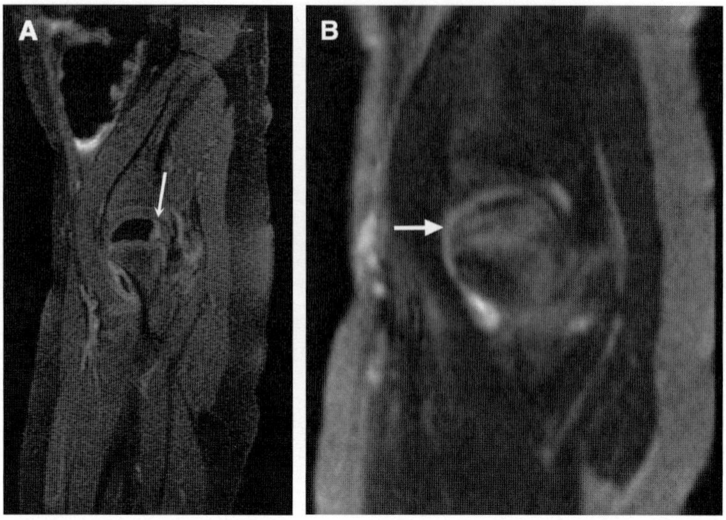


Fig. 15. An 8-year-old boy with left hip LCP. (*A*) Sagittal T1-weighted f/s MR image after gadolinium administration shows only minimal peripheral and lateral enhancement of the femoral head (*arrow*). (*B*) Sagittal apparent diffusion coefficient map of the left hip shows increased diffusion within most of the epiphysis (*arrow*) and the proximal metaphysis. (Courtesy of H. Salamipour, MD, Boston, MA.)

increased risk of early disability by demonstrating osseous bridging across the physis, which leads to growth arrest. Low signal in the femoral head on MR imaging and physeal bridging were statistically significant predictors of growth arrest, whereas epiphyseal abnormalities were not [33]. Extension of physeal cartilage into the metaphysis, similar to that seen in experimental damage to the metaphyseal vasculature, likely reflects the same process responsible for the radiographic finding of metaphyseal radiolucencies (Fig. 16).

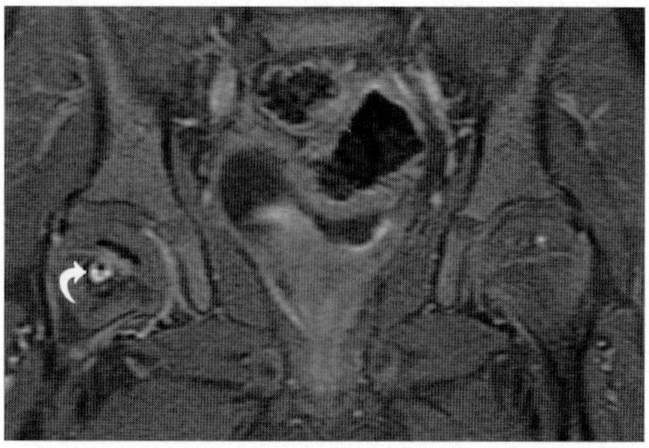

Fig. 16. A 4-year-old boy with right-sided LCP. Coronal T1-weighted f/s MR image after gadolinium enhancement shows a small, predominantly low signal intensity secondary center of ossification and an enhancing metaphyseal abnormality (*curved arrow*).

Treatment options include the use of abduction orthosis and surgical management with femoral varus or innominate osteotomy or shelf arthroplasty. The goal of treatment in LCP is to limit the late onset of degenerative joint disease. Therapy is aimed at maintaining congruence between the developing femoral epiphysis and the acetabulum, thereby limiting stress on the femoral head, preventing lateral extrusion of the femoral epiphysis, and allowing for normal epiphyseal shaping. MR imaging in an open-configuration magnet was found to be comparable to arthrography in the evaluation of femoral head containment and articular congruency [34]. MR imaging provides additional information regarding the degree of cartilaginous coverage of the femoral epiphysis and the extent of femoral epiphyseal deformity.

*Slipped capital femoral epiphysis*

Slipped capital femoral epiphysis (SCFE) is characterized by a Salter-Harris type 1 fracture through the proximal femoral physis. Slippage of the epiphysis occurs posteriorly in 99% and medially in 75% of cases [25]. The term "pre-slip" is appropriate in cases in which there is no radiographic evidence of SCFE but in which physeal and metaphyseal abnormalities may be seen on MR images or CT. SCFE is more common in boys than in girls (2.5:1) and more common in African Americans than in whites. Affected children are frequently obese. In approximately one third of patients, there is bilateral—but not typically simultaneous or symmetric—involvement of the hips. SCFE is most commonly idiopathic; however, it also has been noted in conjunction with renal osteodystrophy and endocrinopathies, including hypothyroidism and hypopituitarism. There is a history of trauma in approximately 50% of patients [25].

Umans and colleagues [35] pointed out that the imaging findings in pre-slip and SCFE represent a continuum. Diffuse or globular physeal widening, in which there is intermediate signal intensity surrounded by linear low signal intensity, is the earliest evidence of SCFE (Fig. 17). Although multidetector CT and MR imaging are able to provide multiplanar images, MR imaging is better suited to evaluating complications such as ischemia and the resultant AVN of the femoral head and can show early changes that are not apparent on either CT or radiographs.

## Pelvic apophyseal avulsions

During the teenage years, apophyses appear in the iliac crest, the anterior superior iliac spine, the anterior inferior iliac spine, the ischium, and the lesser and greater trochanters. Before ossification, the apophyseal growth cartilage constitutes the weakest point in the musculotendinous unit, which renders the apophyses vulnerable to injury during sudden forceful or repetitive traction from the attached muscles. These injuries are most common in sprinters, football players, ballet dancers, and jumpers. Young athletes with a pelvic avulsion injury typically report sudden onset of pain during strenuous activity.

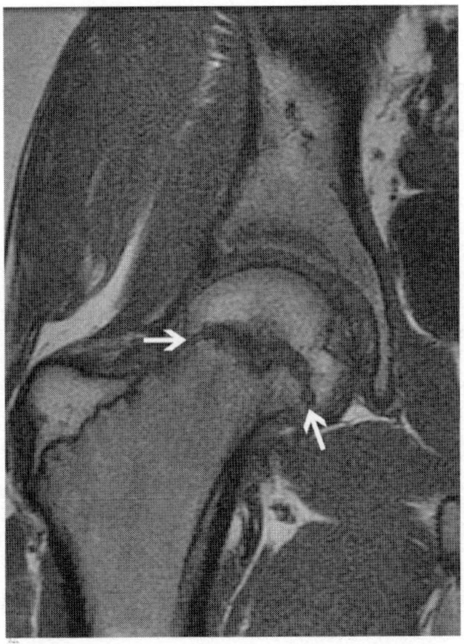

Fig. 17. Teenage boy with a right-sided SCFE. Coronal T1-weighted MR image shows irregular widening of the femoral physis (*arrows*). The foreshortening of the femoral epiphysis is caused by the posterior and medial slip of the femoral epiphysis.

Radiographically, an apophyseal avulsion appears as displacement of an apophyseal center from its normal position. In some cases, there is callus and bony reaction sufficient to suggest a malignancy. On MR imaging, high signal intensity on T2-weighted images indicates bone marrow edema of the apophyseal center and the donor site (Fig. 18). MR imaging may be useful in defining further the avulsed apophyses or, in the occasional difficult case, differentiating an avulsion from a neoplasm. Avulsions of the iliac crest and the anterior inferior iliac spine may show little displacement and escape detection on radiographs. MR imaging may be the first study to suggest the diagnosis in such cases. Apart from apophyseal avulsions, other sites of pelvic injury include the ilium adjacent to the sacroiliac joint and the pubic ramus [36].

## Lumbosacral transitional vertebrae

A lumbosacral transitional vertebra is a common anatomic variant characterized by a large transverse process that follows the contour of the sacral ala and fuses with the sacrum, most often

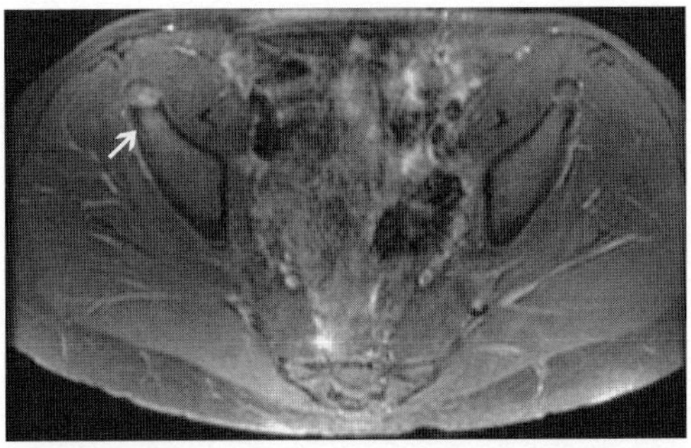

Fig. 18. Teenage girl with low back and right hip pain. Axial T1-weighted f/s MR image after gadolinium administration shows stress changes at the origin of the sartorius muscle on the anterior superior iliac spine apophysis. Enhancing marrow edema within the right anterior superior iliac spine apophysis and the ileum (*arrow*) is shown.

forming a diarthrodial joint but sometimes creating a complete osseous union. The anomaly usually involves one side of a vertebra. Based on the number of non-rib-bearing vertebrae, the affected vertebra is frequently referred to as a sacralized L5 or a lumbarized S1. Because weight is transferred from the upper body through the spinal segment that articulates either directly or indirectly with the ilia, the transverse process-sacral articulation is part of the weight-bearing platform. The altered biomechanics that result from a lumbosacral transitional vertebra can cause stress-related pain, particularly with activities that involve rapid flexion and extension, referred to as Bertolotti's syndrome. The pain associated with a lumbosacral transitional vertebra mimics that which occurs with spondylolysis and is attributable to stress or inflammation at the sacral transverse articulation. It is worth searching for this abnormality, even when it has not been described on prior radiographs, because it may not have been thought to be clinically significant or may have been obscured by overlying bowel gas [37]. MR imaging can help support the diagnosis of stress at the transverse process-sacral articulation by demonstrating periarticular high T2 signal or post-gadolinium enhancement indicative of marrow edema (Fig. 19).

## Sacral stress fracture

Sacral stress fractures are an uncommon but important cause of low back pain in young athletes, among whom distance runners are particularly vulnerable. When a young female athlete presents with a sacral stress fracture in a similar anatomic distribution as an osteoporotic sacral insufficiency fracture, the female athlete triad of disordered eating, amenorrhea, and osteoporosis should be considered [38]. Sacral stress fractures, which result from the transmission of vertical forces through the sacral ala, often escape detection radiographically because of technical factors, such as overlying bowel gas and sacral geometry, and because of the paucity of callus formation that they incite [39]. Alternative methods of diagnosis include CT and MR imaging. MR imaging reveals decreased signal intensity on T1-weighted images and increased signal intensity on T2-weighted images, which enhances after the administration of gadolinium and is caused by bone marrow edema. A discrete line of decreased signal intensity on T1- and T2-weighted images, which represents a fracture line, may or may not be evident (Fig. 20) [40].

## Osteomyelitis

Acute osteomyelitis is a common pediatric problem that may occur at any age, usually is the result of the hematogenous spread of infection, and often is related to an asymptomatic or transient bacteremia. *S aureus* is the infective organism in 70% of cases. One third of neonatal infections are caused by group B β-hemolytic streptococcus. Approximately one third of patients have a history of a recent upper respiratory infection, and one third have a history of recent trauma, the former presumably the source of bacteremia and the latter suggesting that traumatized bone is susceptible to infection. The long tubular bones are involved in 75% of cases. Acute

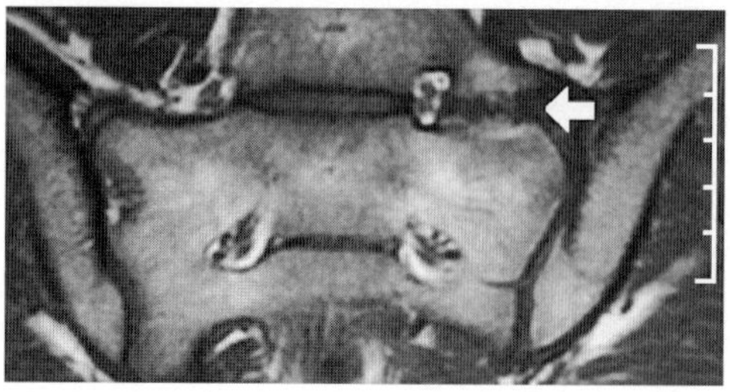

Fig. 19. Teenage boy with low back pain. Coronal T1-weighted MR image after gadolinium administration. The left-sided lumbosacral transitional vertebra has an irregular joint space (*arrow*) and associated mild surrounding enhancing edema, which indicates stress at the lumbosacral transitional vertebra.

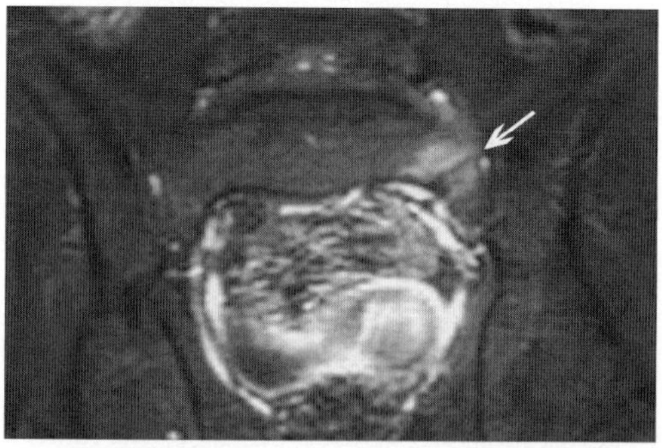

Fig. 20. A 7-year-old soccer player with low back pain. Pertinent medical history includes steroid use for asthma. Coronal T1-weighted f/s MR image after gadolinium administration shows a fracture of the left sacral ala, which is seen as a linear, low signal intensity band (*arrow*) surrounded by enhancing marrow edema.

osteomyelitis of the long bones affects the metaphysis in which blood-borne organisms become lodged because of the high metaphyseal vascularity and the physiologic slowing of blood in the arterial looping vessels and venous sinusoids. Within this metaphyseal microcirculation organisms can incite an exudative response, which causes a local increase in intraosseous pressure and results in further slowing of blood flow. The largest and most rapidly growing long bone metaphyses are involved preferentially, with the distal femur, proximal femur, proximal tibia, distal tibia, proximal humerus, distal humerus, and fibula involved in decreasing order of frequency. In infants and children younger than 18 months of age, the epiphysis is commonly involved because the presence of transphyseal vessels allows spread from metaphysis to epiphysis (Fig. 21). Epiphyseal involvement in a child older than 18 months of age can occur directly across the physis or by spread from septic arthritis or intra-articular osteomyelitis [36,41]. Isolated epiphyseal involvement occurs infrequently.

Acute osteomyelitis involves the flat, irregular, and pelvic bones in 25% of cases and characteristically develops in regions termed metaphyseal equivalents, which are adjacent to cartilage and have a vascular anatomy similar to that of long bone metaphyses. The early diagnosis of acute osteomyelitis is necessary to prevent significant morbidity, such as sepsis, chronic infection, growth arrest, and bone deformity.

At our institution, skeletal scintigraphy is used in children who have suspected osteomyelitis and normal radiographs. This approach can be advocated most strongly when symptoms are either poorly localized or are localized to major long bones [41]. If the response to treatment is slow, MR imaging should be obtained after skeletal scintigraphy shows major long bone involvement. Because of the association of abscesses with pelvic osteomyelitis, MR imaging should be strongly considered after pelvic osteomyelitis is detected and may be substituted for skeletal scintigraphy when symptoms are well localized to the pelvis (Fig. 22). In support of this approach, we recently reviewed our 5-year experience, which included 38 children with pelvic osteomyelitis and a diagnostic MR image. A soft tissue abscess was seen on MR imaging in 21 of 38 children (55%), 10 of 38 (26%) of whom required subsequent drainage [42].

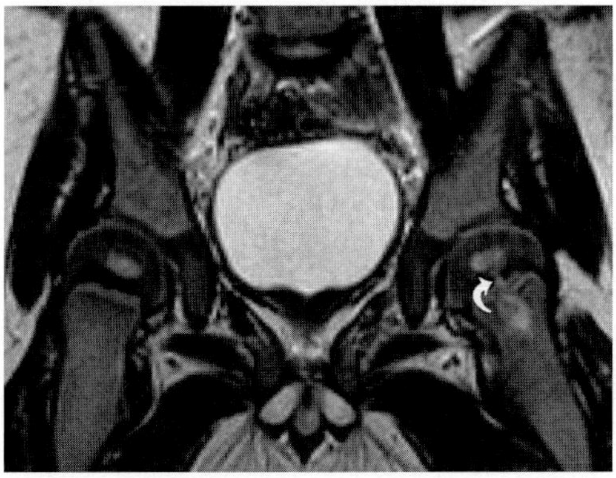

Fig. 21. A 15-month-old infant with transphyseal spread of a left femoral metaphyseal osteomyelitis. Coronal T2-weighted MR image shows the T2 signal abnormality crossing the femoral physis (*curved arrow*).

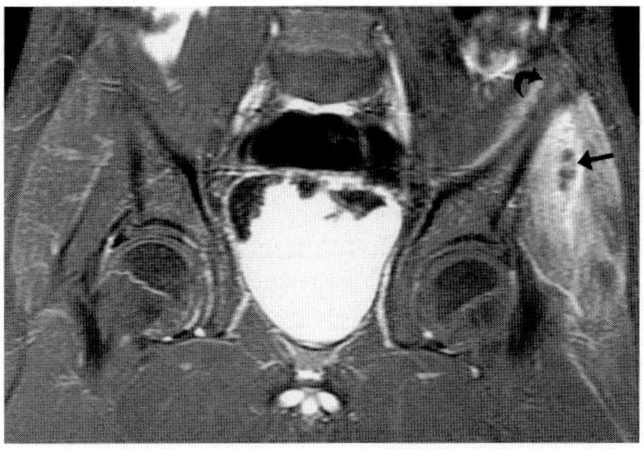

Fig. 22. Teenage boy with left-sided low back and hip pain caused by pelvic osteomyelitis associated with a soft tissue abscess. Coronal T1-weighted f/s MR image after gadolinium administration shows a left gluteal muscle soft tissue abscess (*arrow*) and enhancing bone marrow edema within the left iliac crest (*curved arrow*).

## Summary

This article reviews the MR imaging findings of some of the more common congenital and acquired disorders of the pediatric hip and pelvis, with the intent of increasing the awareness of radiologists and facilitating early and accurate diagnosis and treatment. The importance of MR imaging in the pediatric population is underscored by its ability to evaluate these disorders well and without the use of ionizing radiation.

## Acknowledgments

The authors would like to thank Sherry L. Brec for her expertise in preparation of the manuscript.

## References


[1] American Society of Anesthesiologists Task Force on Sedation and Analgesia by Nonanesthesiologists. Practice guidelines for sedation and analgesia by nonanesthesiologists: an updated report. Anesthesiology 2002;96:1004–17.

[2] Kanal E, Borgstede JP, Barkovich AJ, et al. American College of Radiology white paper on MR safety. AJR Am J Roentgenol 2002;178:1335–47.

[3] Joint Commission on Accreditation of Healthcare Organizations. Standards and intents for sedation and anesthesia care: comprehensive accreditation manual for hospitals. Chicago: Joint Commission on Accreditation of Healthcare Organizations; 2002.

[4] American Academy of Pediatrics Committee on Drugs. Guidelines for monitoring and management of pediatric patients during and after sedation for diagnostic and therapeutic procedures: addendum. Pediatrics 2002;110:836–8.

[5] Court C, Carlioz H. Radiological study of severe proximal femoral focal deficiency. J Pediatr Orthop 1997;17:520–4.

[6] Resnick D, Kransdorf MJ. Bone and joint imaging. 3rd edition. Philadelphia: Elsevier Saunders; 2005.

[7] Shapiro F. Developmental bone biology. In: Shapiro F, editor. Pediatric orthopaedic deformities. San Diego (CA): Academic Press; 2001. p. 142.

[8] Herring J, Cummings D. The limb deficient child. In: Lovell WW, Winter RB, Morrissey RT, et al, editors. Lovell and Winter's pediatric orthopedics. 4th edition. Philadelphia: Lippincott-Raven; 1996. p. 1137–80.

[9] Pavlov H, Goldman AB, Freiberger RH. Infantile coxa vara. Radiology 1980;135:631–40.

[10] Ozonoff M. Pediatric orthopedic radiology. 2nd edition. Philadelphia: WB Saunders; 1992.

[11] DiFazio RL, Kocher MS, Berven S, et al. Coxa vara with proximal femoral growth arrest in patients who had neonatal extracorporeal membrane oxygenation. J Pediatr Orthop 2003;23:20–6.

[12] Dahnert W. Radiology review manual. 5th edition. Philadelphia: Lippincott Williams & Wilkins; 2003.

[13] Brougham DI, Broughton NS, Cole WG, et al. Avascular necrosis following closed reduction of congenital dislocation of the hip: review of influencing factors and long-term follow-up. J Bone Joint Surg Br 1990;72:557–62.

[14] Jaramillo D, Villegas-Medina O, Laor T, et al. Gadolinium-enhanced MR imaging of pediatric patients after reduction of dysplastic hips: assessment of femoral head position, factors impeding reduction, and femoral head ischemia. AJR Am J Roentgenol 1998;170:1633–7.

[15] Laor T, Roy DR, Mehlman CT. Limited magnetic resonance imaging examination after surgical reduction of developmental dysplasia of the hip. J Pediatr Orthop 2000;20:572–4.

[16] Jaramillo D, Villegas-Medina OL, Doty DK, et al. Gadolinium-enhanced MR imaging demonstrates abduction-caused hip ischemia and its reversal in piglets. AJR Am J Roentgenol 1996;166:879–87.

[17] Kim Y, Rodriguez D, Griffey M, et al. Post-closed reduction MRI as a predictor for avascular necrosis in hip dysplasia. Presented at the 36th Annual Conference of the Pediatric Orthopedics Society of North America. St. Louis (MO), April 28–May 1, 2004.

[18] Salter RB, Kostuik J, Dallas S. Avascular necrosis of the femoral head as a complication of treatment for congenital dislocation of the hip in young children: a clinical and experimental investigation. Can J Surg 1969;12:44–61.

[19] Leunig M, Podeszwa D, Beck M, et al. Magnetic resonance arthrography of labral disorders in hips with dysplasia and impingement. Clin Orthop Relat Res 2004;418:74–80.

[20] Klaue K, Durnin CW, Ganz R. The acetabular rim syndrome: a clinical presentation of dysplasia of the hip. J Bone Joint Surg Br 1991;73:423–9.

[21] Kubo T, Horii M, Yamaguchi J, et al. Acetabular labrum in hip dysplasia evaluated by radial magnetic resonance imaging. J Rheumatol 2000;27:1955–60.

[22] Kim YJ, Jaramillo D, Millis MB, et al. Assessment of early osteoarthritis in hip dysplasia with delayed gadolinium-enhanced magnetic resonance imaging of cartilage. J Bone Joint Surg Am 2003;85A:1987–92.

[23] Burstein D, Gray M. New MRI techniques for imaging cartilage. J Bone Joint Surg Am 2003;85-A(Suppl 2):70–7.

[24] Morrissey RT, Weinstein SL. Lovell and Winter's pediatric orthopedics. 4th edition. Philadelphia: Lippincott-Raven; 1996.

[25] Kirks DR. Practical pediatric imaging: diagnostic radiology of infants and children. 3rd edition. Philadelphia: Lippincott Williams & Wilkins; 1998.

[26] de Sanctis N, Rondinella F. Prognostic evaluation of Legg-Calvé-Perthes disease by MRI. Part II: pathomorphogenesis and new classification. J Pediatr Orthop 2000;20:463–70.

[27] Jaramillo D, Treves ST, Kasser JR, et al. Osteomyelitis and septic arthritis in children: appropriate use of imaging to guide treatment. AJR Am J Roentgenol 1995;165:399–403.

[28] Kaplan PA, Helms CA, Dussault R, et al. Knee. In: Musculoskeletal MRI. Philadelphia: WB Saunders; 2001. p. 18.

[29] Lee SK, Suh KJ, Kim YW, et al. Septic arthritis versus transient synovitis at MR imaging: preliminary assessment with signal intensity alterations in bone marrow. Radiology 1999;211:459–65.

[30] Connolly L, Treves S. Pediatric skeletal scintigraphy. New York: Springer-Verlag; 1998.

[31] Hardcastle PH, Ross R, Hamalainen M, et al. Catterall grouping of Perthes' disease: an assessment of observer error and prognosis using the Catterall

classification. J Bone Joint Surg Br 1980;62B: 428–31.
[32] Jaramillo D, Connolly SA, Vajapeyam S, et al. Normal and ischemic epiphysis of the femur: diffusion MR imaging study in piglets. Radiology 2003;227: 825–32.
[33] Kaplan PA, Helms CA, Dussault R, et al. Knee. In: Musculoskeletal MRI. Philadelphia: WB Saunders; 2001. p. 337.
[34] Jaramillo D, Galen TA, Winalski CS, et al. Legg-Calvé-Perthes disease: MR imaging evaluation during manual positioning of the hip: comparison with conventional arthrography. Radiology 1999;212: 519–25.
[35] Umans H, Liebling MS, Moy L, et al. Slipped capital femoral epiphysis: a physeal lesion diagnosed by MRI, with radiographic and CT correlation. Skeletal Radiol 1998;27:139–44.
[36] Connolly L, Treves S. Pediatric skeletal scintigraphy with multimodality imaging correlations. New York: Springer-Verlag; 1997.
[37] Connolly LP, d'Hemecourt PA, Connolly SA, et al. Skeletal scintigraphy of young patients with low-back pain and a lumbosacral transitional vertebra. J Nucl Med 2003;44:909–14.
[38] Johnson AW, Weiss CB Jr, Stento K, et al. Stress fractures of the sacrum: an atypical cause of low back pain in the female athlete. Am J Sports Med 2001;29:498–508.
[39] Connolly LP, Strauss J, Connolly SA. Role of skeletal scintigraphy in evaluating sports injuries of adolescents and young adults. Philadelphia: Lippincott Williams & Wilkins; 2003.
[40] Diel J, Ortiz O, Losada RA, et al. The sacrum: pathologic spectrum, multimodality imaging, and subspecialty approach. Radiographics 2001;21: 83–104.
[41] Connolly LP, Connolly SA, Drubach LA, et al. Acute hematogenous osteomyelitis of children: assessment of skeletal scintigraphy-based diagnosis in the era of MRI. J Nucl Med 2002;43:1310–6.
[42] Connolly SA, Connolly LP, Jaramillo D. Pelvic osteomyelitis: importance of MRI for showing soft tissue abscess. Presented at the 38th Congress of the European Society of Pediatric Radiology. Bergen (Norway), June 17–21, 2002.

ELSEVIER
SAUNDERS

Magn Reson Imaging Clin N Am
13 (2005) 799–809

MAGNETIC RESONANCE IMAGING CLINICS of North America

# Abnormalities in and Around the Hip: MR Imaging Versus Sonography

Theodore T. Miller, MD[a,b,*]

[a]Division of Musculoskeletal Imaging, Department of Radiology, North Shore University Hospital and LIJ Medical Center, 825 Northern Boulevard, Great Neck, NY 11021, USA
[b]New York University School of Medicine, 530 First Avenue, New York, NY 10016, USA

The imaging evaluation of the painful or clinically abnormal hip should always start with radiographs, but advanced imaging is often necessary for further evaluation. MR imaging is the "gold standard," providing an excellent anatomic overview and excellent demonstration of the bony structures, articular surfaces, and surrounding soft tissues. Conversely, sonography is quickly performed, has greater resolution than MR imaging [1], allows dynamic evaluation of tendons and muscles, and can guide percutaneous procedures. An accurate comparison of the two modalities for the evaluation of a particular abnormality requires an evidence-based approach, evaluating the sensitivity and specificity of each modality for the same cohort of patients, but that literature is almost nonexistent. Instead, we are left with anecdotal reports and descriptive series for each of these modalities regarding muscle and tendon injuries, bursitis, and fractures. Although these disease processes and their MR imaging appearances are discussed in depth in other articles, this article concentrates on the MR imaging–sonographic correlations of these entities.

## Muscle and tendon injury

The muscles and tendons about the hip are subject to acute injury and chronic overuse, and sonography and MR imaging can be used to evaluate these conditions. Muscle tears most often occur at the myotendinous junction or at the epimysium. Sonographically, a muscle tear appears as pock-marked hypoechoic or heterogeneous disruption of the normal pennate architecture, linear hypoechogenicity within the muscle, or a frank hypoechoic gap in the muscle (Fig. 1), and on MR imaging, acute muscle tear appears as feathery high signal intensity within the muscle on T2-weighted images (Fig. 2). Hematoma can have a variable sonographic appearance; some authors have reported a hypoechoic appearance acutely that becomes heterogeneously hyperechoic as the hematoma organizes [2,3], some have reported the reverse temporal appearance [4–6], and others have reported no correlation between time course and sonographic appearance [7]. On MR imaging, acute hematoma is typically fluid-like in appearance and develops heterogeneous signal intensity on T1-weighted and T2-weighted images as it organizes, sometimes with a low signal intensity rim of hemosiderin [8].

Adductor muscle injuries are most often encountered in soccer and hockey players [9–12] and are a common cause of groin pain in these athletes. The abnormality may occur at the origin on the symphysis [13], at the musculotendinous junction [14,15], or at the distal insertion on the femur (called "thigh splints") [16,17]. MR imaging may demonstrate high signal intensity edema and hematoma in the muscle or marrow edema at the enthesis and periosteal reaction [13,17,18], whereas sonography may demonstrate similar findings manifested as focal hypoechoic defects or gaps at

* Division of Musculoskeletal Imaging, Department of Radiology, North Shore University Hospital and LIJ Medical Center, 825 Northern Boulevard, Great Neck, NY 11021.

*E-mail address:* tmiller@nshs.edu

1064-9689/05/$ - see front matter 
doi:10.1016/j.mric.2005.08.013

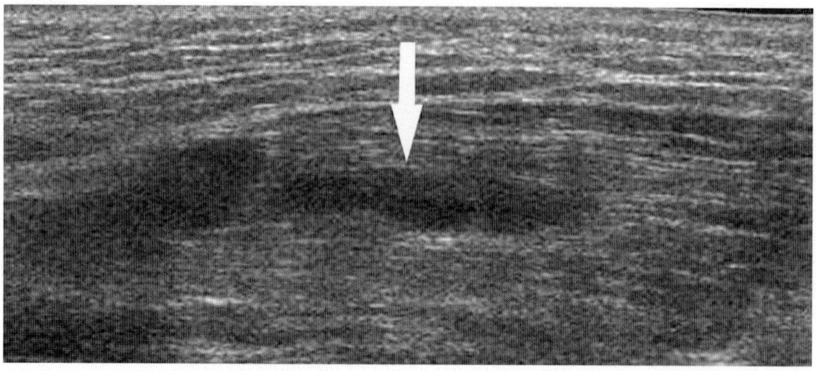

Fig. 1. Tear of the rectus femoris muscle. Longitudinal sonogram shows a hypoechoic region (*arrow*) representing edema and hemorrhage within the tear, with loss of the striated pennate appearance of the muscle fibers in this region. (Courtesy of L. Nazarian, MD, Philadelphia, PA.)

the musculotendinous junction, hypoechoic acute hematoma, and cortical irregularity and hyperemia with color or power Doppler [14–16].

Similarly, other muscles about the hip are subject to tear and enthesopathy. Unilateral enlargement of the tensor fascia lata because of degeneration and overuse has been described with MR imaging [19] and sonography [20]. In Bass and Connell's series of 12 patients [20], all complained of anterior groin pain and point tenderness over the anterior iliac crest and all were engaged in athletic activities. Sonography in all these patients demonstrated enlargement of the tensor fascia lata with a cone-shaped region of hypoechogenicity at its origin and a linear anechoic intrasubstance tear of the muscle in 3 of the patients [20]. Ilaslan and colleagues [19] reported unilateral

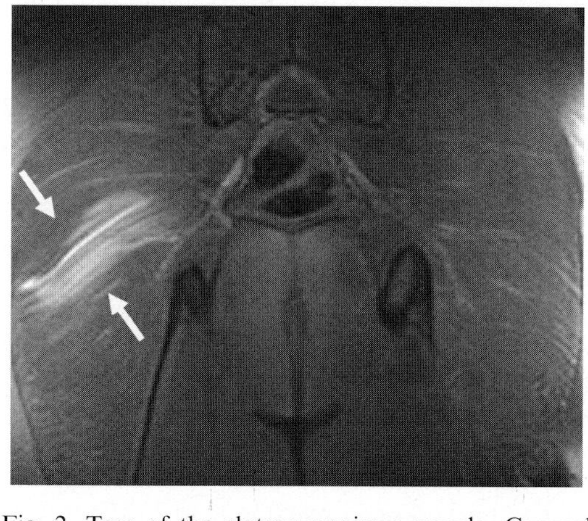

Fig. 2. Tear of the gluteus maximus muscle. Coronal fat-suppressed T2-weighted image shows feathery high signal intensity edema and hemorrhage within the muscle (*arrows*).

enlargement of the tensor fascia lata in 6 patients using MR imaging, all of whom presented with an anterior soft tissue mass, and Asinger and El-Khoury [21] reported two cases of tear of the tensor fascia lata, which presented as a soft tissue mass because of retraction and appeared on MR imaging as avulsed muscle with feathery high signal intensity edema within it on T2-weighted imaging.

In a review of their experience using MR imaging and sonography to evaluate acute hamstring injuries, Koulouris and Connell [22] found that MR imaging correctly identified avulsion from the ischium in 16 of 16 cases, whereas sonography only diagnosed 7 of 12 cases. The deep location of the ischial tuberosity, particularly in heavy or muscular patients, may make sonographic visualization of this area difficult.

In addition to the objective demonstration of muscle injury that can confirm a clinical diagnosis, MR imaging and sonography have been used to predict time to return to activity. In a study of 60 soccer players with an acute hamstring injury clinically, sonography was slightly more sensitive than MR imaging for detecting strain (75% versus 70%), but the length of the strain on MR imaging had the best statistical correlation with time to recovery [23]. Similarly, other studies have found that length and cross-sectional area of muscle injury on MR imaging as well as involvement of the central tendon are important prognostic indicators for time to recovery [24,25].

The "greater trochanteric pain syndrome" is characterized by pain and focal tenderness in the region of the greater trochanter, which is exacerbated with weight-bearing and hip abduction and usually affects middle-aged and older women. It can be caused by tendinosis and tears of the gluteus medius or minimus tendons, inflammation of any of the three subgluteal bursae, or, more commonly, a combination of gluteal tendon injury and gluteal bursitis. Most cases are attributable to chronic degeneration and overuse, with only a few cases caused by prior local trauma [26,27].

An analogy has been made between the gluteus medius and minimus tendons, which are abductors of the hip, and the supraspinatus and infraspinatus tendons, which assist in abduction of the shoulder; thus, the gluteus medius and minimus have been termed the *rotator cuff of the hip* [28]. Similar to the tendons of the rotator cuff, the gluteus medius and minimus tendons are subject to tendinosis, partial tear, and full-thickness tear, and the three intervening bursae may be concomitantly inflamed or merely distended because of an abnormality of the adjacent tendon. The bursa most commonly involved is the subgluteus maximus bursa, also called the greater trochanteric bursa, which is larger than the subgluteus minimus and subgluteal medius bursae and is located over the posterolateral aspect of the trochanter [29].

Abnormalities reported with the greater trochanteric pain syndrome include tendinosis, partial and complete tears of the gluteus medius and minimus tendons, and distention of the subgluteal bursae [26,27,30,31]. Tendinosis is manifest on MR imaging as abnormal signal intensity within the tendon and on sonography as hypoechogenicity within the normal fibrillary appearance of the tendon, with or without thickening of the tendon on either modality (Fig. 3). On MR imaging, a partial tear is a focal discontinuity on the T2-weighted images, whereas it appears as a focal anechoic region with loss of the normal fibrillation or a hypoechoic linear zone within the tendon on sonography. On both modalities, a complete tear involves the full width of the tendon and may or may not demonstrate retraction of the tendon. The fluid-distended bursae appear as discrete high signal intensity collections on T2-weighted images [27,31] and as anechoic collections on sonography (Fig. 4). Using the MR imaging appearances of bursitis, elongation of the gluteus medius tendon, and tendon discontinuity, Cvitanic and coworkers [27] achieved 93% sensitivity and 91% accuracy for diagnosing tears of the abductor tendons, whereas Connell and colleagues [26], using sonography, achieved 90% sensitivity and 95% specificity for diagnosing such tears. Connell and colleagues [26] also reported cortical irregularity of the greater trochanter in 25 of their 53 cases, analogous to that seen on the greater tuberosity of the humerus in rotator cuff tears, and hyperemia on color or power Doppler sonography in only 9 of the 53 hips.

Calcific tendinosis of the gluteus medius tendon was seen in 5 of 53 hips sonographically [26], an appearance that has been described radiographically [32–34] but not reported in MR imaging descriptions of greater trochanteric pain syndrome [27,31]. Possible explanations for lack of detection of calcification in the reported MR imaging series, other than its true absence, are the use of a large field of view and large slice thickness, with resultant decreased resolution and partial volume averaging, respectively, as well as obscuration by adjacent soft tissue edema. Conversely, MR imaging allows evaluation of the hip joint itself and the bone marrow, which are areas that cannot be evaluated sonographically. In the series of Connell and colleagues [26], 12 of the 22 patients with normal sonography underwent subsequent MR imaging, which demonstrated seven instances of degenerative change in the hip joint, three instances of labral abnormalities, and one case of avascular necrosis.

The "snapping hip" syndrome refers to a sudden snapping sensation during hip motion and can be attributable to intra-articular or extra-articular causes [35–37]. Intra-articular causes include loose bodies (from trauma, degenerative arthritis, or synovial osteochondromatosis), labral tears, and femoroacetabular maltracking, whereas extra-articular causes are attributable to abnormal motion of tendons. The extra-articular causes can be further classified as lateral (also called external) snapping attributable to abnormal motion of the iliotibial band or gluteus maximus over the greater trochanter and as medial (also called internal) snapping attributable to abnormal motion of the iliopsoas tendon over the iliopectineal eminence of the pelvis, over the anterior inferior iliac spine, or even over the lesser trochanter [38]. Teenagers and young adults are typically affected and may not have any predisposing occupational or athletic activity [36,37], although four of the eight patients with a snapping iliopsoas tendon reported by Janzen and coworkers [37] had a preceding traumatic event of hip abduction and external rotation. Regardless of a medial or lateral cause, the snapping may or may not be painful [35].

On static imaging using sonography or MR imaging, the offending tendon most often looks normal, although tendinosis, peritendinous fluid, and iliopsoas bursitis have occasionally been

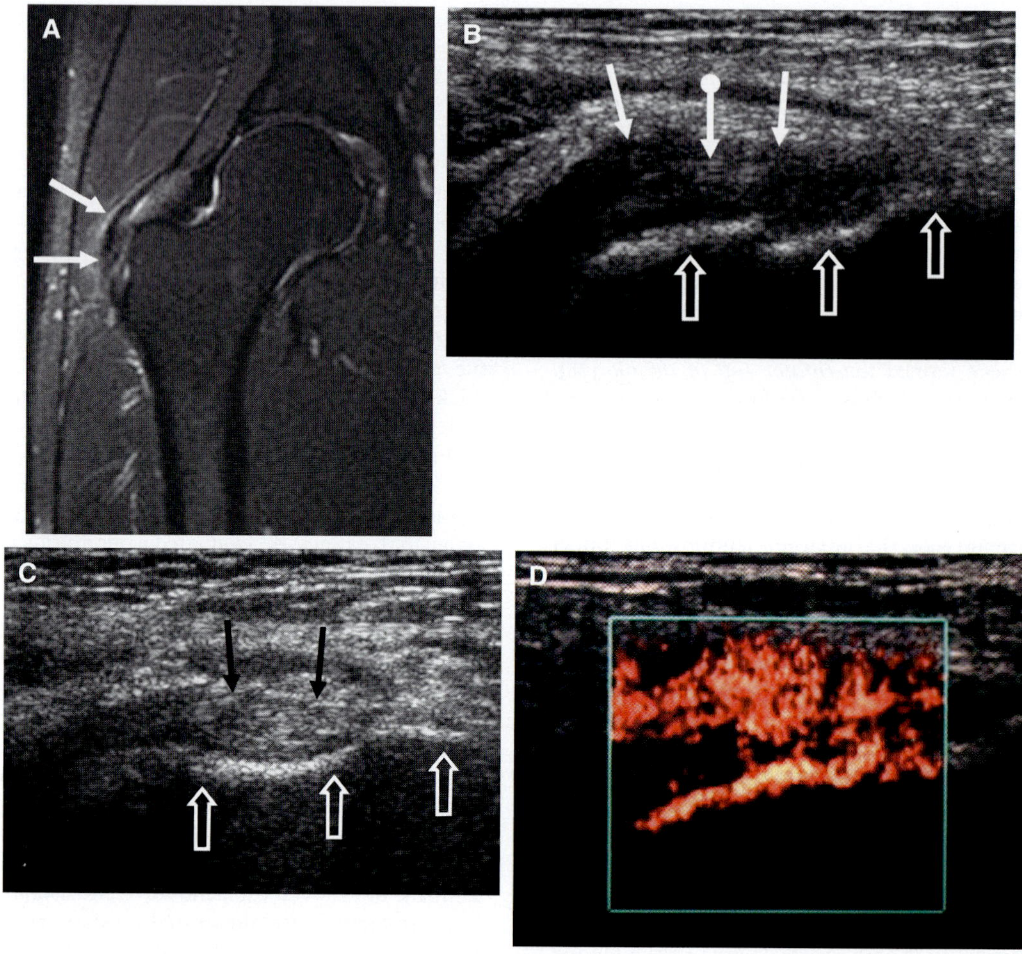


Fig. 3. Gluteal tendinosis. (*A*) Coronal fat-suppressed T2-weighted image shows thickening of and heterogeneous signal within the distal aspect of the gluteus minimus tendon (*arrows*). (*B*) Corresponding longitudinal sonogram shows the thickened, outwardly bowed, and hypoechoic tendon (*straight arrows*). Some of the normal fibrillary appearance of the tendon is still visualized (*round-tailed arrow*). The echogenic cortex of the greater trochanter (*open arrows*) is well seen with mild cortical irregularity between the left and middle open arrows. (*C*) Longitudinal sonogram of the patient's asymptomatic contralateral side shows the distal aspect of the normal gluteus minimus tendon (*black arrows*) overlying the smooth undulating cortex of the greater trochanter (*open arrows*). (*D*) Longitudinal color Doppler sonogram of the symptomatic side shows marked hyperemia. (*E*) Longitudinal power Doppler sonogram of the contralateral asymptomatic side using the same Doppler settings as in *D* shows normal background noise.

described with both modalities [35–37]. The imaging diagnosis is made, however, using dynamic sonography to document the snap or sudden jerk of the tendon. To evaluate a suspected snapping iliopsoas tendon, the transducer is placed transversely over the femoral head or pectineal eminence of the pelvis and the patient, lying prone, is asked to flex, externally rotate, and abduct the femur (producing a frog lateral position) and then to move back to neutral position. A normal iliopsoas tendon has smooth movement but a snapping one shows a sudden jerk, often with a palpable or audible snap. The snap may occur from medial to lateral or vice versa, and may occur during hip flexion to extension or vice versa [35]. To evaluate suspected snapping by the iliotibial band or gluteus maximus, the patient lies in the decubitus position with the affected side up or stands upright, the transducer is placed transversely over the lateral aspect of the greater trochanter, and the patient is asked to flex and extend the hip. Depending on each patient, some

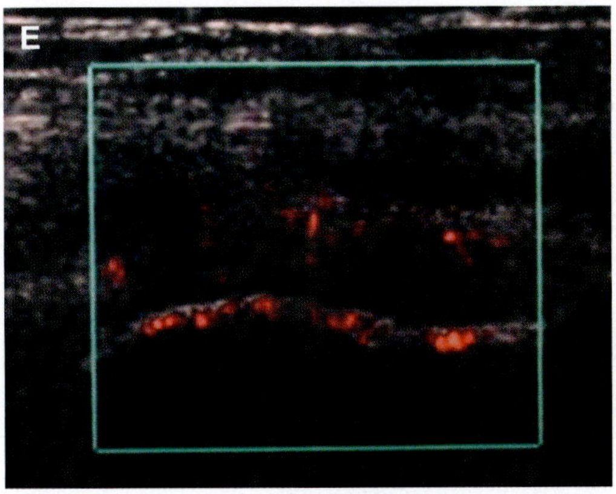


Fig. 3 (*continued*)

degree of internal and external rotation may be needed to elicit that person's symptoms, and the abnormal tendon shows a sudden snap. In their series of 54 patients with symptomatic internal snapping, Wunderbaldinger and colleagues [39] reported that the diagnosis could be made using radiographs and sonography in 83% of the cases; the additional use of MR imaging allowed the correct diagnosis in 100% of the cases, and those authors recommended that radiographs and dynamic sonography be used initially, reserving MR imaging for confusing or unresolved cases.

MR imaging should also be used to evaluate potential intra-articular causes of snapping. Evaluation of a suspected tear of the acetabular labrum is best performed with MR imaging, with [40] or without intra-articular contrast [41]. Anecdotally, labral tears may be seen sonographically as a hypoechoic cleft through the echogenic fibrocartilaginous labrum or as detachment of the echogenic labrum from the bone, similar to tears of the glenoid labrum of the shoulder and tears of the knee menisci. Perilabral cysts are seen sonographically as well-defined anechoic collections adjacent to the labrum (Fig. 5).

## Sportsman's hernia

A sportsman's hernia, seen commonly in soccer and rugby players [42,43], is a tear of the transversalis fascia, which is the posterior wall of the inguinal ring [44], with resultant weakening of this fascia. The term has also been used to describe a wide variety of abnormalities in this region, all of which can cause "pubalgia," such as occult direct and indirect hernias; strain of the internal or external oblique abdominal muscles; and entrapment of the ilioinguinal, obturator, or genitofemoral nerves [44,45]. The pain of a sportsman's hernia is absent at rest, is elicited by exertional activity (especially sudden twisting movements), and may radiate into the thigh or testicles. The diagnosis can be elusive clinically, and these patients often undergo multiple but fruitless imaging examinations to evaluate the pubic region. Dynamic sonography of the inguinal ring is the procedure of choice, demonstrating convex anterior bowing of the transversalis fascia and ballooning of the inguinal canal during the Valsalva maneuver [42]. Albers and colleagues [18] performed MR imaging in 32 athletes with pubalgia and found one case in which a frank defect in the transversalis fascia was present because of a rent from the pubic attachment. MR imaging might be expected to show high signal intensity edema on T2-weighted images in the region of the inguinal canal in acute cases but has not yet been reported to demonstrate the dynamic incompetence of the weakened fascia.

MR imaging and sonography have been used to evaluate direct (medial to the inferior epigastric vessels) and indirect (lateral to the inferior epigastric vessels) inguinal hernias [46]. MR imaging has a reported sensitivity of 85% [47] to 94.5% [48] and a specificity of 96%, whereas sonography has 86% sensitivity and 97% specificity for direct hernias, 97% sensitivity and 87% specificity for indirect hernias [49], and 93% sensitivity and 81.5% specificity overall [48]. Use of color Doppler sonography may be of benefit for identifying the inferior epigastric vessels [50]. Albers and colleagues [18] found a 93% prevalence of bulging and/or attenuation of the abdominal wall musculature, particularly the transversalis and internal oblique fascial layers, in their series of 32 athletes imaged with MR and suggest that these findings are signs of incipient hernia. Van den Berg and coworkers [51] reported the use of dynamic MR imaging in the evaluation of four patients with clinically evident inguinal hernias (three indirect and one direct); although the hernias became more conspicuous on the images during the Valsalva maneuver because of canal enlargement, the nondynamic sequences were also diagnostic.

## Fractures and osteitis pubis

In the skeletally immature pelvis, avulsions of muscles are actually Salter I fractures, and they

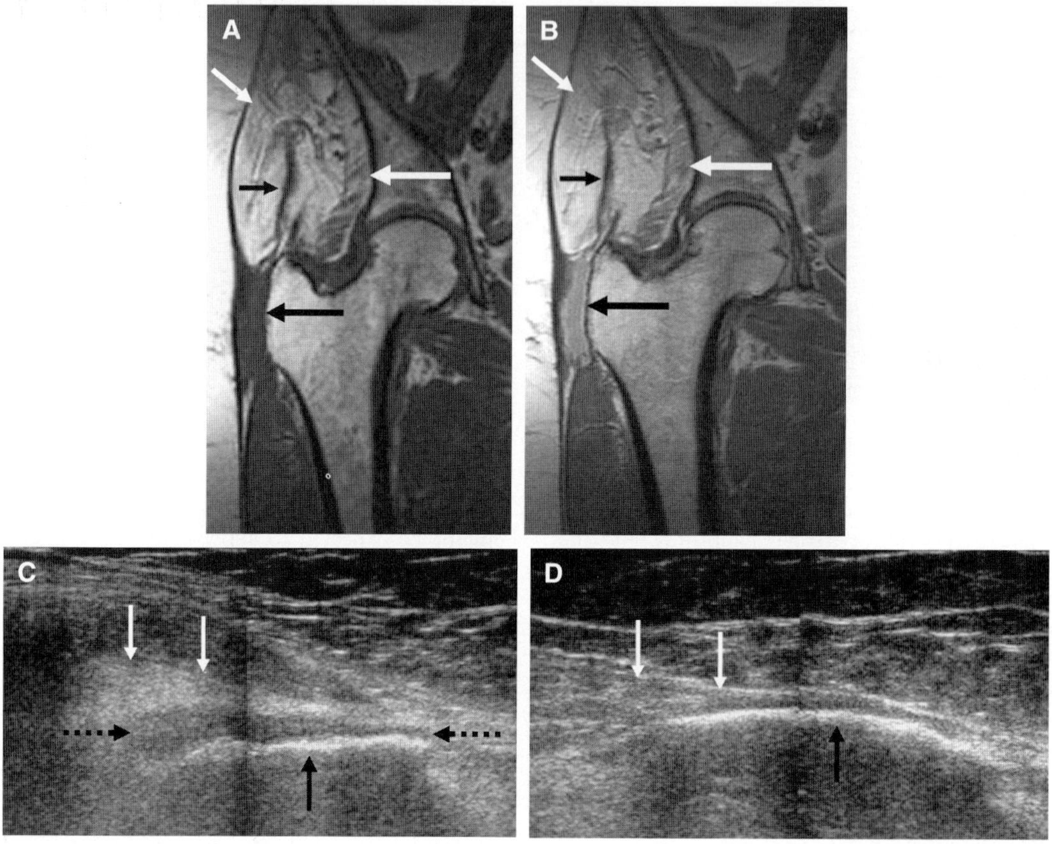


Fig. 4. Chronic rupture of the gluteus medius and minimus tendons. Coronal T1-weighted (*A*) and coronal proton density–weighted (*B*) images show atrophy of the gluteus medius muscle (*short white arrow*), elongation of the gluteus medius tendon (*short black arrow*), atrophy of the gluteus minimus muscle (*long white arrow*), and fluid within a distended greater trochanteric bursa (*long black arrow*). (*C*) Corresponding longitudinal sonogram shows atrophy of the distal aspect of the gluteus medius muscle (*white arrows*), the distended greater trochanteric bursa (*dashed black arrows*), and the underlying echogenic cortex of the greater trochanter (*straight black arrow*). (*D*) Longitudinal sonogram of the patient's asymptomatic contralateral side shows the normal distal aspect of the gluteus medius muscle and tendon (*white arrows*) inserting on the cortex of the greater trochanter (*black arrow*). (*E*) Transverse sonogram over the symptomatic greater trochanter shows the distended greater trochanteric bursa (*short arrow*) overlying the lateral facet (*long arrow*) of the greater trochanter. (*F*) Transverse sonogram of the patient's asymptomatic contralateral side shows the normal appearance for comparison.

can be demonstrated with MR imaging and sonography. Pisacano and Miller [52] reported acute avulsions of the anterior iliac spines in four teenaged boys, demonstrated equally well on MR imaging and sonography. On MR imaging, the injury appears as high signal intensity on T2-weighted images in the widened space between the avulsed apophysis and pelvis, with feathery high signal intensity edema and hemorrhage in the avulsed muscle and surrounding soft tissue, whereas on sonography, the avulsed apophysis is echogenic with posterior acoustic shadowing and is displaced from the underlying pelvis, with anechoic edema and hemorrhage in the gap (Fig. 6).

Osteitis pubis, another cause of anterior groin pain in the athlete, is a stress injury of the symphysis pubis attributable to shear caused by the pull of the rectus abdominus muscles proximally and the adductor and gracilis muscles distally [53]. It is most often associated with sports that involve repetitive twisting of the trunk, cutting or rapid side-to-side movements, and kicking [54,55]. Although radiographs eventually demonstrate sclerosis, irregularity, and erosions of the pubis and widening of the symphysis [53,55],

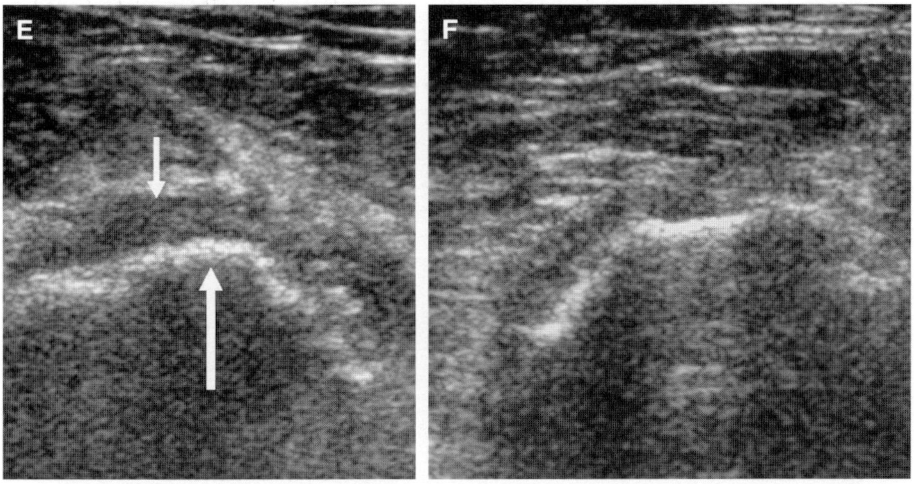


Fig. 4 (*continued*)

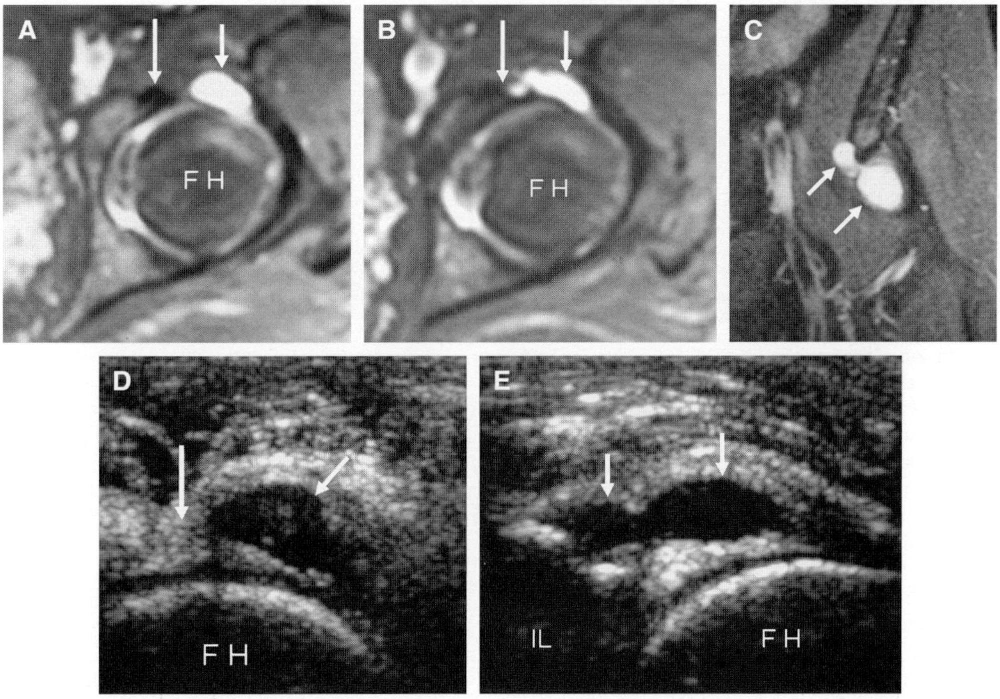


Fig. 5. Perilabral cyst. (*A, B*) Sequential axial fat-suppressed T2-weighted MR images of a painful left hip show a large ganglion cyst (*short arrow*) associated with the anterior aspect of the acetabular labrum (*long arrow*). FH, femoral head. (*C*) Coronal fat-suppressed T2-weighted sequence shows the lobulated nature of this cyst (*arrows*). (*D*) Corresponding transverse sonogram shows the cyst (*short arrow*) adjacent to the echogenic labrum (*long arrow*), both of which are anterior to the FH. (*E*) Corresponding longitudinal sonogram of this region shows the bilobed cyst (*arrows*) overlying the ilium (IL), echogenic labrum and joint capsule, and FH.

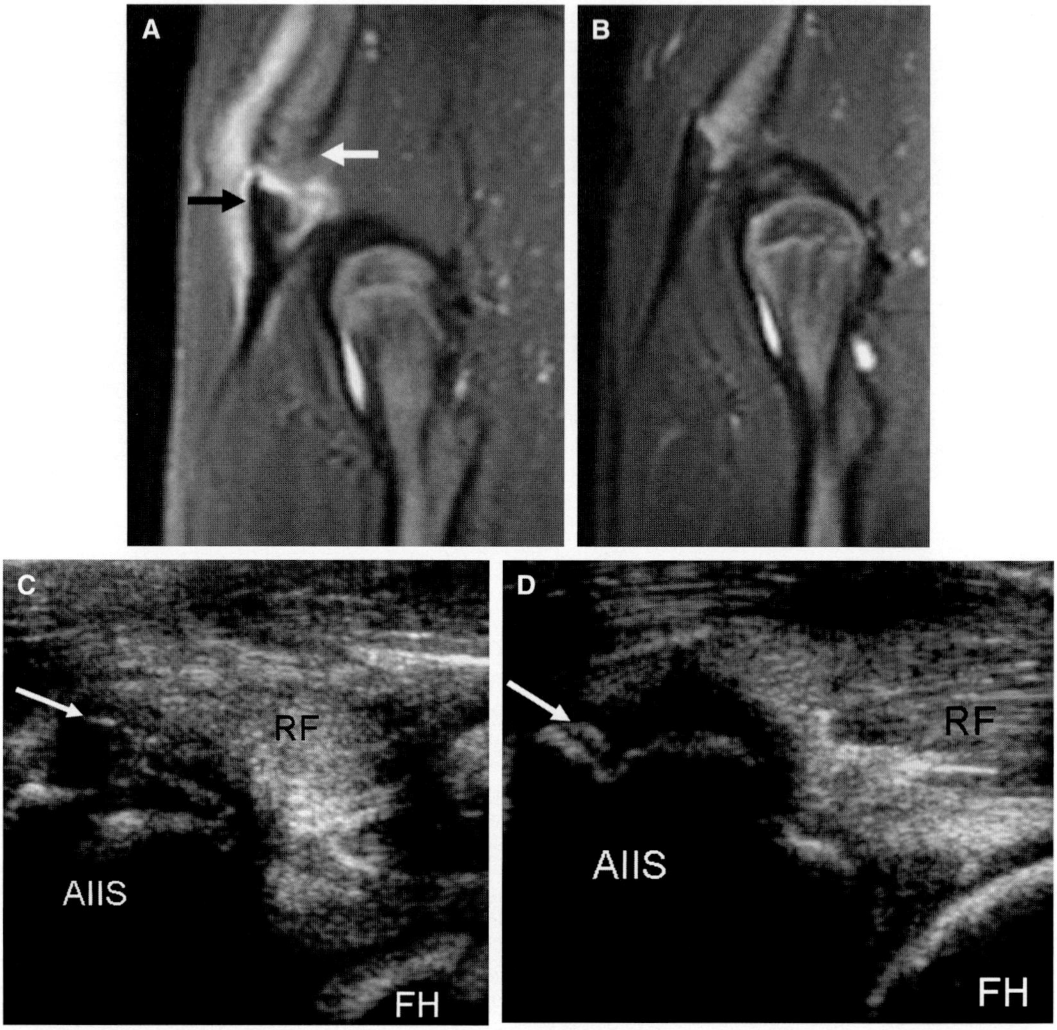


Fig. 6. Avulsion of the apophysis of the anterior inferior iliac spine in a teenager. (*A*) Sagittal fat-suppressed T2-weighted image through the symptomatic side shows the separation of the rectus femoris and apophysis (*black arrow*) from the iliac bone itself (*white arrow*), with intervening and surrounding high signal intensity edema and hemorrhage. (*B*) Sagittal fat-suppressed T2-weighted sequence through the patient's asymptomatic contralateral side shows the normal appearance for comparison. (*C*) Corresponding longitudinal sonogram of the symptomatic side shows the echogenic rectus femoris muscle (RF) and the attached apophysis (*arrow*), which is separated from the anterior inferior iliac spine (AIIS). FH, femoral head. (*D*) Longitudinal sonogram of the patient's contralateral asymptomatic side shows the normal relation for comparison. The arrow points to the normal apophysis.

MR imaging and sonography may demonstrate abnormalities sooner, such as fluid in the symphysis and marrow edema in the pubis on MR imaging [14,18,53,54] and distention of the symphysis caused by effusion, thickening of the joint capsule, and irregularity of the pubis on sonography (Fig. 7). The "secondary cleft sign" has been described on coronal fat-suppressed T2-weighted MR images as high signal intensity that extends from the central cleft of the symphysis and is interposed between the inferior pubic ramus and the adductor and gracilis aponeurosis attachment, and its presence correlates with the presence and side of groin pain [56]. In Brennan and coworker's series [56], four of six patients with osteitis pubis had this secondary cleft, but eight patients with the cleft sign had not yet developed bony changes, suggesting that it is an early indicator of

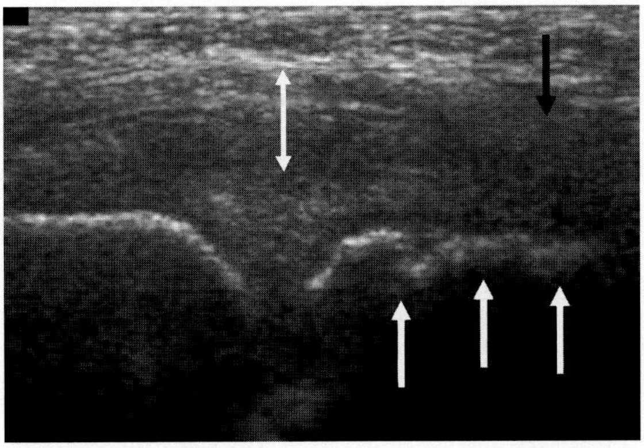

Fig. 7. Osteitis pubis. Transverse sonogram of the symphysis pubis in a patient with left-sided groin pain shows irregularity of the anterior cortex of the superior pubic ramus (*straight white arrows*), adjacent ill-defined hypoechoic edema (*straight black arrow*), and thickening of the joint capsule (*double-tailed arrow*). (Courtesy of L. Nazarian, MD, Philadelphia, PA.)

symptomatic shear stress injury of the symphysis. The sonographic analogy of this cleft sign has not yet been described, nor has the use of power Doppler sonography to demonstrate hyperemia in the symphysis and soft tissues surrounding the pubis.

Fatigue stress fracture of the pubic rami may occur in female long-distance and marathon runners [57] and military recruits, perhaps related to too long a stride [58], and more often affects the inferior pubic ramus than the superior pubic ramus [59]. It is manifested on MR imaging as marrow edema, with or without a discrete fracture line or adjacent soft tissue edema. Sonography of this injury has not been reported.

## Percutaneous intervention

An advantage of sonography is its ability to guide real-time intervention, such as aspiration of hip effusions and other fluid collections (eg, hematomas, abscesses); injection of anesthetics and steroids into the hip joint, bursae, and peritendinous tissues; and percutaneous tenotomy, a procedure in which a needle is passed to and fro through an area of tendinosis or partial tear to stimulate healing. Goh and colleagues [15] reported sonographically guided aspiration of a hematoma associated with tear of the adductor muscles of the groin, followed by two courses of injection of anesthetic and steroid into the tear 7 weeks apart, with complete resolution of groin pain. Sonography can guide selective injection of the gluteal tendons and associated bursitis [26] and has been used to guide injection of iliopsoas tendinopathy [60]. Percutaneous tenotomy, with or without injection of steroid, has had success in treating Achilles and patellar tendinopathies [61–63] but has not yet been reported in the hip.

## Summary

Sonography and MR imaging should be considered complementary rather than competing modalities. They demonstrate similar abnormalities of the soft tissues, but MR imaging is able to demonstrate intraosseous and articular abnormalities and offers a better anatomic overview because of its larger field of view, whereas sonography offers dynamic evaluation and can provide real-time guidance for percutaneous procedures. Both of these modalities have roles in the imaging evaluation of injuries in and around the hip.

## References


[1] Torriani M, Kattapuram SV. Musculoskeletal ultrasound: an alternative imaging modality for sports-related injuries. Top Magn Reson Imaging 2003; 14(1):103–12.

[2] Lohle PNM, Pulaet JBC, Coerkamp EG, et al. Nonpalpable rectus sheath hematoma clinically masquerading as appendicitis: US and CT diagnosis. Abdom Imaging 1995;20:152–4.

[3] Wiggers RH, Rosekrans P. Ultrasound diagnosis of psoas hematoma. Diagn Imaging (San Franc) 1980; 49:98–105.

[4] Maffulli N, So WS, Ahuja A, et al. Iliopsoas haematoma in adolescent taekwondo player. Knee Surg Sports Traumatol Arthrosc Arthroscopy 1996;3: 230–3.

[5] Alanen A, Kormano M. Correlation of the echogenicity and structure of clotted blood. J Ultrasound Med 1985;4:421–5.
[6] Alanen A, Nummi P. Effect of motion on the sonographic and magnetic resonance patterns of ageing blood. Acta Radiol Diagn (Stockh) 1986; 4:455–8.
[7] Aspelin P, Ekberg O, Thorsson O, et al. Ultrasound examination of soft tissue injury of the lower limb in athletes. Am J Sports Med 1992;20(5):601–3.
[8] Rubin JI, Gomori JM, Grossman RI, et al. High-field MR imaging of extracranial hematomas. AJR Am J Roentgenol 1987;148(4):813–7.
[9] Nicholas SJ, Tyler TF. Adductor muscle strains in sport. Sports Med 2002;32(5):339–44.
[10] Emery CA, Meeuwisse WH, Powell JW. Groin and abdominal strain injuries in the National Hockey League. Clin J Sports Med 1999;9(3):151–6.
[11] Ekstrand J, Hilding J. The incidence and differential diagnosis of acute groin injuries in male soccer players. Scand J Med Sci Sports 1999;9:98–103.
[12] Orchard J, Seward H. Epidemiology of injuries in the Australian Football League, seasons 1997–2000. Br J Sports Med 2002;36:39–45.
[13] Robinson P, Barron DA, Parsons W, et al. Adductor-related groin pain in athletes: correlation of MR imaging with clinical findings. Skeletal Radiol 2004;33:451–7.
[14] Kalebo J, Karlsson J, Sward L, et al. Ultrasonography of chronic tendon injuries in the groin. Am J Sports Med 1992;20(6):634–9.
[15] Goh LH, Chhem RK, Wang S, et al. Ultrasonographic features of an adductor longus tear: case report. Can Assoc Radiol J 2001;52(4):252–4.
[16] Weaver JS, Jacobson JA, Jamadar DA, et al. Sonographic findings of adductor insertion avulsion syndrome with magnetic resonance imaging correlation. J Ultrasound Med 2003;22:403–7.
[17] Anderson MW, Kaplan PA, Dussault RG. Adductor insertion avulsion syndrome (thigh splints): spectrum of MR imaging features. AJR Am J Roentgenol 2001;177(3):673–5.
[18] Albers SL, Spritzer CE, Garrett WE Jr, et al. MR findings in athletes with pubalgia. Skeletal Radiol 2001;20:270–7.
[19] Ilaslan H, Wenger DE, Shives TC, et al. Unilateral hypertrophy of tensor fascia lata: a soft tissue tumor simulator. Skeletal Radiol 2003;32:628–32.
[20] Bass CJ, Connell DA. Sonographic findings of tensor fascia lata tendinopathy: another cause of anterior groin pain. Skeletal Radiol 2002;31:143–8.
[21] Asinger DA, El-Khoury GY. Tensor fascia lata muscle tear: evaluation by MRI. Iowa Orthop J 1998;18:146–9.
[22] Koulouris G, Connell D. Evaluation of the hamstring muscle complex following acute injury. Skeletal Radiol 2003;32:582–9.
[23] Connell DA, Schneider-Kolsky ME, Hoving JL, et al. Longitudinal study comparing sonographic and MRI assessments of acute and healing hamstring injuries. AJR Am J Roentgenol 2004;183(4):975–84.
[24] Gibbs NJ, Cross TM, Cameron M, et al. The accuracy of MRI in predicting recovery and recurrence of acute grade one hamstring muscle strains within the same season in Australian Rules football players. J Sci Med Sport 2004;7(2):248–58.
[25] Cross TM, Gibbs N, Houang MT, et al. Acute quadriceps muscle strains: magnetic resonance imaging features and prognosis. Am J Sports Med 2004; 32(3):710–9.
[26] Connell DA, Bass C, Sykes CJ, et al. Sonographic evaluation of gluteus medius and minimus tendinopathy. Eur Radiol 2003;13:1339–47.
[27] Cvitanic O, Henzie G, Skezas N, et al. MRI diagnosis of tears of the hip abductor tendons (gluteus medius and gluteus minimus). AJR Am J Roentgenol 2004;182:137–43.
[28] Bunker TD, Esler CNA, Leach WJ. Rotator-cuff tear of the hip. J Bone Joint Surg Br 1997;79:618–20.
[29] Pfirrmann CWA, Chung CB, Theumann NH, et al. Greater trochanter of the hip: attachment of the abductor mechanism and a complex of three bursae—MR imaging and MR bursography in cadavers and MR imaging in asymptomatic volunteers. Radiology 2001;221:469–77.
[30] Chung CB, Robertson JE, Cho GJ, et al. Gluteus medius tendon tears and avulsive injuries in elderly women: imaging findings in six patients. AJR Am J Roentgenol 1999;173(2):351–3.
[31] Kingzett-Taylor A, Tirman PF, Feller J, et al. Tendinosis and tears of gluteus medius and minimus muscles as a cause of hip pain: MR imaging findings. AJR Am J Roentgenol 1999;173:1123–6.
[32] Gordon J. Trochanteric bursitis and tendinitis. Clin Orthop 1961;20:193–202.
[33] Leonard MH. Trochanteric syndrome: calcareous and noncalcareous tendonitis and bursitis about the trochanter major. JAMA 1958;168(2):175–7.
[34] Schapira D, Nahir M, Scharf Y. Trochanteric bursitis: a common clinical problem. Arch Phys Med Rehabil 1986;67(11):815–7.
[35] Pelsser V, Cardinal E, Hobden R, et al. Extraarticular snapping hip: sonographic findings. AJR Am J Roentgenol 2001;176:67–73.
[36] Choi YS, Lee SM, Song BY, et al. Dynamic sonography of external snapping hip syndrome. J Ultrasound Med 2002;21:753–8.
[37] Janzen DL, Partridge E, Logan PM, et al. The snapping hip: clinical and imaging findings in transient subluxation of the iliopsoas tendon. Can Assoc Radiol J 1996;47(3):202–8.
[38] Schaberg JE, Harper MC, Allen WC. The snapping hip syndrome. Am J Sports Med 1984;12(5):361–5.
[39] Wunderbaldinger P, Bremer C, Matuszewski L, et al. Efficient radiological assessment of the internal snapping hip syndrome. Eur Radiol 2001;11:1743–7.
[40] Czerny C, Hoffman S, Urban M, et al. MR arthrography of the adult acetabular capsular-labral

complex: correlation with surgery and anatomy. AJR Am J Roentgenol 1999;173(2):345–9.
[41] Mintz DN, Hooper T, Connell D, et al. Magnetic resonance imaging of the hip: detection of labral and chondral abnormalities using noncontrast imaging. Arthroscopy 2005;21(4):385–93.
[42] Orchard JW, Read JW, Neophyton J, et al. Groin pain associated with ultrasound finding of inguinal canal posterior wall deficiency in Australian Rules footballers. Br J Sports Med 1998;32:134–9.
[43] Susmallian S, Ezri T, Elis M, et al. Laparoscopic repair of "sportsman's hernia" in soccer players as treatment of chronic inguinal pain. Med Sci Monit 2004;10(2):CR52–4.
[44] Joesting DR. Diagnosis and treatment of sportsman's hernia. Curr Sports Med Rep 2002;1(2):121–4.
[45] Holzheimer RG. Inguinal hernia: classification, diagnosis, and treatment: classic, traumatic, and sportsman's hernia. Eur J Med Res 2005;10:121–34.
[46] van den Berg JC, de Valois JC, Go PM, et al. Radiological anatomy of the groin region. Eur Radiol 2000;10:661–70.
[47] van den Berg JC, de Valois JC, Go PM, et al. Dynamic magnetic resonance imaging in the diagnosis of groin hernia. Invest Radiol 1997;32(10):644–7.
[48] van den Berg JC, de Valois JC, Go PM, et al. Detection of groin hernia with physical examination, ultrasound, and MRI compared with laparoscopic findings. Invest Radiol 1999;34(12):739–43.
[49] Bradley M, Morgan D, Pentlow B, et al. The groin hernia—an ultrasound diagnosis? Ann R Coll Surg Engl 2003;85(3):178–80.
[50] Zhang GQ, Sugiyama M, Hagi H, et al. Groin hernias in adults: value of color Doppler sonography in their classification. J Clin Ultrasound 2001;29(8): 429–34.
[51] van den Berg JC, de Valois JC, Go PM, et al. Groin hernia: can dynamic magnetic imaging be of help? Eur Radiol 1998;8:270–3.
[52] Pisacano RM, Miller TT. Comparing sonography with MR imaging of apophyseal injuries of the pelvis in four boys. AJR Am J Roentgenol 2003;181(1): 223–30.
[53] Major NM, Helms CA. Pelvic stress injuries: the relationship between osteitis pubis (symphysis pubis stress injury) and sacroiliac abnormalities in athletes. Skeletal Radiol 1997;26:711–7.
[54] Verrall GM, Slavotinek JP, Fon GT. Incidence of pubic bone marrow oedema in Australian Rules football players: relation to groin pain. Br J Sports Med 2001;35:28–33.
[55] Le Blanc KE, Le Blanc KA. Groin pain in athletes. Hernia 2003;7:68–71.
[56] Brennan D, O'Connell MJ, Ryan M, et al. Secondary cleft sign as a marker of injury in athletes with groin pain: MR image appearance and interpretation. Radiology 2005;235(1):162–7.
[57] Fon LJ, Spence RAJ. Sportsman's hernia. Br J Surg 2000;87:545–52.
[58] Hill PF, Chatterji S, Chambers D, et al. Stress fracture of the pubic ramus in female recruits. J Bone Joint Surg Br 1996;78(3):383–6.
[59] Kiuru MJ, Pihlajamaki HK, Ahovuo JA. Fatigue stress injuries of the pelvic bones and proximal femur: evaluation with MR imaging. Eur Radiol 2003;13(3):605–11.
[60] Wank R, Miller TT, Shapiro JF. Sonographically guided injection of anesthetic for iliopsoas tendinopathy after total hip arthroplasty. J Clin Ultrasound 2004;32(7):354–7.
[61] Koenig MJ, Torp-Pedersen S, Qvistgaard E, et al. Preliminary results of colour Doppler-guided intratendinous glucocorticoid injection for Achilles tendonitis in five patients. Scand J Med Sci Sports 2004;14(2):100–6.
[62] Fredberg U, Bolvig L, Pfeiffer-Jensen M, et al. Ultrasonography as a tool for diagnosis, guidance of local steroid injection and, together with pressure algometry, monitoring of the treatment of athletes with chronic jumper's knee and Achilles tendinitis: a randomized double-blind, placebo-controlled study. Scand J Rheumatol 2004;33(2):94–101.
[63] Testa V, Capasso G, Benazzo F, et al. Management of Achilles tendinopathy by ultrasound-guided percutaneous tenotomy. Med Sci Sports Exerc 2002; 34(4):573–80.

ELSEVIER
SAUNDERS

Magn Reson Imaging Clin N Am
13 (2005) 811–825

MAGNETIC
RESONANCE
IMAGING CLINICS
of North America

# Cumulative Index 2005

*Note:* Page numbers of article titles are in **boldface** type.

## A



1064-9689/05/$ - see front matter 
doi:10.1016/S1064-9689(05)00120-0

## B

## I

## N



## O

## *Changing Your Address?*

Make sure your subscription changes too! When you notify us of your new address, you can help make our job easier by including an exact copy of your Clinics label number with your old address (see illustration below.) This number identifies you to our computer system and will speed the processing of your address change. Please be sure this label number accompanies your old address and your corrected address—you can send an old Clinics label with your number on it or just copy it exactly and send it to the address listed below.

We appreciate your help in our attempt to give you continuous coverage. Thank you.

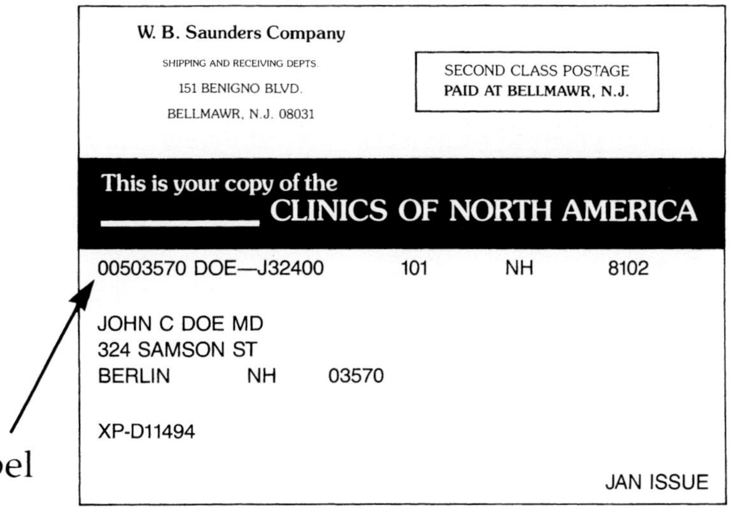

W. B. Saunders Company
SHIPPING AND RECEIVING DEPTS.
151 BENIGNO BLVD.
BELLMAWR, N.J. 08031

SECOND CLASS POSTAGE
**PAID AT BELLMAWR, N.J.**

**This is your copy of the**
**________ CLINICS OF NORTH AMERICA**

00503570 DOE—J32400 101 NH 8102

JOHN C DOE MD
324 SAMSON ST
BERLIN NH 03570

XP-D11494

JAN ISSUE

Your Clinics Label Number

Copy it exactly or send your label along with your address to:
**W.B. Saunders Company, Customer Service**
Orlando, FL 32887-4800
Call Toll Free 1-800-654-2452

Please allow four to six weeks for delivery of new subscriptions and for processing address changes.

United States Postal Service

**Statement of Ownership, Management, and Circulation**

| 1. Publication Title | 2. Publication Number | 3. Filing Date |
|---|---|---|
| Magnetic Resonance Imaging Clinics of North America | 1 0 6 4 - 9 6 8 9 | 9/15/05 |
| 4. Issue Frequency | 5. Number of Issues Published Annually | 6. Annual Subscription Price |
| Feb, May, Aug, Nov | 4 | $190.00 |

7. Complete Mailing Address of Known Office of Publication (*Not printer*) (*Street, city, county, state, and ZIP+4*)

Elsevier Inc.
6277 Sea Harbor Drive
Orlando, FL 32887-4800

Contact Person: Gwen C. Campbell
Telephone: 215-239-3685

8. Complete Mailing Address of Headquarters or General Business Office of Publisher (*Not printer*)

Elsevier Inc., 360 Park Avenue South, New York, NY 10010-1710

9. Full Names and Complete Mailing Addresses of Publisher, Editor, and Managing Editor (*Do not leave blank*)

Publisher (*Name and complete mailing address*)

Tim Griswold, Elsevier Inc., 1600 John F. Kennedy Blvd., Suite 1800, Philadelphia, PA 19103-2899

Editor (*Name and complete mailing address*)

Barton Dudlick, Elsevier Inc., 1600 John F. Kennedy Blvd., Suite 1800, Philadelphia, PA 19103-2899

Managing Editor (*Name and complete mailing address*)

Heather Cullen, Elsevier Inc., 1600 John F. Kennedy Blvd., Suite 1800, Philadelphia, PA 19103-2899

10. Owner (*Do not leave blank. If the publication is owned by a corporation, give the name and address of the corporation immediately followed by the names and addresses of all stockholders owning or holding 1 percent or more of the total amount of stock. If not owned by a corporation, give the names and addresses of the individual owners. If owned by a partnership or other unincorporated firm, give its name and address as well as those of each individual owner. If the publication is published by a nonprofit organization, give its name and address.*)

| Full Name | Complete Mailing Address |
|---|---|
| Wholly owned subsidiary of | 4520 East-West Highway |
| Reed/Elsevier Inc., US Holdings | Bethesda, MD 20814 |

11. Known Bondholders, Mortgagees, and Other Security Holders Owning or Holding 1 Percent or More of Total Amount of Bonds, Mortgages, or Other Securities. If none, check box → ☐ None

| Full Name | Complete Mailing Address |
|---|---|
| N/A | |

12. Tax Status (*For completion by nonprofit organizations authorized to mail at nonprofit rates*) (*Check one*)
The purpose, function, and nonprofit status of this organization and the exempt status for federal income tax purposes:
☐ Has Not Changed During Preceding 12 Months
☐ Has Changed During Preceding 12 Months (*Publisher must submit explanation of change with this statement*)

(*See Instructions on Reverse*)

PS Form **3526**, October 1999

13. Publication Title: Magnetic Resonance Imaging Clinics of North America

14. Issue Date for Circulation Data Below: August 2005

| 15. Extent and Nature of Circulation | | Average No. Copies Each Issue During Preceding 12 Months | No. Copies of Single Issue Published Nearest to Filing Date |
|---|---|---|---|
| a. Total Number of Copies (*Net press run*) | | 5075 | 4700 |
| b. Paid and/or Requested Circulation | (1) Paid/Requested Outside-County Mail Subscriptions Stated on Form 3541. (*Include advertiser's proof and exchange copies*) | 3093 | 2949 |
| | (2) Paid In-County Subscriptions Stated on Form 3541 (*Include advertiser's proof and exchange copies*) | | |
| | (3) Sales Through Dealers and Carriers, Street Vendors, Counter Sales, and Other Non-USPS Paid Distribution | 714 | 739 |
| | (4) Other Classes Mailed Through the USPS | | |
| c. Total Paid and/or Requested Circulation [*Sum of 15b. (1), (2), (3), and (4)*] | | 3807 | 3688 |
| d. Free Distribution by Mail (*Samples, compliment-ary, and other free*) | (1) Outside-County as Stated on Form 3541 | 116 | 119 |
| | (2) In-County as Stated on Form 3541 | | |
| | (3) Other Classes Mailed Through the USPS | | |
| e. Free Distribution Outside the Mail (*Carriers or other means*) | | | |
| f. Total Free Distribution (*Sum of 15d. and 15e.*) | | 116 | 119 |
| g. Total Distribution (*Sum of 15c. and 15f.*) | | 3923 | 3807 |
| h. Copies not Distributed | | 1152 | 893 |
| i. Total (*Sum of 15g. and h.*) | | 5075 | 4700 |
| j. Percent Paid and/or Requested Circulation (*15c. divided by 15g. times 100*) | | 97% | 97% |

16. Publication of Statement of Ownership
☐ Publication required. Will be printed in the **November 2005** issue of this publication. ☐ Publication not required

17. Signature and Title of Editor, Publisher, Business Manager, or Owner

Jean M. Fanucci – Executive Director of Subscription Services — Date: 9/15/05

I certify that all information furnished on this form is true and complete. I understand that anyone who furnishes false or misleading information on this form or who omits material or information requested on the form may be subject to criminal sanctions (including fines and imprisonment) and/or civil sanctions (including civil penalties).

**Instructions to Publishers**

1. Complete and file one copy of this form with your postmaster annually on or before October 1. Keep a copy of the completed form for your records.
2. In cases where the stockholder or security holder is a trustee, include in items 10 and 11 the name of the person or corporation for whom the trustee is acting. Also include the names and addresses of individuals who are stockholders who own or hold 1 percent or more of the total amount of bonds, mortgages, or other securities of the publishing corporation. In item 11, if none, check the box. Use blank sheets if more space is required.
3. Be sure to furnish all circulation information called for in item 15. Free circulation must be shown in items 15d, e, and f.
4. Item 15h., Copies not Distributed, must include (1) newsstand copies originally stated on Form 3541, and returned to the publisher, (2) estimated returns from news agents, and (3), copies for office use, leftovers, spoiled, and all other copies not distributed.
5. If the publication had Periodicals authorization as a general or requester publication, this Statement of Ownership, Management, and Circulation must be published; it must be printed in any issue in October or, if the publication is not published during October, the first issue printed after October.
6. In item 16, indicate the date of the issue in which this Statement of Ownership will be published.
7. Item 17 must be signed.

***Failure to file or publish a statement of ownership may lead to suspension of Periodicals authorization.***

PS Form **3526**, October 1999 (*Reverse*)